The North American Guide to
COMMON POISONOUS
Plants and Mushrooms

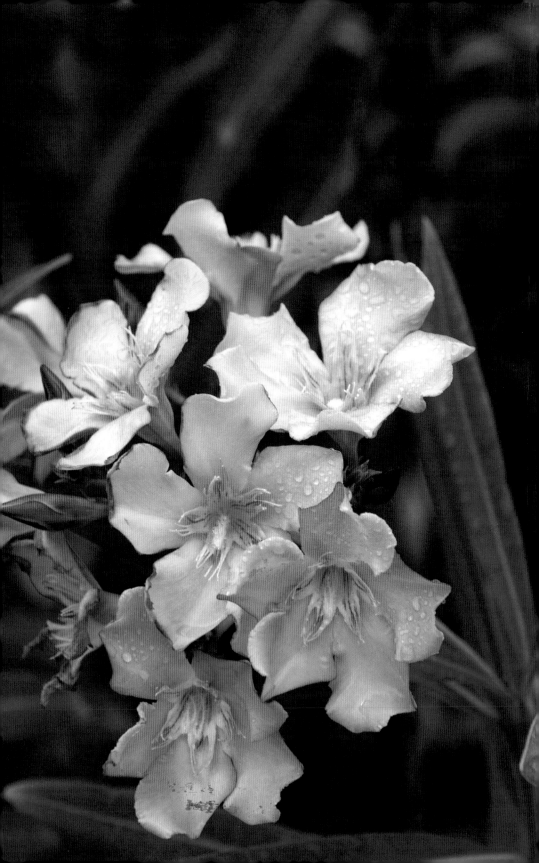

The North American Guide to
COMMON POISONOUS
Plants and Mushrooms

Nancy J. Turner, Ph.D., F.L.S., O.B.C., F.R.S.C.
and
Patrick von Aderkas, Ph.D., F.L.S.

TIMBER PRESS
Portland · London

This book is a revision of *Common Poisonous Plants and Mushrooms of North America* by Nancy J. Turner and Adam F. Szczawinski, published in 1991 by Timber Press, Inc. **It cannot replace the expertise of qualified medical personnel, whose immediate advice and assistance should be sought. In the United States, in all cases of suspected poisoning by plants (or any other substance), call 1-800-222-1222, the national hotline of the American Association of Poison Control Centers.**

Unless otherwise credited, photographs are by Robert D. Turner and Nancy J. Turner. Frontispiece: *Nerium oleander.*

Published in 2009 by Timber Press, Inc.

The Haseltine Building
133 S.W. Second Avenue, Suite 450
Portland, Oregon 97204-3527
www.timberpress.com

2 The Quadrant
135 Salusbury Road
London NW6 6RJ
www.timberpress.co.uk

Printed in China
Second printing 2010
Text designed by Susan Applegate

Library of Congress Cataloging-in-Publication Data

Turner, Nancy J., 1947–
    The North American guide to common poisonous plants and mushrooms/Nancy J. Turner and Patrick von Aderkas.
      p. cm.
      Includes bibliographical references and index.
      ISBN 978-0-88192-929-4
      1. Poisonous plants—Identification. 2. Poisonous plants—Toxicology.
3. Mushrooms, Poisonous—Identification. 4. Mushrooms, Poisonous—
Toxicology. 5. Poisonous plants—North America—Identification. 6. Mushrooms,
Poisonous—North America—Identification. I. Aderkas, P. von. II. Title.
      QK100.A1T87 2009
      581.6'59097—dc22   2008035095

A catalog record for this book is also available from the British Library.

To
Adam Szczawinski
(1913–2006),
botanist, friend, and mentor

CONTENTS

IN CASE OF POISONING

If a poisonous or unknown plant (or other poisonous substance) has been swallowed:

• **If patient is unconscious, call 911.** Otherwise . . .

• **Call your local Poison Control Center (PCC) immediately,** and seek professional medical aid and advice. In the United States, in all cases, call **1-800-222-1222,** the national hotline of the American Association of Poison Control Centers, which will connect you directly with your local or state poison control center. If you are unable to reach a PCC, take patient to a hospital immediately.

• **Do not panic.** Keep patient as comfortable as possible. Remember that there are very few really serious poisonings from plants, and even fewer fatalities. Most plant ingestions don't require active treatment.

• **Watch breathing** closely, and if necessary, apply artificial respiration (CPR).

• **Keep a sample** of the plant or substance. (Sample should be whole and uncooked ideally, but any sample is better than none.) Place mushroom samples in a paper bag or cardboard box; they will deteriorate in plastic. If vomiting has occurred, save a sample of the vomit for further identification.

• **DO NOT induce vomiting without medical help, or give anything to drink IF patient is under 12 months old, or extremely drowsy, unconscious, or convulsing.**

• **If patient is awake and not convulsing, give them milk to drink.** This will adsorb many poisons, reducing how much is taken up by the stomach lining, until they can get to a hospital, where they will likely be given activated charcoal. Gastric lavage may be indicated but should be done *only* by a qualified physician.

• **Vomiting may occur spontaneously, but do not try to induce vomiting,** especially if patient is unconscious, under 12 months old, or is not showing symptoms of poisoning. Ipecac syrup was formerly widely used as an emetic in cases of suspected poisoning, but its use *is no longer recommended*. If vomiting occurs, save vomit for hospital laboratory.

• **If patient is convulsing or clenching teeth,** place a piece of rolled cloth between the jaws to prevent damage to teeth or tongue.

• **For eye contamination** by plant irritants, gently flush the eyes with a stream of slightly tepid water or saline solution for five minutes.

• **For skin contamination** by plant irritants, wash skin immediately with a large amount of running water; use soap if available; remove and thoroughly wash contaminated clothing.

HOW TO PREVENT POISONING

• Never eat any part of an unknown plant or mushroom. If you are trying a "new" food, eat only a small amount at first, and do not mix it with other "new" foods.

• Carefully supervise babies and young children. Keep poisonous houseplants out of their reach. Remove poisonous berries from house- and garden plants. Remove mushrooms from lawns and play areas. Store bulbs and seeds out of sight and out of reach.

• Teach children about poisonous plants and mushrooms just as they are taught about busy roads and hot stoves. Train them never to put any plants or parts of plants or mushrooms into their mouths. Even babies and toddlers can learn about "bad" plants.

• Learn to identify poisonous plants in the house, yard, and neighborhood. Eliminating all poisonous plants is not practical; knowing about them is.

• Teach children to recognize poison ivy, poison oak, and poison sumac and any other plants in the locality causing skin injuries, or dermatitis.

• Do not assume a plant is safe because birds or other wildlife eat it. What is poisonous to humans is not necessarily harmful to other animals.

• Do not assume, just because the fruits or roots of a plant are edible, that other parts of the plant can also be eaten. Many plants with edible parts also have poisonous parts.

• Do not count on heating or cooking a plant or mushroom to destroy any toxic substances it contains.

• Avoid breathing or coming in contact with smoke from burning plants, including poison ivy.

• Do not use unknown plants as skewers for toasting marshmallows or grilling meat and vegetables, as decorations, or as playthings for children.

• Anyone using herbal medicines or teas, wild edible plants, or wild mushrooms, should be *positive* of the identifications of the plants they use and know how to prepare them properly. Each year many people are poisoned, some fatally, from mistaken identifications or misuse of herbal remedies.

• Do not use edible plants or mushrooms gathered from roadsides or from areas where herbicides or insecticides may have been applied.

FOREWORD

For an authoritative yet easily read reference on the subject of poisonous plants and mushrooms to which North Americans can be exposed in home, urban, and rural environments, one need look no further than this revision of the classic book of Turner and Szczawinski. Although wearing a slightly different title and having a change in the second author, this book retains the basic format and tone of the previous edition. Some changes involve simple but critical updates in scientific information; others reflect new attitudes in modern toxicology, especially in the management of the poisoned patient and in the field of herbal medicine.

The North American Guide to Common Poisonous Plants and Mushrooms can be used as a field guide because of its size, descriptive accuracy, and the quality of the illustrations; but it is not simply a field guide. The introduction—with its historical references, background information, and perspective—provides interesting and informative reading for those seeking something more than facts about the plants themselves. The sections on the plants are accurate, clear, and mixed with enlightening case histories and anecdotes. Useful medical information throughout the book is given in a clear and simple fashion and has been updated to keep current with modern therapeutic practices. It provides good insights into overall management principles but never intends to do more than provide guidance to the public for initial management until proper medical care can be accessed. The Appendices offer very useful summaries for quick reference. Most of the plants in this book are toxic in doses that can be easily ingested in small quantities, but other, less toxic plants—although they are not designated as poisons—can be dangerous if eaten in larger quantities. The overall message is clear: one must be totally familiar with any plant or mushroom that is to be ingested, not only the ones included in this book.

BRIAN A. SAUNDERS, B.Sc., M.D., F.R.C.P.(C)
Clinical Professor
Department of Anesthesiology,
Pharmacology, and Therapeutics
Faculty of Medicine
University of British Columbia

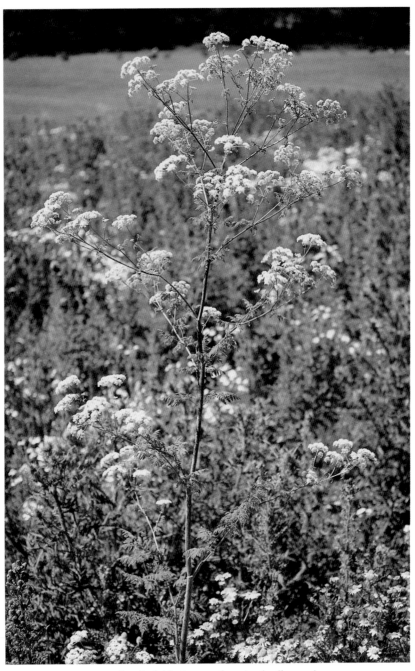

Poison hemlock (*Conium maculatum*), a deadly member
of the carrot family and a common weed.

PREFACE

In April 1980, a five-year-old girl was fatally poisoned in Victoria, British Columbia, from eating poison hemlock (*Conium maculatum*) while at play with her sisters. The little girl felt sick and would not eat. She lay down and within an hour fell into a deep coma. It was only at this point that her sisters related that she had eaten the roots of a plant, pretending they were carrots; she was rushed to the hospital, where she died six days later. In February 1987, a six-year-old girl, also of Victoria, became paralyzed and stopped breathing after eating poison hemlock, but the hospital staff were able to save her by using a respirator and pumping out her stomach.

These are only two out of hundreds of incidents in which humans have been poisoned from eating toxic plants or mushrooms or drinking teas made from harmful plants. Many involve young children at play, "pretending" to eat better-known edible look-alikes. In fact, statistics show that children aged five and under are most vulnerable to accidental poisoning. The carrot-like taproots of poison hemlock, the pea-like pods of golden chain tree (*Laburnum anagyroides*), the onion-like bulbs of daffodils (*Narcissus* spp.), and the attractive, colorful berries of climbing nightshade (*Solanum dulcamara*), Jack in the pulpit (*Arisaema triphyllum*), daphne (*Daphne mezereum*), and European lily of the valley (*Convallaria majalis*) have all severely poisoned children.

It is impossible to remove poisonous plants from our environment. The best way to prevent poisoning is for people to learn which plants are harmful and to teach their children not to play with plants and never to put them in their mouths. We hope that this book will be useful to parents, pet owners, outdoors people, gardeners, and people who keep houseplants, helping them to identify, in advance, the poisonous plants around them. If this book can prevent a single poisoning, we will feel it was worth our efforts.

This is an updated revision of a book first published in 1991. Although the poisonous qualities of plants and mushrooms and the incidences of poisoning have changed little since, there have been changes in our knowledge of the toxic compounds and in the classification of poisonous species, especially in some of the mushrooms. Furthermore, recommended treatments for poisoning have changed over time: ipecac syrup, which was almost universally recommended by physicians and health care workers in the 1980s, has been questioned for its safety and efficacy and is no longer recommended. Gastric lavage is less often used; activated charcoal, as an absorbing agent for toxins, is the current method-of-choice by ER physicians. The references have, of course, been updated: a number of excellent and authoritative books on poisonous plants and mushrooms have been published since 1991, and the major ones are cited here. Above all, the Internet is now a major and highly convenient source of information on toxic plants and mushrooms. Although Internet users should be cautious about accepting everything they find on the Web, they can trust online peer-reviewed journals and Web sites based in universities, hospitals, poison control centers, and professional societies to provide sound, up-to-date information, including detailed species descriptions and, in many cases, spectacular color illustrations.

What hasn't changed? This book is not intended to replace the advice of trained medical personnel but to provide general information about potentially poisonous plants and mushrooms; in all cases of suspected poisoning by plants or any other substance, medical advice should be sought from the family physician or local poison control center.

ACKNOWLEDGEMENTS

Many people helped to produce *Common Poisonous Plants and Mushrooms of North America* by Nancy J. Turner and Adam F. Szczawinski. These include Dr. Walter H. Lewis (now Professor Emeritus), Department of Biology, Washington University, St. Louis; Dr. George H. Constantine, Associate Dean and Head Advisor (now Professor Emeritus), College of Pharmacy, Oregon State University, Corvallis; Dr. Bettina Dudley and the late Dr. T. R. Dudley; Dr. Robert Bandoni (now Professor Emeritus), Department of Botany, University of British Columbia, Vancouver; Dr. Scott A. Redhead, Biosystematics Research Institute, Agriculture Canada (now Agriculture & Agri-Food Canada), Ottawa; Dr. Al Funk and John Dennis, Pacific Forest Science Research Centre, Victoria; Dr. J. N. C. (Ian) Whyte, Pacific Biological Station, Nanaimo, B.C.; Dr. Eugene Anderson, University of California, Riverside (now of Seattle); Dr. Denis R. Benjamin, Director of Laboratories, Children's Hospital and Medical Center, Seattle; Dr. Philip Chambers, of Nanaimo, B.C.; Dr. Adolf Ceska (now retired) and Dr. Richard Hebda, Royal British Columbia Museum, Victoria; Dr. Amadeo Rea, San Diego Natural History Museum; the late Dr. R. E. Schultes, Director Emeritus, Harvard University Botanical Museum; the late Dr. G. N. Towers, Department of Botany, University of British Columbia; Ken O'Connor, Victoria, B.C.; and Krista Thie, White Salmon, Wash. We have lost touch with some of these people, but we gratefully acknowledge their contributions, reviews, and suggestions, which continue through this revision.

For the present revision, Dr. Brian Saunders, M.D., kindly reviewed the entire set of galleys and agreed to contribute a foreword, for which we are most grateful. Dr. Les Vertesi, M.D., also reviewed the medical information for us, and mycologist and *Amanita* expert Dr. Rodham E. Tulloss reviewed the chapter on poisonous mushrooms and offered many valuable suggestions and updated information. Mycologist Dr. Michael W. Beug, Professor

Emeritus at Evergreen State College, Olympia, Washington, also read the mushroom chapter and provided important insights. Many other friends and colleagues contributed in various ways, and we are grateful to them all: Mark Blumenthal (founder and executive director, American Botanical Council, Austin); Dr. Alain Cuerrier (Montreal Botanical Garden); Dr. James A. Duke (USDA Maryland, retired); Dr. Lucile A. Housley (Oregon State Bureau of Land Management); Dr. Glen S. Jamieson (Pacific Biological Station, Nanaimo, B.C.); Dr. Timothy Johns (McGill University, Montreal); Dr. Leslie Main Johnson (Athabasca University, Edmonton); Dr. Kendrick Marr (Royal BC Museum, Victoria); Maurice L. Oates (Terrace, B.C.); Dr. Alain Touwaide (Smithsonian Institution, Washington, D.C.); and Douglas Trainor (Phoenixville, Pa.). Heather Anholt, a very capable summer research assistant, provided organization and information.

Mycologist Paul Kroeger of Vancouver (and through him and Trudy Greif, the late Stan Czolowski) and Dr. Michael Beug (and through him, Kit Scates Barnhart) provided several mushroom photographs for this book. Other photographers who contributed photographs include Dr. Larry K. Allain (USGS, National Wetlands Research Center), Allan Armitage, G. A. Cooper (courtesy of Smithsonian Institution, Rusty Russell and Deborah Bell, U.S. National Herbarium), Jan Dauphin, Dr. Richard Hebda, and Dr. James Miller. We are deeply grateful to all these people, and particularly to Robert D. Turner, for his photographic contributions, and to Robert D. Turner and Elizabeth von Aderkas for their unending support and encouragement. We also acknowledge Alan Szczawinski and Barbara Lund and their family for encouraging us to produce the book you hold in your hands, in memory of Alan's late father.

Finally, we would like to thank our friends at Timber Press, past and present, Richard Abel and Jane Connor (publishers), Dale Johnson and Franni Bertolino Farrell (editors), and Michael Dempsey (production coordinator), for publishing our work and for their help and support.

HOW TO USE THIS BOOK

The table of contents shows the overall organization of the book. In Chapter 2, poisonous mushrooms are listed in alphabetical order by scientific name, since their common names are variable and their scientific names often well known. For the succeeding chapters, within the broad categories indicated in the table of contents, plants are listed alphabetically by their prevalent common names, with scientific names and family names also provided. In cases where a plant could potentially be included in more than one category (for example, either as a wild plant in Chapter 3 or a garden plant in Chapter 4), we have tried to place it in its most relevant context—that is, where a reader would be most likely to encounter the plant. If there is any doubt about where to find a reference to a particular plant, or if only the scientific name is known, please consult the index. In the main plant entries, we have tried to keep technical terminology, either botanical or medical, to a minimum. Some specialized botanical terms are defined and illustrated in the glossary.

We have generally followed the USDA Natural Resources Conservation Service (http://plants.usda.gov/index.html) for plant nomenclature and classification. We have cited commonly used synonyms; we have not provided archaic family names but only the accepted modern ones (i.e., Fabaceae, not Leguminosae; Asteraceae, not Compositae). For the more technical aspects of plant identification, and for descriptions of plants that are poisonous to livestock but not to humans, other references are provided, many of which contain complete literature citations for various plant species and families and groups of plant toxins.

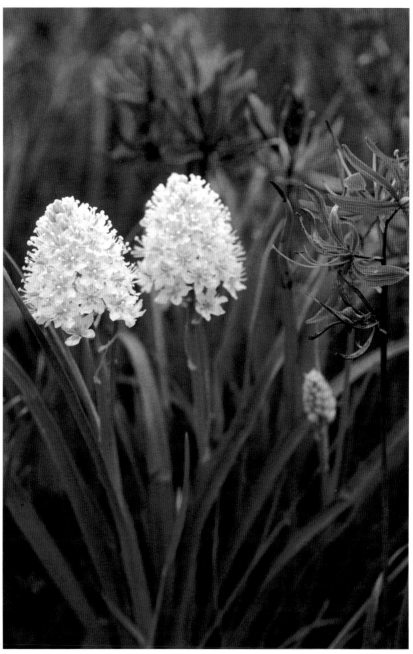

Poisonous plants are sometimes taken for edible species. Here, meadow deathcamas (*Zigadenus venenosus*) (left, with cream-colored flowers) is growing together with blue camas (*Camassia quamash*), whose bulbs are edible.

CHAPTER 1
Introduction

POISONOUS PLANTS AND MUSHROOMS: AN OVERVIEW

Any plant or mushroom that contains known toxic compounds in concentrations high enough to be dangerous if touched or consumed is considered poisonous. There are therefore literally thousands of poisonous plants and probably hundreds of poisonous mushrooms in the world. In this book we describe the most common and dangerous plants and groups of toxic mushrooms to be found in the temperate regions of North America: in homes and buildings, in gardens and urban areas, and in the wild. We give emphasis to plants and mushrooms known to have caused poisoning to humans, but many of the same types have also caused injury to animals, including household pets and grazing or browsing livestock.

It is important to remember that "natural" and "organic" do not necessarily mean "safe" and "wholesome." Some of the most virulent poisons known are derived from plants, which are, of course, both "natural" and "organic." Many medicinal plants, and even many food plants, contain chemicals that can be harmful. Our bodies are adept at handling and eliminating small amounts of many potentially harmful substances. In large concentrations, however, these same substances, when ingested, can affect our digestive, circulatory, or nervous systems, can cause irreparable damage to our liver or kidneys, can lower blood sugar, interfere with normal blood clotting, prevent cell division, or affect our immune systems. Other substances found in plants can cause skin reactions—pain, redness, blistering, swelling—or can harm the eyes, simply from contact.

Poisonous substances in plants are often considered to be byproducts of essential plant functions. For many of these chemical compounds, scientists have not determined any obvious role in the functioning, or metabolism of the plants containing them. Some may simply be waste products. Some may serve as reservoirs of carbon compounds that can be recycled into other compounds as metabolic necessity dictates. As well as being poisonous, many such compounds are bad-tasting or have an unpleasant odor. These protect the plant against plant-eating insects and other browsing animals, or possibly even harmful microbes.

Often, individual plants or local populations of plants vary in the relative concentrations of toxic compounds they contain. This natural variation has helped plant breeders over many centuries to select and develop plant varieties with low concentrations of poisonous substances. In fact, some of the vegetables we most enjoy were derived from ancestral plants too toxic to eat in any quantity. The potato is a good example. Even the edible tubers contain traces of solanine, which is found in higher concentrations throughout the potato plant, rendering the green leaves, sprouts, and green, light-exposed tubers very poisonous.

Tubers of the potato's wild ancestors are also poisonous. It was only through focused and continued selection of less toxic potato varieties that the native farmers of the South American highlands were able to develop such a delicious and globally treasured vegetable tuber. Selection would have been quite straightforward in this case, as solanine is an alkaloid whose bitterness gives away its presence. The less bitter the potato, the less poisonous. Johns and Kubo (1988) describe some of the means people have devised to render otherwise poisonous plants edible.

Can a plant be called poisonous if it has never poisoned anyone? The answer is yes. Some plants can only be inferred to be toxic for humans, either because they are known to be poisonous to some animal species, or because chemical studies have revealed the presence of dangerous compounds. Controlled feeding studies with laboratory animals are sometimes used to determine potential toxicity, although many people feel this is an unacceptable and inhumane means of acquiring such information. At least one hybrid begonia, the flowers of *Gladiolus gandavensis*, and species of drag-

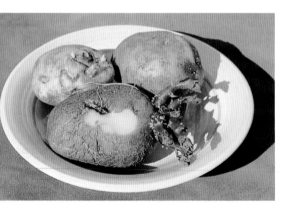

Green-skinned and sprouting
potatoes are poisonous.

ontree (*Dracaena*), prayer plant (*Maranta*), *Peperomia*, snake plant (*Sansevieria*), *Selaginella*, and goosefoot plant (*Syngonium*)—all received positive toxicity scores in such tests (Der Marderosian and Roia 1979). Because there is no evidence since against these plants, they are not described in detail in this book, but people should be wary of them nonetheless.

Herbicides and pesticides used on house- and garden plants or in forests can render otherwise edible species dangerous, causing unpleasant reactions that may not be distinguishable from plant poisoning. Never harvest plants, berries, or mushrooms along roadsides or highway rights-of-way: toxic heavy metals and other contaminants from vehicle exhaust can accumulate in plant structures and mushrooms. People seeking aquatic or marine edible plants, such as cattail (*Typha latifolia*), watercress (*Nasturtium officinale*), or seaweeds, should ensure that there are no pollutants in the waters where the plants are harvested. Some molds and mildews growing on foods can also render them poisonous due to the presence of mycotoxins; moldy or rotting foods should be strictly avoided, and foods such as nuts and grains should be stored in cool, dry places to reduce the chances of them being infected with harmful fungi or bacteria.

Some plants, including many range species that might normally be edible for animals, have the capacity to absorb and concentrate nitrates, selenium salts, lead, molybdenum, and other naturally occurring compounds. This sometimes leads to large-scale poisoning of livestock. Beets, turnips, and kale, for example, may accumulate excessive amounts of nitrates if they are overfertilized. The nitrates may then be converted by bacteria in the digestive tracts of livestock to much more toxic nitrites. Since relatively large amounts of the plants must be consumed for toxic reactions to occur, and because many of the plant species involved are not normally eaten by people, human poisoning has seldom been a problem in these cases.

Prevalence of plant and mushroom poisonings

Poisonous species are everywhere, found among virtually all groups of plants—algae, mosses, ferns, coniferous trees, and flowering plants—as well as in most groups of fungi and lichens. Many of our most prized and admired garden flowers, ornamental trees, and houseplants are poisonous, and some can be deadly.

Each year, throughout North America, newspapers, Web sites, and medical journals describe hundreds of instances of poisoning from ingestion of plants and plant parts, or fungi. Babies and toddlers are often involved, especially in poisoning by philodendrons and other ornamental houseplants; dieffenbachia, or dumbcane, is one of the most commonly ingested houseplants, and we have heard of at least three instances of adults, who should have known better, inadvertently chewing on the stems. Older children at play may eat poisonous plants, in imitation of real foods. Adult poisonings generally result from misidentification of "edible" wild plants or mushrooms, or misinformed use of herbal remedies. A general survey of family, friends, and students while we were preparing this book revealed that almost everyone we talked to had had some kind of personal experience, or knew someone who had, with poisonous plants or fungi. The instances of poisonings by plants in a group of students surveyed was almost entirely restricted to when they were children, which is borne out in statistics on poisonings in many parts of the world.

Many instances of poisoning may not even be reported. As authors of books on edible wild plants and lecturers on this subject, as well as in interviewing indigenous elders and oldtimers, we hear many accounts of poisoning, some very serious, which are not necessarily officially documented. At least a dozen people told us they tried to eat western skunkcabbage (*Lysichiton americanus*) leaves because they "looked good" or "must be like cabbage." The resulting intense and prolonged burning of the lips and mouth usually prevents ingestion of more than a bite, but one man was hospitalized for several days, and experienced a swollen, raw throat "as if I had swallowed a whole cup of scalding coffee." A staff gardener at a well-known botanical garden once decided to taste the berries of red baneberry (*Actaea rubra*) because they looked so beautiful; he became dizzy, suffered from stomachache, and had to go home (but fortunately recovered without further problems). Another incident, which could have been disastrous but fortunately was not, occurred when a man attending a banquet, in a fit of boredom during a lengthy after-dinner speech, reached out and plucked a daffodil out of a vase in the center of the table, and ate it. He assumed it was edible—a foolish assumption indeed.

The red theme runs deep with childhood poisonings. One colleague told us about his five-year-old son, who had consumed the berries of climbing nightshade (*Solanum dulcamara*), which was trailing across the lawn; the result was a trip to the emergency room. Another friend recalled as a child eating the bright red berries of Jack in the pulpit (*Arisaema triphyllum*) and crying from the burning pain to his mouth these berries caused. To make matters worse, some college students who were rooming with his family assumed that it was simply that he did not like hot food. They, foolishly, ate

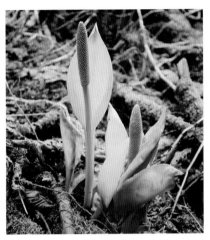

Western skunkcabbage (*Lysichiton americanus*): eating any part of the plant causes intense burning of mouth and throat.

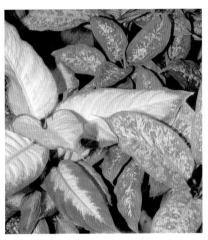

Dumbcane (*Dieffenbachia seguine*, top, and *D. picta*, below).

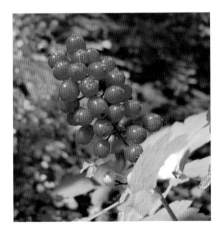

Red baneberry (*Actaea rubra*) berries are attractive but poisonous.

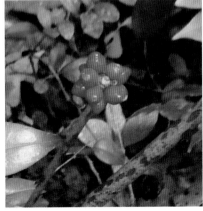

Jack in the pulpit (*Arisaema triphyllum*), berries.

the berries because they liked spicy food. Of course, they all ended up in the emergency room.

Not uncommonly, Christmas is a time when many children run into problems after eating red berries of holly, red leaves of poinsettias, and other festive plants. Red color is a plant adaptation for better dispersal of seeds by mammals and birds, but many of these animals do not chew the berries as thoroughly or digest them as efficiently and suffer little ill effect compared to human children.

Some indigenous people, and more than one outdoor recreationist, have been seriously, sometimes fatally, poisoned from mistaking highly toxic water hemlocks (*Cicuta* spp.) for similar-looking waterparsnips (*Sium* spp.). One of the worst cases of mistaken identity occurred along the Owyhee River, Oregon, in April 1984. A young river rafter and outfitter guide mistook water hemlock roots for waterparsnip, which are considered edible. He and five of his six clients ate the roots. He and one of the five who ate a large quantity started having seizures within 45 minutes of their meal. The guide died in under two hours; the others all survived, but needed medical assistance (Naegele 2006).

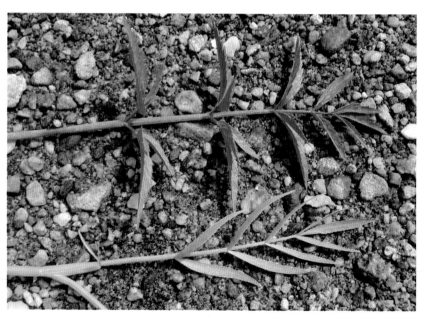

Leaves of the deadly Mackenzie's water hemlock (*Cicuta virosa*) (top) and waterparsnip (*Sium suave*).

Many edible and poisonous species are look-alikes. Confusion between edible blue camas (*Camassia quamash*), whose bulbs were a staple food for many indigenous peoples of western North America, and deathcamas (*Zigadenus* spp.), whose generic common name speaks for its lethal qualities, has sometimes occurred. The risk is heightened because species of these two genera often grow together. Other species growing in similar habitats (in this case, wetland areas) and sometimes confused are the edible cattail (*Typha latifolia*) and some flags (*Iris* spp.), which are toxic.

Another common and potentially deadly mistake is made by wild mushroom harvesters who confuse the choice edible species *Tricholoma magnivelare* (pine mushroom, or American matsutake) with toxic amanitas, notably Smith's lepidella (*Amanita smithiana*), with identification made more difficult because people may cut off the stem above the bulb that characterizes amanitas. Sometimes people attempting to harvest the shoots of false lily of the valley (*Maianthemum racemosum*; syn. *Smilacina racemosa*) as a springtime green vegetable have inadvertently harvested the shoots of the deadly green false hellebore (*Veratrum viride*). Others have been poisoned from attempting to use green false hellebore or other dangerous species as medici-

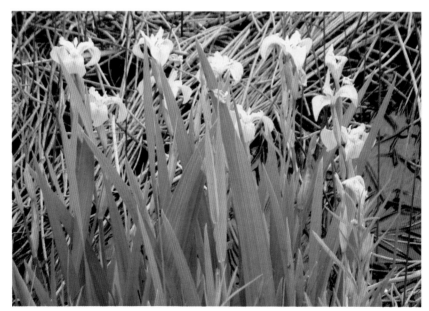

Yellow iris (*Iris pseudacorus*) is sometimes confused with cattail (*Typha latifolia*) by edible wild plant seekers.

nal remedies. Many potentially poisonous plants are used medicinally by Native Americans, but only because they are guided by the immense knowledge and experience of medicinal specialists. No one should attempt to use herbal medicine without professional advice. We heard of a case where a hospitalized pregnant woman, anxious to proceed with her delivery and return home to her older children, secretly took a preparation of blue cohosh root (*Caulophyllum thalictroides*) to bring on labor; her baby was delivered prematurely, at great risk to both mother and infant.

One unexpected reaction to the irritant properties of buttercups was experienced by one of us (NT) and her students, when they were oven-drying samples of sagebrush buttercup (*Ranunculus glaberrimus*) for phytochemical analysis in a friend's kitchen. They noticed their eyes starting to sting about 30 minutes after placing the buttercups on a tray in the oven at low heat. Their eyes started streaming, and they started coughing, with a choking sensation. At this point they realized that their discomfort was caused by the drying buttercup plants. They aired out the house thoroughly and took showers to wash their eyes, but the stinging remained for many hours. It is no wonder that children of the nearby indigenous communities were taught never to play with or handle this buttercup (Turner et al. 1980).

In the past, human poisonings occurred in epidemic proportions from such substances as the grain fungus ergot (*Claviceps* spp.) and milk from cows feeding on white snakeroot (*Ageratina altissima*) (Fyles 1920). These types of poisonings have been virtually eliminated, but at the same time more and more people are seeking outdoor recreation, living in suburbs, and bringing new and exotic plants into their homes and gardens. The increasing popularity of herbal medicines and teas and of eating wild plants has resulted in a greater exposure of people to potentially harmful plant substances; and hence, despite more advanced knowledge and education on toxic plants, poisonings from plants and

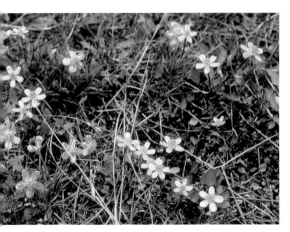

Sagebrush buttercup
(*Ranunculus glaberrimus*).

fungi continue to plague us. Fortunately, despite the thousands of cases of plant and mushroom poisonings that occur in North America each decade, very few actually result in serious illness or death.

Studies of hospital visits related to poisonings show that plant and mushroom poisonings are among the major classes of poisonings (the others being household chemicals and medicines). People seek medical attention most often for children, who are often too young to disclose accurately what it is they have consumed, causing great anxiety for their parents. This partially explains the fact that one of the most common reasons to take children to North American emergency rooms is suspected poisoning by chili peppers. Children's suite of taste buds differs from adults; they are probably more sensitive, which only adds to their misery when they mistakenly take in too much chili.

Identifying poisonous plants and mushrooms

The best time to identify plants or mushrooms that might be poisonous is before any poisoning has occurred. Correct identification can be critical, and people tempted to harvest wild plants or mushrooms for eating should take exceptional care to identify, or have an expert identify, any plant before it is consumed. Parents of young children, preschool teachers, or anyone else caring for youngsters should also take special precautions to identify ornamental plants they keep indoors or have planted in yards. Never buy a plant for the house unless its identity is known, and its potential for harm understood. Florists and plant nursery workers may not volunteer information about potential toxicity of the plants they sell, but if asked, they will provide this information or at least the name of a plant so that the buyer can find out more about it. Frohne and Pfänder (2005) discuss the problems of labeling cultivated toxic plants and educating people about them.

Information about plant identification and poisonous plants and mushrooms can be obtained in many places and from many people who are willing and able to help. Libraries, nature centers, natural history museums, universities, medical centers, poison control centers, veterinary clinics, forest research facilities, horticultural centers, and botanical gardens are all places where people can go to find out more about poisonous plants. Many of these institutions employ botanists who are pleased to help people identify plant specimens. Many communities and institutions offer courses in plant or mushroom identification for the nonspecialist, and these are an excellent way to learn the basics of plant identification—and to avoid accidental poisoning by toxic plants or fungi.

Many Web sites provide helpful and authoritative information on poisonous plants and mushrooms. These include university Web sites, poison control centers, and government Web sites. We have listed some of these in our reference section, but there are many more out there.

Toxic properties and life cycles

The complexity of plants in evolution is reflected in their biochemistry. The embryophyta, as land plants are generally known, are divided, in evolutionary order, into mosses, ferns, gymnosperms (e.g., conifers), and angiosperms (flowering plants). Biochemically, mosses are far less complex than flowering plants; they share many basic housekeeping pathways, but in the rich biochemistry of secondary metabolites, flowering plants are infinitely more complex. Mosses, ferns, and conifers have archegoniate life cycles: the distinguishing feature is that the female gamete, or egg, is located in an archegonium, which is located in a gametophyte (gamete-bearing plant). Gametophytes of mosses and ferns are physically separate organisms; spores are released from the spore-bearing generation (the sporophyte). When the spores find a suitable substrate and sufficient water, they germinate to produce gametophytes that form male and female gametes, or sperm and egg, respectively. Mating occurs in water. Gymnosperms differ from mosses and ferns by the very significant fact that the gametophyte never leaves the sporophyte but is encased within an ovule. Angiosperms take this to a different level: the gametophyte is now a simplified structure called the embryo sac within an ovule, and even fertilization is different, with male gametes producing the embryo and the nutritive tissue of the seed, or endosperm.

The reproductive cycles of these plants do not in any way account for the differences in biochemical complexity, as reproduction via embryos is a conserved feature that unites all higher plants. Where life cycle has played an important role, however, is in the chemistry of attraction and reward of animals that serve as pollen vectors. Mosses and ferns reproduce in puddles of water, requiring no other organisms, and gymnosperms are wind-pollinated. The flowering plants, in contrast, evolved mechanisms to attract and reward pollinators. This depends on biochemistry of volatile compounds in scent, as well as chemistry of rewards, be they fat, protein, or carbohydrate. The diversity of compounds involved in attracting pollinators is astonishing. Attraction of animals is not limited to flowers but can extend to fruit and seeds. The compounds that the plant produces in these situations can have single or dual functions. Single functions include attraction or reward. Dual function would be attraction of insects but defense against microbes. In this case, what is a reward for one kind of organism is a growth inhibitor, or worse, for another organism. And this brings us back to poisons.

Plant biochemistry has many universal pathways; for example, terpene synthesis is found in all groups. However, plants differ in how much biochemistry they do, which is reflected in differences such as the low caloric value of mosses versus the high caloric value of flowering plants, to pick the two extremes in plant evolution. Here life cycle differences come out quite clearly: spores of mosses and ferns have very high fat storage (50% of their dry weight), as do seeds of gymnosperms and flowering plants. However, the biochemistry of these calorically rich stages is not very complex. The real complexity is found in the organism bearing the seeds or spores, which may not be particularly rich in stored products.

This is because other major factors that have influenced biochemical complexity come into play, especially those related to abiotic (from the physical environment) stresses and biotic stresses (those from other living organisms). Seeds and spores are, after all, propagules and are in a dormant or quiescent state. At the moment of dispersal, they aren't doing much. Only upon germination do they renew their activities. The spore- or seed-bearing plant needs to photosynthesize, grow new organs and tissues, and defend itself against abiotic (drought, extremes in temperature) and biotic (animal and microbial attack) stresses. The investment strategy of mosses—low caloric value, small size (a consequence of missing much of the pathway required for lignification, a prerequisite for upright growth above a few centimeters), and unpalatability—requires little complexity compared with flowering plants, which are larger and more varied both ecologically and morphologically. The interrelationships that flowering plants have formed with other organisms are largely a consequence of natural selection in biochemical pathways.

The life cycle stage that requires the most protection, simply put, is the one that is biochemically active the longest. In the case of mosses, it is the gametophyte, but for ferns, gymnosperms, and angiosperms it is the sporophyte. It is tempting to believe that plants that live longest are also more likely to have developed more complex defenses, but there is no indication that trees differ fundamentally from annuals in their defenses, as can be seen in groups of plants such as legumes, where every kind of plant—from minuscule annuals to forest-dominating perennials and all sizes in between, including vines—is found. The reason that this is true is that plants evolved in ecological situations in which animals have also evolved, resulting in adaptations of animals to plant defenses, which have resulted in natural selection of more effective defenses—a biochemical arms race. Each time an animal develops an enzymatic or physiological response that allows it to survive some plant toxins, the plant must respond by creating novel defense compounds. This is reflected in the multiplication of classes of catabolic enzymes in animals and the parallel evolution of biosynthetic enzymes in plants. Since plants and animals evolved onto the land surface, there has been an explosion in enzymes (e.g., cytochrome P450s) that are related to the creation of defense compounds in plants and, in animals, to their modification and elimination. Flowering plants, with their more than 250,000 species, are the most prevalent plants on earth; not surprisingly, this group has the most compounds, many of which are defense compounds. There is overlap in how plants respond to biotic stresses such as insect, bacterial, and fungal attack, and abiotic stresses such as drought and cold, so that pools of metabolites that can build up poisons are also potential building blocks for compounds that can reg-

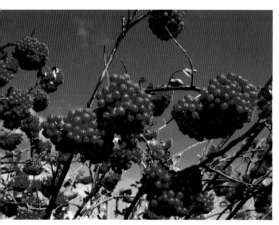

Mountain ash, or rowan fruits (here of *Sorbus aucuparia*) are commonly eaten by birds; seeds contain cyanogenic glycosides.

ulate cold tolerance. The plant is flexible, but in general and in short, many poisonous compounds exist because they ward off predators. Plants do not have the ability to flee. They must stand and fight, and among their best weapons are poisonous compounds.

This brings us to one of the paradoxes of poisons: why do plants have poisonous fruits? Fleshy fruits attract predators, which may be potential seed dispersers, so why do some fruits contain toxins? This question can be considered in a number of ways. The first is by dosage: cyanogenic glycosides are common in bird-dispersed fruit. Cedar waxwings, for example, can consume over five times the quantity that would be a lethal dose for a mammal, such as a rat. This would indicate that dispersers (birds) are favored over predators and poor dispersers (mammals). Some fruits contain sorbitol and other laxatives that speed the passage through the animal, in essence, ensuring the passage of the seed before the animal can digest it. This view, that there is some advantage to the chemical composition of fruit, is met with some skepticism. Most plants that are generally toxic are also producers of toxic fruit, so there may be no paradox: the plant is simply toxic in all parts. Surprisingly, there is little work on this aspect of plants; answers are expected in the future.

Foods, poisons, medicines

Again, many plants we routinely eat contain some potentially harmful compounds. What may not be as well appreciated is just how many of our food plants are also considered to have medicinal properties, and, in turn, how many medicinal plants may also be toxic if used in too high a dosage or wrongly prepared and administered. Indigenous and local peoples familiar with their local plant and fungus resources often have no difficulty in maneuvering within the "food/medicine/poison triangle." In one study by Turner (2008), 375 traditional food and medicine plants, fungi, lichen, and algal species, as well as those species reported to be toxic by indigenous knowledge holders, were surveyed across 12 First Nations groups of British Columbia, each with distinct languages, for overlaps across the categories of food, medicine, and poison. She found significant numbers of food species with reported healing properties, many food species that have also been used as medicine, and a notable proportion of both food and medicinal species recognized as harmful or toxic under some circumstances. Even most of those species considered extremely poisonous have been taken internally as medicines in some way. It takes a tremendous base of knowledge and experience, however, to be able to rely on such a complex of species for safe nutrition and health care without incurring harm through inadvertent poisoning. Unfortunately, this type of knowledge, embedded within entire indigenous systems known collectively as traditional ecological knowledge (TEK), is eroding as local people succumb to the forces of acculturation and globalization. Several recent anecdotal accounts of poisoning from traditional medicinal plants and from mistaken identity or lack of proper preparation of traditional food plants can be traced to loss of this knowledge, often because barriers of one sort or another have prevented knowledgeable elders from passing what they know to the younger generations.

A common concern in North America is what happens when people use polymedicine, which is mixing modern pharmaceutical drugs and different types of medicines, such as alternative, TEK, natural health products, or traditional Chinese medicine (TCM). Interactions between drugs and herbs can alter absorption, distribution, and elimination of either drug or herb. Physicians are quick to point out that patients often fail to tell them that they are taking herbal medicines (and patients are equally quick to suggest that physicians don't take the time to ask). In such situations, adverse interactions can be expected; for example, herbs that affect liver enzymes can alter drug metabolism. The different types of medicine trace some of their roots and practices to some common plant medicines, and so they are hardly mutually exclusive; however, the fact that consumers often speak as if they are choosing one form of medicine over another means that communication is hampered. Fortunately, there are excellent sources that concern themselves with potential interactions between active herbal constituents and pharmaceutical drugs. Using these sources to find possible drug-herb interactions is not difficult. Consumers should be encouraged to investigate such sites, because it will make them more informed patients who will be likely to supply better information to their physicians and healers and ask more relevant questions.

Allergies

Some types of plants and plant products cause allergic reactions in people and animals. This is when individuals have or develop unusual sensitivities to substances that may be harmless to others. Allergy-causing materials, or allergens, include airborne spores of fungi and pollen grains from many different plant species, which produce hay fever in susceptible individuals. Although hay fever is not usually life-threatening, it does cause cold-like symptoms including stuffy nose, watering eyes, and sneezing, leaving hay fever sufferers miserable during flowering season. Furthermore, if left untreated, hay fever can lead to asthma and other serious complications. Many, many plants, including grasses and numerous members of the aster family, such as ragweeds (*Ambrosia* spp.) and goldenrods (*Solidago* spp.), cause widespread allergies. It is not within the scope of this book to describe the many hay fever plants (but details can be found in Lewis et al. 1983). If hay fever is suspected, a physician or allergy specialist should be consulted.

Other plants can cause even more serious allergies in some individuals. Some people, for example, are violently allergic to peanuts, buckwheat, or any number of other specific types of plants and plant products. These

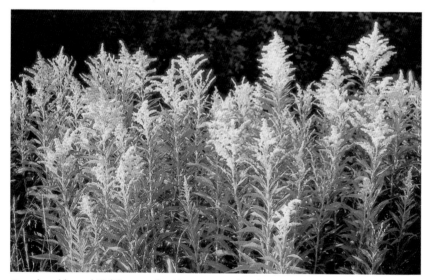

Canada goldenrod (*Solidago canadensis*), a common hay fever plant.

allergies can be life-threatening for some; reactions to ingesting even minute quantities of an allergen can be severe, with vomiting, swelling of the throat, and restricted breathing. For people suffering from an allergy of this type, even certain common and normally edible plants can be deadly. It is impossible here to deal with such plant allergens because they are so diverse and so specific to individuals. Suffice to say, even if you have no known allergies, you could be allergic to a new food, drug, or herb you try for the first time, or even subsequently. If you develop any unusual symptoms after tasting a new type of food or mushroom, or a new herb, stop taking it immediately and consult a physician or allergist. If you experience difficulty breathing, call 911 immediately, as you may be experiencing anaphylactic shock, a violent allergic reaction. In its most severe form, it can prove fatal if not promptly treated.

Another common type of allergy is caused by skin contact with certain plants. The best-known contact plant allergens are poison ivy and its relatives, poison oak and poison sumac. On average, seven of every ten people are immediately allergic to these plants, and almost everyone is after prolonged or continuous exposure; for some the reaction is severe enough to

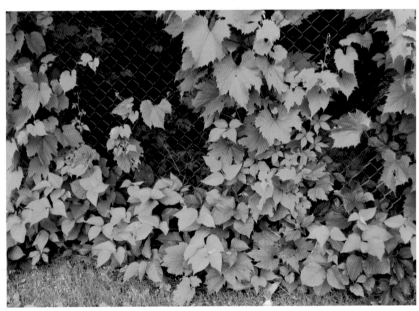

Poison ivy (*Toxicodendron radicans*) growing along a fence,
with wild grape and Virginia creeper.

require hospitalization. These wild plants are described in detail in Chapter 3; several others that commonly cause injury to the skin (dermatitis), through allergic reaction or chemical irritation, are listed in Appendix 3. See Mitchell and Rook (1979) for a more thorough treatment of plants causing skin allergies and of other types of plants injurious to the skin.

Poisoning of pets and livestock

Household pets, especially puppies and kittens, are as vulnerable to poisoning from plants and mushrooms as young children. In a report on mushroom poisonings in 2004 (an exceptionally prolific year for mushrooms in the western United States), mycologist Michael Beug (2004) described over 50 dog poisoning cases. Eight dogs, some of them puppies, died or were euthanized after mushroom consumption in this survey. Pet owners should watch their animals closely around dangerous plants and mushrooms, whether indoors or out. If poisoning is suspected, prompt attention, just as with a child, can mean the difference between survival and death or lasting damage. As with human poisoning, samples of the plants or mushrooms eaten, or vomited materials, can aid significantly in the identification process, and hence, in the treatment given.

Different types of animals have different levels of tolerance to poisonous plants. Cattle, sheep, goats, and other ruminants can often eat larger quantities of toxic plants without noticeable symptoms than single-stomached animals, such as horses, pigs, dogs, cats, and humans. Some animals have developed special enzymes that enable them to break down some toxic compounds into harmless ones. For example, some rabbits possess an enzyme that allows them to eat belladonna (*Atropa bella-donna*) in quantities that would be fatal to other animals. Squirrels have often been observed eating poisonous *Amanita* mushrooms, and deer are said to be able to feed on yew and rhododendron. Deer and bears eat western skunkcabbage leaves and rhizomes with impunity, in amounts that would cause excruciating pain for humans.

Because of their general unpalatability, many poisonous plants are avoided by browsing or grazing animals except in times of extreme hunger and food shortage, which, for range animals, often occur in the winter and early spring months. At such times an animal may develop a taste for a poisonous plant not normally eaten, and become addicted to it, still seeking it when other feed is available. Hence, in animals once poisoned there are often recurring episodes, and this can be a serious problem for farmers and ranchers.

A major problem in animal poisoning is that it often takes place away from human observation, and the only indication that poisoning has occurred is when symptoms appear. Since most poisonous plant manuals classify by plant species rather than by exhibited symptoms, it is often difficult to pinpoint which plant or plants have caused the problem and what the best treatment would be.

Some types of animal poisoning are chronic and difficult to detect. They are manifested in high rates of miscarriage, stillbirths, and infant mortality, lowered milk or wool production, slow growth, and general listlessness. All of these result in severe economic losses to farmers and ranchers as well as untold suffering to the animals.

The best means of preventing acute or chronic poisoning in animals, as well as obtaining the healthiest and most productive livestock, is to maintain high quality pasturage and grazing lands, provide supplemental feed-

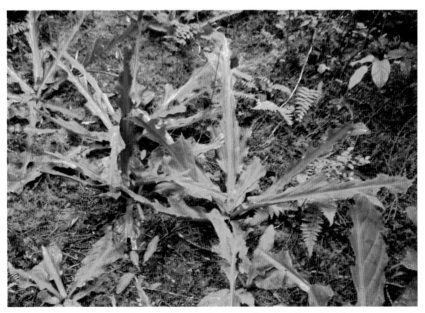

Deer-browsed leaves of western skunkcabbage (*Lysichiton americanus*).

ing whenever required, ensure adequate intake of essential minerals such as calcium and magnesium, and offer a good supply of fresh, clean water. Overgrazed lands lead to underfed livestock far more likely to consume any plant, even a poisonous plant, available to them. For further information on animal poisoning by plants, see Burrows and Tyrl (2006); Frohne and Pfänder (2005); and Knight and Walter (2001).

History of poisoning

As long as humans have been around, we have had to face the challenge of sorting poisonous plants from nonpoisonous plants. In this, we do not differ from any other animal. We have many adaptations that allow us to make these decisions, including the presence of many nerves in the mouth and lips, and taste buds that select for salt, sweet, sour, bitter, and umami (the deeper protein taste in foods). If a plant tastes good, it doesn't mean, at all, that it is good. Some of the most poisonous plants in this book would easily pass any palatability test, which is precisely why they are so insidious. The stomach will expel poisons that are recognized. Should a plant be chewed up in the mouth, digested in the gut, and its poisonous constituents enter the body, there is still the liver that detoxifies such compounds on a regular and daily basis. The liver's large size is a testament to its importance in breaking down compounds.

This begs the question that has puzzled many, which is how did humans sort out the poisonous from the palatable and harmless? Was it one endless Hobbesian nightmare before agriculture was invented? The answer is a clear no. As Richard Ford, an eminent ethnobotanist, would have it, we give too little credit to our powers of observation. Humans were very much aware of their environment and observed animals closely. Domestication of pets and food animals is a legacy of this ability, but prior to this, humans surely observed other omnivorous mammals with diets similar to their own to see what was preferred or what was rejected. In this way, many lives were spared, and the selection of edible plants was not only reinforced by human cultural activities but by further and more refined observation of other animals. Prehistoric poisoning can only be inferred, but given that human structure—eyes, mouths, hands, and GI tract—have been relatively unaltered in the last 100,000 years, the implication is that the early humans had the same organs and appendages integrated into a central nervous system that likely responded the same way; in short, early humans were probably just as observant as modern humans, which, given our visual abilities, is very observant indeed.

The history of poisoning would be a history of mistakes, were it not for the simple fact that we use plants for more than food. Animals immediately ancestral to humans have very primitive forms of culture, that is, learned and transmitted knowledge. Studies of chimpanzees and bonobos over the last 50 years have shown that different populations of these animals do things (how they use tools to extract termites from nests, how they hunt other animals) differently from one another. It is clear that they can learn and transmit behavior. This has contributed to a complex picture of each animal population, which is partly defined by what they pass on in knowledge to one another. People, unlike chimps, use plants in many more ways, including ritual, dance, shelter, religion, and many other social interactions. This tends to structure how poisonings occur.

According to polls that one of us (PvA) took of the undergraduates he regularly teaches, alcohol poisoning is common (25% of the students admitted to having poisoned themselves with alcohol). The prehistory of alcohol poisoning is likely to overlap with the first archaeological artifacts that are unique to alcoholic beverage production. There is ongoing debate in this field, as evidence is scattered, but it has been argued that alcohol consumption may predate cereal cultivation: beer may well have predated bread.

Guessing at the history of alcohol is relevant to any ideas about early poisoning, because alcohol use slipped in on the coattails of plant usage. Mammals other than humans, including chimpanzees, elephants, and bears, are known to use plants for medicinal reasons. For early hominids and early humans, plants played a medicinal role.

Medicine arose independently from a number of different sources, such as the Indo-Germanic, Egyptian, Chinese, and Babylonian traditions. The Greek tradition provides the best chain of ideas that link lore through philosophy to medicine and then modern medicine. The history of this tradition in medicine begins with Anaximander of Miletus, the first known philosopher to pay attention to living things. He did not differentiate between plants and animals: both originated from the moist element of the earth. His writings indicate a clear idea that animals and plants evolved and changed. The 6th century B.C. was a time of great intellectual and social upheaval in Greece. Ideas developed rapidly. About 50 years after Anaximander, Empedocles of Akragas systematized the world into water, earth, air, and fire, and the attraction and repulsion between these elements. Plants, in his opinion, were the first organisms on the earth. Empedocles had a lasting influence because he developed coherent ideas about plants, plant nutrition, and plant evolution. This created a strong base for the great interest in plants that occurred in the next century. A body of writing attributed to Hippocrates of Cos is the first extensive picture of medicine in ancient Greece. This work, detailing observations and recorded medical experiences, lists over 200 plants that are found as ingredients in remedies, and 100 plants that are of dietary importance, which was considered a part of therapy. Hippocrates' principal contribution was that lessons in medicine must be drawn from experience. This formed the basis for rational medicine. Medical practitioners who practice rational medicine were differentiated from those who practiced nonrational medicine, such as magic-based, priest-controlled groups, or specialized cults, such as that of Asclepias.

Ideas generated from philosophers of natural history influenced both rational and nonrational medicine. Echion's idea that the shape of a plant organ might provide an indication of potential use in human medicine was embraced, in various forms, by both sides in the centuries that followed. Herbals both of pharmocognosy (Diocles) and later, illustrated herbals (Crateaus) created a longstanding tradition in botany of compendia of information. By the 4th century B.C., rationalist physicians were divided into two camps: Aristotelians, who created a theoretical basis for plant use, and empiricists, who believed in experience.

The next leap in medicinal use of plants, and one that would have an impact for a millennium, was Dioscorides' compilation of all possible components—animal, mineral, and vegetable—of medicines. He traveled, did field work, inquired from locals about plant use, made comparisons to establish what was universally accepted, and performed trials on the efficacy of plant drugs on particular diseases.

We can look back at the lists of drugs current in the ancient world, analyzing the various ancient medical treatises housed in libraries and archives, and try to understand how they were used—looking, for example, at the chemical evidence from archaeological samples. If a survey of the medical treatises from the 5th century B.C. to the 2nd century A.D. is made, then we can compare the number of prescriptions with the types of plants that are used. According to medical historian and classicist Alain Touwaide, as many as a few thousand plants are listed as ingredients of formulas or prescriptions, but these prescriptions can be roughly divided into two types: those with many ingredients and those with few ingredients. The formulas that require many ingredients—and these are the bulk of the ancient prescriptions—tend to use the same small subset of plants, approximately 45 to 60 common plants. All these medicinal plants were common garden plants, not wild weeds. Garlic, parsley, leek, flax, cauliflower, oregano, and other plants were represented dozens of times in ancient prescriptions.

Medicinal poisoning, through from ancient times and all the way to Renaissance Europe, ought to have been low, as most historical medical formulations for which we have records are relatively harmless. However, this does not take into account the complexities of ancient medicine in regard to poisons. Poisons are not unique to plants but are well known from snakes and other animals. The impressive lethality of animal and plant poisons was considered in two books written by Nicander of Colophon in 130 B.C. In the first, *Theriaca*, he describes snakes, their poisons, and the potential antidotes. In the second, *Alexipharmaca*, he listed other animal poisons, as well as mineral and plant poisons. Remedies are also itemized, and these are almost always herbal. Experimentation in the interests of discovering antidotes occupied infamous ancient kings such as Mithridates of Pontus and Attalus III of Pergamon, both of whom experimented on prisoners. In short, a branch of medicine was obsessed with poisons and how to overcome their effects. This is difficult to appreciate, since we live in an age when we have a microbial explanation of many diseases, not to mention genetic and molecular understanding of the basis for numerous illnesses. Ancient practitioners had few reliable treatments, so it is not surprising that powerful poisons should occupy a prominent position in medical thinking.

The first mention of dosage is in Dioscorides, in which the effects of belladonna are given in a graded series based on one, two, or three drachmas' worth, with the first being good, the second with psychoactive effects for up to three days, and the third, deadly. Medicine from the time of the Greeks to the Romans and later to the Middle Ages was an evolving set of traditions that experienced the occasional flowering, as it did in the 6th century B.C., and again in the 2nd century A.D. However, for long periods, this knowledge was simply copied, often unreliably, so that errors crept in and were perpetuated. The field stagnated until modern medicine began its rise in the early Renaissance with the rediscovery of Greek and Roman documents.

Today, with approximately 120 prescription drugs derived from plants (less than 100 plant species supply these drugs), medicinal use remains one of the major causes of poisoning, whether attributable to incorrect dosages, drug-drug interactions, or individual reactions to dosages that were unforeseen or unpredicted.

A history of poisonings would not be complete without mention of memorable deliberate poisonings. State killings are interesting examples where humans normally appalled by murder will agree on a death for the greater good, including political execution. The state poison of ancient Athens was poison hemlock (*Conium maculatum*); both Phokion and, most famously, Socrates were executed by being forced to drink it. A more recent example of state execution—or rather assassination—was the 1978 murder of Georgi Markov, who was injected with ricin from castorbean (*Ricinus communis*) while he stood at a London bus stop (a pellet containing the toxin was pushed into his leg by the tip of an umbrella carried by a Bulgarian secret agent). The attack on Markov was one of three such attacks in the same year in different European capitals. From killing individuals to finishing off your enemies is a small step. The ancient Greek general Solon besieged Cirrha, then diverted a stream that flowed into the city, forcing the besieged to drink well water and collected rainwater until these supplies gave out. The general then directed the stream back to its original course, but dipped hellebore plants in the water. The thirsty Cirrhaeans drank deeply and suffered general diarrhea. Stricken guards left their posts just long enough for Solon and his troops to enter and take the city.

Medicinal applications

Just because a plant is considered poisonous or harmful in some way does not mean that it cannot be useful or valuable. Many poisonous plants are beautiful and decorative, offering "food for the soul," if not for the body. Aside from their ornamental value, though, many provide important compounds widely used in traditional and modern medicine. The very actions that render them poisonous—their effects on the heart and circulatory system, the nervous system, the blood, or on cell division, for example—make them useful in treating certain conditions. Pharmacognosy is the science dealing with the knowledge of natural drugs and their biological, chemical, and economic features. By definition, this science also includes the study of the poisonous properties of medicinal plants.

Purple foxglove (*Digitalis purpurea*) is one of the best known and most widely used poisonous medicinal plants. It was known to be poisonous but was used for centuries by illiterate farmers and housewives in England and Europe for treating dropsy, a condition of massive fluid retention in the body, known more recently to be brought about by poor heart function. The link between foxglove, heart activity, and dropsy was first proposed in the late 1700s by prominent British physician William Withering. We now know that foxglove contains a mixture of cardiac glycosides, including digitoxin, gitoxin, and gitaloxin, which have a strong effect on the heart muscles. When used in correct dosages they change the rhythm of the heartbeat, lengthening the time between heart contractions and thus allowing the ventricle to be emptied more completely. They also improve general circulation, relieve fluid buildup, or edema, and help kidney secretion. The dosage must be carefully controlled, however, because the effective therapeutic dose may be as high as 70% of the toxic dose. Today, millions of people take some form of digitalis to help regulate and strengthen their heartbeat—proof that poisonous plants can be life-savers as well as life-takers.

There are many other examples of useful yet toxic plants. Opium poppy (*Papaver somniferum*) yields, among other compounds, the potent but habit-forming painkiller morphine, as well as the milder, usually non-habit-forming analgesic codeine. Both are alkaloids, isolated from opium. A third opium alkaloid, papaverine, is used mainly in the treatment of internal spasms, particularly of the intestines.

Green false hellebore (*Veratrum viride*), which has been used medicinally by North American indigenous peoples for generations, yields a number of important alkaloids, particularly the ester alkaloids germidine and germitrine, which have been used in the treatment of high blood pressure. May-apple (*Podophyllum peltatum*) contains lignans having anticancer and anti-viral properties and provides a drug of choice for treating human vene-real warts. Pacific yew (*Taxus brevifolia*), well known to Northwest Coast indigenous peoples as a strong, resilient wood and a source of medicine, is renowned as the original source of the anticancer drug Taxol, derived from its bark. Many other toxic plants have been used in folk medicine in various parts of the world, and some are still marketed in health food and herbal

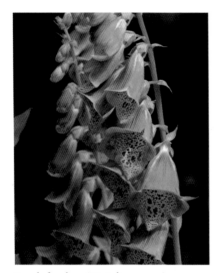

Purple foxglove (*Digitalis purpurea*).

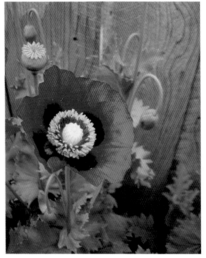

Opium poppy (*Papaver somniferum*).

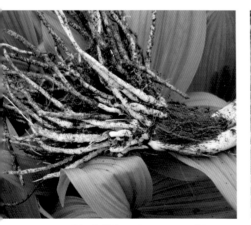

Green false hellebore (*Veratrum viride*) roots: an important but potentially dangerous traditional medicine.

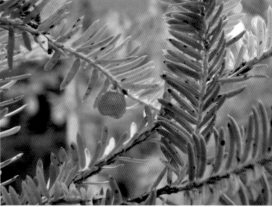

Pacific yew (*Taxus brevifolia*).

healing stores. Most are safe if used correctly, but a very few products that have been bought and used as directed have resulted in serious illness or death for the user.

Many herbs sold as teas or for medicinal use are labeled only by common names on their packages, and this can be misleading, since the same common name may be used for two or more distinct types of plants. Sometimes, too, people have a violent allergy to herbal medicines that may be safe for others. Since laws to guide the use of herbal medicines are not well established, the onus is on the user to ensure that the herbal medicines taken are safe. Appendix 6 lists some herbal medicines with potentially harmful effects, as well as providing a short discussion on safety and efficacy of herbal remedies. The American Botanical Council is dedicated to effective and safe use of herbal medicine; its journal, *HerbalGram*, is a good source of information on herbal medicines.

TREATMENTS: WHAT TO DO, WHAT TO EXPECT

Digestive tract irritants

The most common type of internal poisoning by plants is irritation of the mouth, throat, stomach, and intestines due to the ingestion of toxic substances. Although the actual toxins and their means of action vary considerably, the general treatment for such irritation is relatively uniform. The simple suggested procedures provided here are as outlined by the *Poison Management Manual* (Kent et al. 1997).

For mouth and throat irritation, caused by chewing on plants such as *Dieffenbachia* and other plants in the arum family (Araceae) containing calcium oxalate crystals that burn and irritate the mouth and throat, give milk or ice cream, or allow the patient to suck on a popsicle or ice chips. Observe for swelling of the mouth and throat, which may block air passage. Antihistamines may relieve the swelling.

After ingestion of stomach irritants, including wisterias (*Wisteria* spp.) and daffodils (*Narcissus* spp.), vomiting usually occurs spontaneously. Antacids may provide relief. Ingestion of intestinal irritants usually results in vomiting, abdominal pain, and diarrhea within an hour. Other systemic effects occur only if large amounts have been ingested. In this group are saponin plants such as horse chestnuts and buckeyes (*Aesculus* spp.); resin-containing plants such as daphnes (*Daphne* spp.), irises (*Iris* spp.), and American pokeweed (*Phytolacca americana*); taxine-containing yews (*Taxus* spp.); and miscellaneous plants including oaks (*Quercus* spp.), English holly (*Ilex aquifolium*), mistletoes (*Phoradendron* spp.), poinsettias and spurges (*Euphorbia* spp.), European privet (*Ligustrum vulgare*), and common snowberry, or waxberry (*Symphoricarpos albus*).

Some plants cause intense digestive reactions that may be delayed for an hour or up to two days following ingestion. These include such violent toxins as colchicines in autumn crocus (*Colchicum autumnale*) and glorylily, or flame lily (*Gloriosa superba* and its relatives); oxalates and other toxins in rhubarb (*Rheum rhabarbarum*); solanine in nightshades, potato sprouts and green tubers, tomatoes, and Jerusalem cherries (*Solanum* spp.); and poisonous proteins in castorbean (*Ricinus communis*), rosarypea (*Abrus precatorius*), and black locust (*Robinia pseudoacacia*).

For all these plants, activated charcoal may be administered by medical staff, followed by appropriate supportive care and observation.

Skin and eye irritation

Skin irritations are of various types, including mechanical injury caused by spines, thorns, or barbs, chemical irritation, allergic skin reactions, and photodermatitis, which occurs when exposure to the plant is followed by exposure to sunlight. Plants that irritate the skin and eyes are listed in Appendix 3, and some of the more serious dermatitis-causing plants (poison ivy, poison oak, and poison sumac) are treated in Chapter 3. Irritation, itching, burning, blistering, and/or excessive pigmentation may result from touching or rubbing against these plants, and sometimes there is danger from secondary infection if the skin is broken.

For mechanical injury to the skin, remove thorns, spines, or barbs, and treat the wound with a disinfectant. Small cactus spines can sometimes be removed by dripping candle wax over the affected area, allowing the wax to harden by immersing the area in cold water, and then peeling off the hardened wax. For other types of dermatitis, wash the skin thoroughly with soap and water. Remove any contaminated clothing and wash prior to reuse. For poison ivy or its relatives, application of calamine lotion, Burow's solution (containing aluminum acetate), or an antiperspirant containing aluminum salts may provide relief. Severe itching may be treated with diphenhydr-

amine given orally or by muscular injection, or with topical or systemic cor-
ticosteroids. Maintain close observation for bacterial or fungal infections.

To treat eye irritations, gently flush the eyes with a stream of slightly
tepid water or saline solution for five minutes. If the irritation persists, an
ophthalmologist should be consulted. For further information on treatment of skin and eye irritations caused by plants, see Kent et al. (1997).

It's mainly about adsorption: activated charcoal

Suspected plant poisoning is now treated more simply than it was in the
past. Formerly, emetics were considered necessary to induce vomiting, but
studies showed that most poisonous substances could be rendered physiologically inactive by adsorption (binding them onto surfaces). One way
to increase the surface area of an adsorbing substance was to use chemical-
binding compounds that have enormous surfaces. The most commonly
used adsorptive substance is activated charcoal, the adsorptive surface of
which is infinitely larger than the absorptive surface of the stomach and
intestines. As a result the dangerous compounds attach themselves to the
most abundant surface available, which is the charcoal.

Activated charcoal is not likely kept in most home medicine cabinets,
as ipecac syrup was, and just as well: its administration is not easy, as it is
unpleasant to ingest. However, a patient on his/her way to a hospital can
attempt to minimize poisons by drinking milk, which has a highly adsor-
bent protein suspension. Once in hospital, the patient is given activated
charcoal, provided with appropriate supportive care, and put under observation—a "wait and see" approach. Again, most plant ingestions don't
require active treatment involving plant identification and the complexities of dealing with a list of suspected biochemical compounds. Immediate
analysis is often inadequate if not impossible.

Beyond activated charcoal and observation

Poisons that require more than activated charcoal and observation, according to Dr. Les Vertesi, are classified according to the following criteria.

1. Simple gastrointestinal and mucous irritants, such as saponins, which
   need only supportive care.
2. Hallucinogens, which require only supportive care.

3. Belladonna derivatives, which may require specific pharmaceutical antagonists (such as physostigmine). These are often present with delirium (which can be difficult to distinguish from 2), but there are other physical signs. Most of these can be managed with supportive care, but severe overdoses can be fatal even in professional hands.

4. Cardiac glycosides, such as those found in foxglove, have complex effects on the heart that essentially stop it from beating. Treatment can involve cardiac pacing. An antidote—Digi-bind—is kept on hand in most emergency rooms.

5. Cyanides are not found free in plants but are sometimes generated after ingestion. Without a good history of what plants were consumed, diagnosis can be tricky. If cyanide is suspected, there is a specific antidote kit available (inhaled amyl nitrite and intravenous sodium nitrite and sodium thiosulfite).

6. *Amanita phalloides* is most feared as there is generally little that can be done. It causes extensive damage, ultimately destroying bowel, liver, and kidneys. Rapid dialysis can be effective, but few hospitals have the necessary equipment.

Safety of ipecac?

It is commonly mentioned in past books on poisonous plants, and consequently on the Web, that inducing vomiting by using an emetic (in particular, widely available ipecac syrup) is a useful treatment. Since the first edition of this book was published in 1991, the safety and effectiveness of ipecac syrup has been called into question by the American Academy of Clinical Toxicology and European Poison Centres (1997). In their position paper on ipecac syrup (*Journal of Clinical Toxicology* 35:699–709), they submit that there is no evidence that ipecac syrup actually helps improve the outcome in cases of poisoning and argue that administering this emetic can delay the administration of more effective treatments such as activated charcoal and/or antidotes. They note that ipecac syrup can change one's neurological status, making it difficult to distinguish the effects of the poisoning from the effects of the ipecac, and that ipecac administered at home could result in an accidental overdose. Finally, they cite serious cases of abuse of this substance by people with eating disorders such as bulimia. Other poison control centers advise against using ipecac under most circumstances, unless as a last resort when there is no alternative therapy available and when it would not adversely affect more effective treatment that might be provided at a hospital in the immediate future. The Rocky Mountain Poison and Drug Center, for one, suggests that the routine stocking of ipecac in all households with young children is neither necessary nor advisable; for summary recommendations, see http://www.guidelines.gov/summary/summary.aspx?doc_id=8052#s23

Gastric lavage

Gastric lavage, a standard procedure in most cases of serious poisoning in the past, is seldom used, having been superseded by activated charcoal in most situations. It is a procedure done *only* by a physician or qualified medic, involving the passage of a tube into the stomach, removal of the stomach contents through gravity or suction, and careful replacement of the contents with water or normal saline solution. The procedure is usually repeated until the washings are clear and free of toxic materials and is generally followed by a dose of activated charcoal and a saline cathartic. Unless the patient is in a coma, sedation is usually required before gastric lavage is carried out: it is an uncomfortable and somewhat frightening procedure. It has saved many lives, however; one of us (PvA) had his stomach pumped when as a three-year-old he consumed a bottle of some kind of medicine.

Cathartics

Cathartics—substances that speed up elimination of materials through the digestive tract—can be very useful in treatment of poisoning but should be given only under medical supervision. They are usually given at the same time as activated charcoal: after the patient has vomited, or after gastric lavage has been performed. By hastening the passage of toxic materials through the digestive tract, they help to decrease the body's absorption of harmful compounds. They also help to disperse the activated charcoal more evenly and prevent it from becoming cemented into hard lumps. Cathartics include such substances as magnesium sulfate (epsom salts), sodium sulfate, sodium phosphate-biphosphate complex (Fleet Enema), and sorbitol. These can be given orally or through a tube. The first three are salts, which are dissolved in water, juice, or sweetened fluid. The last can be given straight or mixed with activated charcoal. A table of dosages is given in the

Poison Management Manual (Kent et al. 1997). Cathartics should *not* be used for poisoning by corrosive substances, or if a patient's electrolyte balance is disturbed. If the patient is suffering from kidney failure, magnesium-containing cathartics should not be used. Castor oil or mineral oil are not recommended because they may increase absorption of fat-soluble poisons.

PLANT POISONS AND THEIR EFFECTS

Classification of plant poisons

Many types of potentially harmful substances are to be found in plants. Biochemists classify them according to their chemical structures, as well as their effects on people and animals. Many poisonous plants contain more than one kind of toxic substance, and sometimes the major classes of toxic compounds overlap by virtue of sharing certain chemical structures. In spite of all that is known about the chemistry of toxic plants, there is still much more to learn. As already indicated, many plant toxins can be put to use by people as medicines, and undoubtedly many more medicinal uses are yet to be discovered.

Alkaloids and glycosides comprise two major classes of plant toxins, both highly complex and diverse. They are difficult to characterize in more than a general way, and in each case several subclasses are recognized based on chemical structure and physiological action. Some other poisonous principles found in plants are oxalates, tannins, phenols, alcohols, aldehydes, volatile oils, and poisonous proteins. Following is a brief overview of these classes. For further, more detailed information, the reader is referred to Frohne and Pfänder (2005).

Alkaloids

Alkaloids are a major group of organic compounds. Over 4000 alkaloid compounds have been identified, and they occur in about 15 to 20% of vascular plants and at least 40% of plant families. They are found in roots, seeds, leaves, bark, and stems. Many plant species contain several different alkaloids similar in structure. Alkaloids are mostly basic in nature, as implied by their name, meaning "alkali-like." Derived from amino acids, they have a complex molecular structure, with at least one nitrogen (N) atom included within a heterocyclic ring. By definition they have a specific pharmacological activity, especially on the nervous systems of animals. This makes them both potentially toxic and potentially medicinal. Most are bitter-tasting.

Many alkaloids bear names based on the scientific name of their plant sources, with the ending -*in*, or -*ine* (e.g., solanine, from nightshade, *Solanum*, and lupinine, from lupine, *Lupinus*). Some are named from their physiological actions, such as morphine ("sleep-inducing") from opium poppy (*Papaver somniferum*).

Plant families with many alkaloid-containing species include the aster family (Asteraceae), spurge family (Euphorbiaceae), pea family (Fabaceae), lily family (Liliaceae), poppy family (Papaveraceae), buttercup family (Ranunculaceae), coffee or madder family (Rubiaceae), and nightshade family (Solanaceae). Two very poisonous groups of alkaloid-type compounds, however, are from yews (*Taxus* spp.) in the yew family (Taxaceae) and poison hemlock (*Conium maculatum*) in the carrot family (Apiaceae); these families are otherwise poorly represented by alkaloids. Examples of some major subclasses of alkaloids and representative plants containing them are given in Table 1.

Once ingested, alkaloids may be chemically altered by enzyme reactions in the liver. Sometimes they are rendered harmless; in other cases they become even more deadly. This is apparently the case with the pyrrolizidine alkaloids found in ragworts (*Senecio* spp.). It has been suggested that the ragwort alkaloids themselves are not harmful to the liver, but compounds produced from them are. They cause irreversible liver damage in humans and animals for which there is no satisfactory treatment. People drinking herbal teas from ragwort species, or even consuming milk or honey contaminated with ragwort, are at risk even if the quantities consumed are minor.

Structural similarities have been shown between various alkaloids and nerve transmitter substances produced by the human body, including acetylcholine, norepinephrine, dopamine, and serotonin. It is thought that the toxicity of many alkaloids is due to their mimicking or blocking the action of such substances. Symptoms common to acute poisoning by these alkaloids include excess salivation, dilation or constriction of the pupils, vomiting, abdominal pain, diarrhea, lack of coordination, convulsions, and coma. Treatment is with drugs that counteract the central nervous system effects of alkaloids.

Table 1. Some major subclasses of alkaloids and examples
of plants and fungi containing them.

ALKALOID SUBCLASS	ALKALOID NAME	PLANT OR FUNGI CONTAINING ALKALOID
pyrrolizidine	senecionine and others	ragworts (*Senecio* spp.), heliotropes (*Heliotropium* spp.)
piperidine	coniine	poison hemlock (*Conium maculatum*)
	lobeline	Indian-tobacco (*Lobelia inflata*)
tropane	atropine	belladonna (*Atropa bella-donna*)
	hyoscyamine	black henbane (*Hyoscyamus niger*)
	scopolamine	jimsonweed (*Datura stramonium*)
quinolizidine	lupinine	lupines (*Lupinus* spp.)
	cytisine	golden chain tree (*Laburnum anagyroides*), Scotch broom (*Cytisus scoparius*)
pyridine-piperidine	nicotine	tobaccos (*Nicotiana* spp.)
	anabasine	tree tobacco (*Nicotiana glauca*)
indole	psilocybin	magic mushrooms (*Psilocybe* spp.)
	ergot alkaloids	ergots (*Claviceps* spp.), morning-glory, or grannyvine (*Ipomoea tricolor, I. violacea*)
	gelsemine	evening trumpetflower (*Gelsemium sempervirens*)
isoquinoline	berberine	barberries (*Berberis* spp.)
	emetine	ipecac (*Psychotria ipecacuanha*)
	protopine series	opium poppy (*Papaver somniferum*) and other poppy species, celandine (*Chelidonium majus*), bloodroot (*Sanguinaria canadensis*)
steroidal	solanine	nightshades, potatoes (*Solanum* spp.)
	buxine complex	common box (*Buxus sempervirens*)
	germidine and others	false hellebores (*Veratrum* spp.)
	zygadenine	deathcamases (*Zigadenus* spp.)
diterpenoid	aconitine	monkshoods (*Aconitum* spp.)
	delphinine	larkspurs (*Delphinium* spp.)
purine	caffeine	coffee (*Coffea arabica*), tea (*Camellia sinensis*), chocolate (*Theobroma cacao*), hollies (*Ilex* spp.)

Cyanogenic glycosides

Glycosides are compounds that consist of one or more sugar molecules, combined with an aglycone, or non-sugar component. When ingested, glycosides are readily broken down by enzymes or acids into sugar and aglycone units. The poisonous qualities of glycosides are determined by their aglycones, and the properties of the latter are often used to classify glycoside compounds.

Cyanogenic glycosides release hydrogen cyanide as a byproduct of their breakdown, which may occur when the plants are bruised, wilted, or ingested. Trace amounts of cyanogenic glycosides are found in many types of plants. Altogether, some 800 species in 80 different families contain them. However, relatively high concentrations leading to cyanide poisoning occur in only a few species, mainly in the rose family (Rosaceae) and pea family (Fabaceae). Cyanide-producing plants possess an enzyme system which, when it comes in contact with the cyanogenic glycoside, breaks down the glycoside into sugar, cyanide, and an aldehyde or ketone.

The digestive system is capable of breaking down small quantities of cyanides, but in larger doses they cause anxiety, confusion, dizziness, headache, and vomiting, with an odor of bitter almonds on the breath or vomit. Cyanides inhibit oxygen uptake in the body's cells, and thus poisoning may occur very suddenly if the ingested amounts are able to overwhelm the body's detoxification mechanism. Difficulty in breathing, fluctuations of blood pressure and heart rate, and possible kidney failure may also occur. Coma, convulsions, and death from respiratory arrest may happen suddenly and rapidly.

Glucosinolates

Another important group of glycosides is the goitrogenic glycosides, mustard oil glycosides, or glucosinolates. They are responsible for the hot, pungent flavor of radishes, cresses, cabbages, and other members of the mustard family (Brassicaceae). They may be present in all parts of a plant, but the highest concentration is usually in the seeds. Goitrogenic glycosides break down with an associated enzyme into a glucose sugar, a sulfate fraction, and irritant mustard oils, or goitrogens, which interfere with the uptake of iodine by the thyroid gland and ultimately limit thyroxine production. In small quantities they are harmless to people eating a balanced diet, but if eaten in excess over long periods of time they could lead to lowered thyroid activity. Mustard oils should not be confused with mustard gas, the greenish-colored poisonous chlorine gas used in chemical warfare.

Cardiac glycosides

Cardiac glycosides, also known as cardioactive and cardiotonic glycosides, are a group characterized for their direct action on the heart. Over 400 have been isolated, the best known being the digitalis glycosides present in purple foxglove (*Digitalis purpurea*). Besides their effect on the heart muscle, cardiac glycosides can produce severe digestive upset with nausea, vomiting, abdominal pain, diarrhea, blurred and disturbed color vision, and other symptoms relating to decreased heart function.

Saponins

Saponins are glycosides of terpenoid compounds; their aglycone component is a compound termed a sapogenin. They are water-soluble, bitter-tasting, and soap-like, even at low concentrations. They are seldom harmful in small amounts, but if consumed in large doses their effects can be serious. Symptoms may include irritation of the mucous membranes, increased salivation, nausea, vomiting, and diarrhea, and in severe cases, dizziness, headache, chills, heart disturbances, and eventually convulsions and coma. Saponins alter the permeability of cell membranes and break down red blood cells; hence a saponin injected into the bloodstream can be fatal. They are highly toxic to cold-blooded animals and have been used around the world as fish poisons.

Examples of these and other major classes of toxic glycosides are given in Table 2.

Other classes of poisonous plant compounds

Plant toxins other than the alkaloid and glycoside classes form a diverse chemical mixture of many different types of compounds, some defined by their chemical composition and some by their effects on humans and other animals.

Oxalic acid and oxalates. Oxalic acid and its salts, called oxalates, occur in nearly all organisms, but in certain plant families such as the goosefoot family (Chenopodiaceae) and the buckwheat family (Polygonaceae), relatively

Table 2. Some major classes of toxic glycosides and examples of plants containing them.

GLYCOSIDE SUBCLASS	GLYCOSIDE NAME	PLANT CONTAINING GLYCOSIDE
cyanogenic	amygdalin, prunasin	leaves, bark, and seed kernels of apricots, cherries, plums (*Prunus* spp.) and apples (*Malus* spp.)
	sambunigrin	elderberries (*Sambucus* spp.)
	vicia group	vetches (*Vicia* spp.)
goitrogenic	glucosinolates	black mustard (*Brassica nigra* and related spp.), horseradish (*Armoracia rusticana*)
cardiac	digitalis group	purple foxglove (*Digitalis purpurea*)
	cymarin	Indianhemp (*Apocynum cannabinum*)
	helleborin	black hellebore (*Helleborus niger*)
	convallatoxin	European lily of the valley (*Convallaria majalis*), star of Bethlehem (*Ornithogalum umbellatum*)
	evomonoside	burningbush (*Euonymus alatus* and related spp.)
	oleandrin	oleander (*Nerium oleander*)
saponin	githagoside	corncockle (*Agrostemma githago*)
	aescin	horse chestnuts and buckeyes (*Aesculus* spp.)

large and potentially toxic amounts occur in a number of species. The sour taste of rhubarb stalks and sorrels is from the acid itself. Other plants contain high concentrations of the salts, including sodium oxalate and potassium oxalate, both water-soluble, and calcium oxalate, which is not. When large quantities of plants containing oxalic acid or soluble oxalates are eaten, the oxalate component (oxalate ions) may combine with free calcium in the digestive tract to form insoluble calcium oxalate. This "tying up" of free calcium can lead to a calcium deficiency, especially if the diet is already poor in calcium. Additionally insoluble calcium oxalate crystals may be deposited in the kidneys and other organs, causing mechanical damage.

Oxalate content varies considerably with the plant's age, and with seasonal, climatic, and soil conditions. Under normal circumstances, oxalates in moderate amounts can be broken down by bacteria in an animal's digestive tract. Usually oxalic acid salts must comprise 10% or more of a plant's dry weight to be seriously toxic. Several range plant species in the goosefoot family are particularly notorious for their accumulation of large amounts of oxalates. These include saltlover (*Halogeton glomeratus*), greasewood (*Sarcobatus vermiculatus*), and Russian thistle (*Salsola kali*). Of plants eaten by people, rhubarb (*Rheum rhabarbarum*) stalks (the leaves contain other severe toxins), beets (*Beta vulgaris*), sorrels and woodsorrels (*Rumex* spp., *Oxalis* spp.), and purslane, or little hogweed (*Portulaca oleracea*) should all be used only moderately and not in large amounts due to their potential for accumulating oxalic acid and oxalate salts.

Additionally, certain plants, mostly in the arum family (Araceae), contain calcium oxalate in bundles of minute but sharp, needle-like crystals that cause intense burning, swelling, and discomfort to the lips, mouth, and throat if ingested, by puncturing the sensitive mouth tissues. This physical damage and irritation can become even more serious if the breathing passage is constricted by swelling. Many of our common houseplants—philodendrons, dieffenbachias, caladiums, and calla lilies, for example—are in the arum family and contain these irritating crystals (see Chapter 5).

Tannins and other phenols. Phenols are acidic and form salts with alkaline compounds. Probably the most notorious types of phenols are those of the various species of *Toxicodendron* (formerly in the genus *Rhus*), poison ivy, poison oak, and poison sumac, which cause serious allergic skin reactions in most people. Tannins are complex, astringent phenols, the active part being gallic acid. They are used commercially in tanning leather. They bind up proteins, including enzymes, and thus can quickly stop all cell functions. They occur in many tree barks and other plant structures but are seldom a problem for humans. They are, however, present in the acorns and leaves of oaks (*Quercus* spp.), making them extremely bitter and potentially toxic. Even edible types of acorns, before they can be safely consumed, usually must have their tannins removed through leaching.

Alcohols. These carbohydrate derivatives are best known to people in the form of ethyl alcohol, the active ingredient of wine, beer, and other alcoholic beverages that is produced by fermentation of carbohydrates. We do not normally consider this type of alcohol to be poisonous, but the first definition of "intoxication" (the term that usually covers the abnormal state of "being drunk") is "essentially a poisoning." According to compilations of emergency room records, alcohol poisoning in northern temperate countries accounts for the highest percentage of self-poisonings.

Polyacetylene compounds. Water hemlocks (*Cicuta* spp.), probably the most violently poisonous plant genus of the north temperate zone, contain highly unsaturated polyynes, cicutoxin and cicutol, as their main toxic principles.

Aldehydes and ketones. Aldehyes and ketones are carbohydrate derivatives and are not commonly associated with plant poisoning. When a person has eaten an inky-cap (*Coprinopsis atramentaria*), followed by an alcoholic beverage, coprine in the mushroom causes the body's metabolism of the alcohol to be slowed down. This results in the accumulation of acetaldehyde, a toxic aldehyde, and in the symptoms of coprine poisoning as described under this mushroom.

Ketones are rarely toxic. One that is reputed to be harmful is found in pennyroyal (*Mentha pulegium*), making this mint potentially unsafe for use as a medicinal herb or tea. Another toxic compound is tremetone, an aryl ketone that occurs in white snakeroot (*Ageratina altissima*) and some of its relatives.

Proteins, peptides, and amino acids. Proteins are essential constituents of all living cells. Composed of 20 different types of amino acids linked together, proteins play a major role in cell structure and metabolism. Peptides are less complex combinations of two or more amino acids. Longer peptide chains are known as polypeptides. Many different types of proteins, peptides, and amino acids occur in plants, and some are toxic.

Over 250 different amino acids are known, but only 20 occur in proteins. The others occur in a free state in living cells and are derived from chemical alteration of the protein amino acids. Lathyrogens, amino acids found mainly in the seeds of sweetpea (*Lathyrus odoratus*) and its relatives (*Lathyrus* spp., *Vicia* spp.), are responsible for lathyrism, a chronic disease.

Toxic polypeptides are relatively rare, although cyclic polypeptides are responsible for the most deadly types of mushroom poisoning. They are found in death cap (*Amanita phalloides*), destroying angel (*A. bisporigera* and several related species in the *A. verna-virosa* complex), galerinas (*Galerina* spp.), several small *Lepiota* species, including *L. subincarnata*, and some corts (*Cortinarius* spp.), as well as in some poisonous cyanobacteria (bluegreen algae). European mistletoe (*Viscum album*) and akee (*Blighia sapida*) seeds also contain toxic polypeptides.

Poisonous proteins were previously called toxalbumins because of their solubility properties. Most of these proteins exhibit lectin-like characteristics, such as agglutinization of red blood cells. One such lectin, ricin, is said to be the most toxic naturally occurring compound. Found in castorbean (*Ricinus communis*), it inhibits protein synthesis in the cell wall and agglutinates red blood cells. Other toxic lectins include abrin, found in rosarypea

(*Abrus precatorius*); robin, found in black locust (*Robinia pseudoacacia*); and a lectin found in American pokeweed (*Phytolacca americana*), which is a mitogen affecting the activity of white blood cells.

Thiaminase, the thiamine-destroying enzyme found in brackenfern (*Pteridium aquilinum*) and horsetails (*Equisetum* spp.), is an example of a protein that is toxic not because of its structure, but rather in consequence of its activity.

In addition to these toxic proteins, others are responsible for the specific allergic reactions some people have toward certain types of plants. In these cases, the intensity of the reaction depends not on the quantity of the toxic protein but on the sensitivity of the affected person.

Resins and volatile oils. Resins and volatile, or essential, oils are complex and diverse compounds widely produced by plants. They tend to be secondary compounds—substances that apparently play no role in the primary or fundamental physiology of the plant. Resins are fat-soluble mixtures of volatile and nonvolatile terpenoids and/or phenolic compounds, which occur widely in woody plants. Resins and volatile oils are derived from terpenes, the largest class of organic compounds in the living world, which are hydrocarbons with multiples of isoprene units (molecular formula C_5H_8). According to their complexity, these compounds are divided into mono-, sesqui-, di-, and triterpenes. Resins are usually secreted in specialized structures located either within or on the surface of a plant. Sometimes they are produced when a plant is injured, and they help to protect the plant while it is repairing the damage. Resins and volatile oils often occur together in mixtures, or oleoresins. Turpentine, for example, is an oleoresin obtained from sapwood ducts of certain pines (*Pinus* spp.). Resins are widely harvested for a host of industrial applications. For those who want to learn more about plant resins, we recommend the book by Jean Langenheim (2003).

Mayapple (*Podophyllum peltatum*) contains a complex of toxic compounds known in commerce as podophyllum resin. These are bitter, irritant, and strongly purgative. Podophyllotoxin and its derivatives have medicinal potential in cancer therapy. Only the ripe fruit of mayapple is edible.

Spurges (*Euphorbia* spp.), including christplant, or crown of thorns, poinsettia, and other ornamental species, contain phorbol, an irritant compound, as a major toxic component of their latex. Many members of the heather family (Ericaceae), including rhododendrons and azaleas (*Rhododendron* spp.), mountain, sheep, and alpine laurels (*Kalmia* spp.), and Japanese pieris (*Pieris japonica*), contain andromedotoxins, terpenes that affect the heart and circulatory system and are potentially deadly. Other toxic terpenes are found in daphne, or paradise plant (*Daphne mezereum* and related spp.), irises (*Iris* spp.), marijuana (*Cannabis sativa*), and chinaberrytree (*Melia azedarach*).

Ester derivatives of some resins, including phorbol from the spurges and their relatives, and mezerein from *Daphne*, are known to present another hazard in addition to being directly poisonous. They are cocarcinogens, acting as potent cancer-causing agents when applied after a low-dosage application of a carcinogen. The initial carcinogen may initiate a latent tumor cell, which may remain normal in appearance for a long period; when the cocarcinogen is applied, the cell rapidly becomes cancerous. The cocarcinogen however, does not cause malignant growth itself, even when applied repeatedly.

Volatile oils are almost all mixtures of compounds, usually a liquid and one or more solid components. They are strongly scented and, as their name suggests, they evaporate rapidly when exposed to air. They occur in various plant tissues, depending on the plant family. These are the compounds responsible for the many scents of flowers, herbs, and spices. Some, such as bitter almond oil and mustard oil, are produced from glycosides, and hence are often classed together with glycosides.

Many volatile oils are fragrant and pleasant flavorings of our foods and beverages. In larger amounts, however, they can be harmful. Some are irritants, and some may be tumor-inducing. Thujone is a volatile oil occurring in various cedars, cypresses, and junipers (*Thuja* spp., *Chamaecyparis* spp., *Juniperus* spp.), and also found in various species of the aster family (Asteraceae), including wormwoods (*Artemisia* spp.), common tansy (*Tanacetum vulgare* and related spp.), and yarrow (*Achillea millefolium*). If used repeatedly, thujone can cause serious personality changes, and in large quantities it can produce convulsions and brain cortex lesions. Other potentially harmful volatile oils include umbellulone, from the leaves of California laurel (*Umbellularia californica*); asarone, from the roots of some strains of sweetflags (*Acorus* spp.) and wildgingers (*Asarum* spp.); menthol, from peppermint oil (*Mentha* ×*piperita*); camphor, from the camphortree (*Cinnamomum camphora*) and synthetic sources; myristicin, from nutmeg and mace (*Myristica fragrans*); and safrole, from sassafras (*Sassafras albidum*) and other spicy flavorings.

Phototoxins. Some plants contain phototoxins, or photosensitive agents, chemical substances that can make the skin extremely sensitive to ultraviolet radiation in sunlight. Some compounds in this diverse group can cause cell damage simply on contact with the skin. These include the furanocoumarins in various plants in the carrot family (Apiaceae), including giant hogweed (*Heracleum mantegazzianum*), and the thiophene compounds in marigolds (*Tagetes* spp.) and other members of the aster family (Asteraceae); such compounds give primary photosensitization effects. Other phototoxic substances (e.g., naphthodianthrones) travel to the skin after being eaten and absorbed into the blood stream. In this category are phototoxins in St. Johnswort (*Hypericum perforatum*), buckwheat (*Fagopyrum esculentum*), knotweeds and smartweeds (*Polygonum* spp.), and lambsquarters (*Chenopodium album*).

A secondary type of photosensitization, occurring in livestock, results from any type of damage to the liver that prevents the normal excretion of phylloerythrin, a common pigment produced in the digestive tract as a breakdown product of chlorophyll. The phylloerythrin accumulates in the blood and tissues and causes skin reactions in sunlight (Knight and Walter 2001).

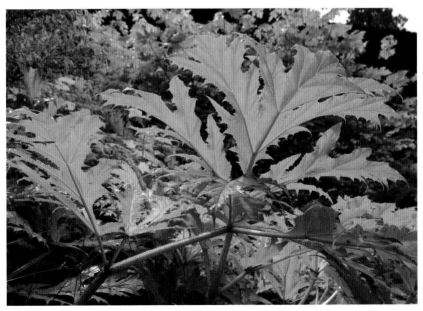

Leaves and stems of giant hogweed (*Heracleum mantegazzianum*) have phototoxic properties, which can cause severe skin irritation (redness, soreness, blistering, and discoloration) when contact is followed by exposure to sunlight.

Symptoms of photosensitization resulting from cell damage to the skin include itchiness, redness, heat, swelling, and blistering that may last for many days, weeks, or even months. Excessive pigmentation, or hyperpigmentation, of the skin in the affected area may remain for a year or more. Photodermatitis is sometimes difficult to distinguish from skin reactions caused by poison ivy and its relatives, which are allergens. The condition, being activated by ultraviolet light, occurs only if the skin of the person or animal is exposed to sunlight (or to artificial UV light) after exposure to a phototoxic substance. Light-skinned people and animals are more likely to be affected by phototoxins than dark-skinned individuals.

The reactivity of some furanocoumarin phototoxins with UV light has been exploited with success in treating psoriasis. The phototoxins, given orally and followed with exposure to certain wavelengths of ultraviolet radiation, prevent the excessive cell division of skin cells that is characteristic of psoriasis.

Cancer-causing plant substances. Many plant substances are known to increase the likelihood of the growth of abnormal or cancerous cells in laboratory animals such as rats and mice. Humans can be expected to have similar reactions to these substances, although in most cases their hazards can only be assumed. A review of naturally occurring, tumor-inducing substances is provided by the American Cancer Society on their Web site (www.cancer.org). Although cancer-causing plants must certainly be considered toxic, it is not within the scope of this book to treat the various types in detail. We do know that some substances statistically increase the risks of contracting cancer, and for this reason certain plants and foods definitely should be avoided.

Fungi, especially molds, are known to produce many tumor-inducing substances. For example, aflatoxins, potent cancer-causing substances acting mainly on the liver but also on other tissues, are produced by certain molds (mainly *Aspergillus flavus*) growing on peanuts and some other foods. It has been suggested that there is a direct link between high rates of liver cancer and consumption of mold-contaminated peanuts in various parts of the world. The grain-contaminating fungus ergot (*Claviceps* spp.) contains many alkaloids and other physiologically active substances, and has also been found to induce tumors in laboratory animals. As well as occurring on wheat, rye, and other domesticated grains, ergot also grows on the grains of wild grasses, including sweet vernalgrass (*Anthoxanthum odoratum*), reed canarygrass (*Phalaris arundinacea*), orchardgrass (*Dactylis glomerata*), and various bromegrass (*Bromus*) and fescue (*Festuca*) species. People preparing grains from wild species should be aware of this hazard.

Pyrrolizidine alkaloids, occurring in ragworts (*Senecio* spp.), heliotropes (*Heliotropium* spp.), and rattleboxes (*Crotalaria* spp.), are potent liver and lung toxins and are also suspected of being carcinogenic under some circumstances.

Safrole, a volatile oil, is present in several different flavorings and spices, especially the root bark of sassafras (*Sassafras albidum*), a favorite wild tea. With prolonged ingestion of large concentrations, it has caused the growth of liver tumors in laboratory rats; because of this, safrole is no longer used as a flavoring agent in root beers.

Cycad or sago palm (*Cycas revoluta*) and other cycads or seedferns (*Cycas* spp.) and their relatives are commonly grown as houseplants and greenhouse ornamentals, as well as outdoors in warmer areas. The bluegreen cyanobacteria that grow in special root structures of cycads produce a highly toxic compound, beta-methylamino-L-alanine (BMAA), a nonproteinogenic amino acid. This neurotoxin becomes concentrated in the seeds. Humans and animals eating these seeds accumulate high amounts of BMAA in their bodies and risk developing a neurological degenerative disease very similar to amyotrophic lateral sclerosis (ALS), or Lou Gehrig's disease. These plants also contain a series of toxic glycosides, the principal one being cycasin. Their seeds, produced on large, cone-like structures, have been found to be highly carcinogenic when fed to rats and other animals. Cycads have been used as an emergency and staple food by native peoples in the tropics, but their use is not recommended under any circumstances.

Brackenfern (*Pteridium aquilinum*), whose green fiddleheads and black-skinned rhizomes have been widely eaten by certain ethnic groups, have been found to contain several cancer-causing substances, as well as other toxins. It has been suggested that the high incidence of stomach cancer in Japan, New Zealand, and the United States may be partially linked to eating bracken shoots.

Numerous other substances have been linked with cancers in laboratory studies and surveys, but how closely laboratory conditions simulate ordinary living conditions for people is still the subject of much speculation.

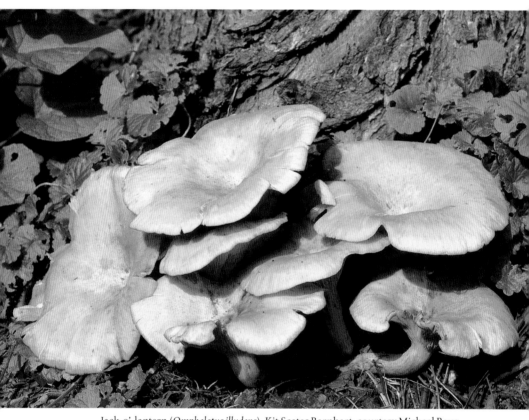

Jack-o'-lantern (*Omphalotus illudens*). Kit Scates Barnhart, courtesy Michael Beug

CHAPTER 2
Poisonous Mushrooms

WHAT ARE MUSHROOMS?

Mushrooms are fleshy, spore-bearing structures that are easily visible. They are familiar to adults and children alike from their most characteristic shape, a rounded, bell-shaped, or conic cap on a central stalk. Mushrooms belong to the kingdom Fungi, a large, complex group of organisms, all of which lack chlorophyll, the green substance that enables green plants to manufacture their own food through photosynthesis. Lacking chlorophyll, fungi obtain their food from decaying plant and animal remains, from symbiosis, or, in the case of parasitic fungi, from living plants or animals. Mushrooms are only the reproductive parts of their organism—analogous to the fruit of a tree. The main part of a mushroom-producing fungus is a seldom-seen mass of tiny, branching thread-like growths, or hyphae, called the mycelium. Ever present but usually inconspicuous, mycelia may penetrate soil or the tissues of plants, animals, or other fungi. One common form of symbiosis involving fungi is a mutually beneficial relationship developing between fungal mycelia and the roots of higher plants, among which are many woody species. The fungus-plant interfaces in such associations, mycorrhizae, consist of a merger of fungal mycelium and (for example) the fine root hairs of some trees. Some fungi also develop special, close relationships with particular kinds of algae; the two-species organisms that result are lichens, or lichenized fungi.

Mushrooms make up only a small fraction—about 10,000 to 20,000 or perhaps more—of the total number of fungi, which includes an estimated 1,500,000 (Hawksworth 1991) or more species (less than 80,000 named), the majority being inconspicuous or microscopic. The number of species in the mushroom genus *Amanita* alone is estimated at 900 to 1000 (Bas 2000;

Tulloss 2000), and the genera *Russula* and *Cortinarius* are also very large, each with a similar number of species.

Although many fungi are edible or useful to people in some way, many are potentially harmful. Of these, the smaller, less visible toxic fungi are discussed elsewhere, in Chapter 3. Poisonous mushrooms, or toadstools, are treated here as a distinct group. Only general descriptions are provided. Exact identifications of many species must be carried out at a microscopic level and usually require the skills of a fungus expert, or mycologist.

MUSHROOM POISONING

There are many safe, edible, even choice, species of wild mushrooms in North America, but some are poisonous to varying degrees. It is estimated that of approximately 5000 named mushroom species in the United States, about 100 are considered poisonous; in the genus *Amanita* alone, the number of potentially deadly species is probably close to a dozen (Bas 2000; Tulloss 2000). The actual number of edible or poisonous species is impossible to determine because most mushrooms are not collected for food, and most have not been analyzed for toxins. One-third to one-half of the mushroom taxa of the United States remain unnamed and undescribed, and this includes many toxic species. Due to the very small number of mycologists specializing in agarics, the continued misapplication of European names in North America, and the limited state of disseminated knowledge of mushrooms, the numbers provided here are most likely underestimates.

In recent years the number of cases of mushroom poisoning in North America has increased considerably, and poison control centers everywhere are called on to cope with this problem, especially in the fall. In the year 2006, for example, there were nearly 400 calls about mushroom poisoning to PCCs in California alone. New information on the identification and distribution of toxic mushrooms, and on the treatment of mushroom poisoning, is appearing all the time. Kidney dialysis and, rarely, organ transplants are now being used to save the lives of some mushroom poisoning victims who would have died with more conventional treatment; according to mycologist Michael Beug (pers. comm. 2008), with prompt hospitalization in North America, 90% survive eating deadly mushroom species. Untreated, however, and in less developed parts of the world, the death rate from these same species is in excess of 50%.

As might be expected, children under the age of six are the group most vulnerable to mushroom poisoning. This is at least in part because they absorb a larger dose of toxins per unit of body weight. Furthermore, their ability to deal with toxins is not yet fully developed. Elderly people, too, are more susceptible to poisoning, as they are losing their ability to deal with toxins due to underlying illnesses and infirmities. Immigrants are also frequent victims of mushroom poisoning. People moving from one part of the world to another need to be extremely careful when they attempt to harvest wild mushrooms, because they may encounter new species or strains that resemble those they considered edible but are not the same; mushrooms that may seem familiar to people from their homelands in Finland, Japan, Mexico, Turkey, or Laos may actually be highly toxic look-alikes. Many people have been poisoned, some fatally, because of such confusion over mushroom identity. Another reason, Beug suggests, may be that in some cultures, people tend to take more chances with wild mushrooms, whereas those of Anglo-Saxon background have traditionally had considerable fear of eating wild mushrooms (mycophobia) and may use more caution to start with.

The fall of 2004 was a record-breaking season for mushrooms, and there was a matching increase of reports of mushroom poisonings. Beug (2004) reported on 148 individuals poisoned by mushrooms in the western half of the United States, including about 40 children and youth. For the first time in several years, in 2004 there were documented deaths from eating mushrooms: one from ingestion of death cap (*Amanita phalloides*) and two from destroying angel (*A. bisporigera*). Over half the poisonings by *Amanita* species involved Asian immigrants, who mistook the young, button stage of these mushrooms for the pink-spored *Volvariella volvacea* (paddy straw mushroom), or an edible Asian amanita such as *A. chepangiana*, favorites in various southern and eastern Asian cuisines.

Collectors sometimes neglect to check for the form of the stem base on mushrooms they harvest; moreover, they cut the stems off above the ground so that the identifying feature—such as the presence of a volva or uniquely formed stipe bulb—may be lost. Other distinctive marks can vary with the age of the mushroom and its locality, making identification problematic. One woman on southern Vancouver Island learned about this the hard way. She mistook another amanita for the delicious and highly valued pine mushroom, or American matsutake (*Tricholoma magnivelare*), which also has a white spore print and distinctive (though different) odor. She cut the mushroom stems off above ground, took them home, and cooked and ate them with Japanese noodles and vegetables at about two o'clock in the afternoon. Around ten o'clock that night, she started feeling nauseated and started to vomit, first infrequently and then, by midnight, every 15 minutes. By this time she knew she had done something foolish and recognized the symptoms as being similar to those of amatoxin poisoning, including the characteristic five- to eight-hour delay in any noticeable effects. She went to the emergency department of the hospital, where they tentatively identified the mushroom as *Amanita smithiana* (Smith's lepidella), a common mushroom of Douglas-fir woods of the Pacific Northwest; it has been confused with pine mushrooms on a number of other occasions (Tulloss and Lindgren 1992; Pelizzari et al. 1994; Kuo 2006a, b; Tulloss and Yang 2007). This woman was lucky. Her kidneys failed completely, and she needed dialysis treatments immediately and thereafter every two days for three weeks. After many weeks, her energy gradually returned, and there were no lasting effects. She is even able to enjoy some kinds of mushrooms again but does not pick her own.

Sometimes species widely considered edible can cause poisoning under some circumstances. One example, surprising to us, is the angel's wing mushroom (*Pleurocybella porrigens*; syn. *Pleurotus porrigens*), a common species on rotten stumps and logs throughout North America and generally considered edible; one of us (NT) has eaten it on many occasions. In fact, Beug (2004) had no records of this species ever causing poisoning in North America. However, in 2004, over 45 people in Japan developed severe encephalopathy with dizziness two to three weeks after ingesting a different, more toxic strain of angel's wings. There was a tremendous fruiting of this sugihiratake (as it is known in Japan) that season, and people ate large quantities, repeatedly. All the victims had a history of kidney failure, most having undergone hemodialysis at some point prior to eating the mushrooms. Fourteen of these people died, one as long as 29 days after the onset of symptoms—a clear demonstration that a mushroom that might be safe in small amounts can be seriously poisonous when eaten in large amounts and repeatedly, and is especially harmful to those already compromised with kidney ailments. Other poisonings have been documented recently in Europe and Japan from species of *Tricholoma* and *Clitocybe* considered by most to be edible (Lincoff 2005).

Three other mushrooms that come highly recommended as edible species (Lincoff 2007) but that have been known to cause problems in isolated instances are blewit (*Lepista nuda*; syn. *Tricholoma nudum*), honey mushroom (*Armillaria mellea* complex), and fairy ring mushroom (*Marasmius oreades*). In a case described by Michael Beug (2004), a retired physician in Washington and his wife fried some blewits from their backyard and ate them for lunch. Fourteen hours afterward, he suffered severe upper abdominal cramps and diarrhea but recovered quickly. He didn't associate this episode with his meal of mushrooms at the time, but a few weeks later, they again picked and ate blewits, and he experienced similar and even more severe symptoms, which persisted for about two and a half days. This man had food allergies to cherries, some plums, and hazelnuts. His wife had no problems with the mushrooms. Beug also reported on cases of stomach upset, cramps, nausea, and diarrhea experienced by several people from eating honey mushrooms from conifer logs or stumps, and we have heard of others who have become sick from eating honey mushrooms growing under oak trees. Beug suspects, however, that it was just one species out of nine or so closely related species of the *Armillaria mellea* group, *A. ostoyae*, which is the culprit in these poisonings; this species, he notes, is easily mistaken for its edible relatives and seems to be a problem no matter what kind of tree it is growing on or under. A child in Colorado became sick after eating mushrooms from her yard; fairy ring mushrooms were implicated because they were the only mushrooms to be found there. Her parents induced vomiting and she recovered well (Beug 2004). Lessons to be drawn from these cases are that people who have a preexisting kidney condition or other medical condition (including food allergies) should be extra careful in consuming any kind of wild mushrooms, and everyone should eat mushrooms only in moderation (Lincoff 2005).

Another group of individuals who are sometimes victims of mushroom poisoning are those seeking a hallucinogenic experience from psilocybes and other psychotropic mushrooms, and either overdosing or misidentifying these mushrooms or suffering food poisoning from decayed material sold to them by ignorant or dishonest purveyors.

Typical symptoms of mushroom poisoning include nausea, cramps, vomiting, and diarrhea, usually between 15 minutes and two hours after the meal. In some cases these symptoms are accompanied by a sense of anxiety, rapid heartbeat, drowsiness, hallucinations, or even coma. Depending upon the toxins involved, different combinations of these symptoms may be exhibited. In some mushroom poisonings, symptoms can be delayed for eight hours or more after ingestion. There is a great deal of variation among individuals in their response to the less toxic mushrooms. We know that some people react adversely to species that are harmless to most, and some may experience unpleasant effects from a mushroom they had eaten on previous occasions without any bad reaction. Children may be affected from rapid loss of fluids associated with vomiting. People can be allergic to certain mushrooms just as they can to other types of foods such as peanuts or wheat products. People sick with infections or flu may react to eating mushrooms. Some become upset after eating mushrooms out of fear alone, from nervousness about eating a species they have never tried before. In many cases, gastrointestinal upset caused by mushrooms is simply overindulgence, especially if the dish is cooked with butter, sour cream, or bacon. In most circumstances, mushroom poisoning symptoms will resolve spontaneously within eight to 12 hours. However, for the more serious toxins, symptoms vary little and can be fatal.

The poisonous qualities of mushrooms can vary with state of maturity, geographical location, and other environmental and genetic factors. Some species are considered poisonous in one region, and edible and completely safe in another; however, such cases may be ones of misidentification. Much of the world lacks a detailed understanding of local fungi, and local researchers rely upon inappropriate literature (usually intended for application in Europe or North America). It is a good idea never to rely for identification upon field guides originally published for a geographic region other than that in which one is collecting (Bhatt et al. 2003). Furthermore, new fungi may be imported to an area when nursery stock or forest trees are imported from distant places. This happened in Scotland, where *Chlorophyllum molybdites* was imported to the Edinburgh area from Florida, evidently through soil brought in with a tree. *Cortinarius rubellus* has become more frequent in Scotland due to importation of North American Sitka spruce (*Picea sitchensis*) as a plantation tree. Any edible mushroom species can become harmful if infected by toxic organisms such as certain molds or bacteria. Avoid mushrooms growing alongside busy roads, or on golf courses, powerline rights-of-way, or industrial sites, where they can become contaminated with herbicides or pesticides, or can absorb poisonous metals such as mercury, lead, or cadmium.

POINTS TO REMEMBER FOR MUSHROOM GATHERERS

1. There are no rules of thumb or simple tests for determining if a mushroom is edible or poisonous.
2. Before eating any wild mushroom, be absolutely certain of its identification and edibility. Collect only firm, fresh mushrooms without insects or worms. Store mushrooms in paper bags, or in waxed paper, in a cool place. It is best to cook all wild mushrooms; do not eat them raw.
3. When eating for the first time a wild mushroom that has been identified as an edible species, consume only a small portion, and do not drink any liquor. Do not eat more than one kind of mushroom at a time (eating mixtures complicates identification of stomach contents). If no side effects occur within 48 hours, try a slightly larger portion the next time, but never eat a very large quantity, no matter how often a particular species has been eaten; moderation is a key to safe use of mushrooms as food.
4. When trying a new mushroom, save one or two whole specimens to provide positive identification and proper treatment should any ill effects occur.
5. Do not eat any *Amanita* species (even though some are edible) and carefully identify amanita look-alikes. It is a good idea to avoid any mushroom with warty spots on the cap, white caps, white gills, a ring on the stem, and/or a globular, carrot- or turnip-like, or cup-like structure at the base of the stem.
6. Avoid LBMs (little brown mushrooms) and large brownish mushrooms, especially those with pinkish, brownish, purple-brown, or blackish gills; these can be confused with the highly toxic galerinas (*Galerina* spp.) or with some of the toxic *Cortinarius* species.
7. As with gilled mushrooms, do not eat any boletes (with pores rather

than gills beneath the cap) unless identification is certain. Above all, avoid species in which the pore surface is red or orange and those in which the cut flesh turns quickly to blue.

Should poisoning occur from eating mushrooms, prompt treatment can make the difference between recovery and death. **If patient is unconscious, call 911.** In the United States, in all cases, call **1-800-222-1222,** the national hotline of the American Association of Poison Control Centers, which will connect you directly with your local or state poison control center; poison control will guide you as to what actions to take. If you fail to reach a PCC, take the patient to a hospital immediately. Bring a sample of the mushroom, ideally whole and uncooked and *not* in a plastic bag, but even a processed and cooked sample (in any container) is far better than nothing. Save any stomach contents from vomiting to help in identification. The physician should request immediate identification of the mushroom through the authorities known to the poison control center, or through an appropriate mycologist. Often, a microscopic examination of the mushroom is required to make a positive identification.

A well-written, well-illustrated mushroom identification book is vital (we recommend Lincoff 1981). Paul Stamets (1996) provides descriptions of *Psilocybe* mushrooms, as well as the deadly look-alike genera, *Galerina* and *Conocybe* (formerly *Pholiotina*). For a thorough, technical treatment of toxic mushrooms, see Benjamin (1995). In particular, his Chapter 6 ("Guidelines for Would-be Mycophagists") provides excellent advice for those wishing to pick wild mushrooms; physicians and others treating victims of mushroom poisoning will find his Chapter 11 ("Diagnosis and Management of Mushroom Poisoning") particularly helpful.

WEB SITE REFERENCES TO MUSHROOM POISONING

There are many. Check for authoritative sources, such as government or university Web sites, or those maintained by mycological associations. One excellent, continually updated source is eMedicine, a site designed primarily for use by qualified physicians and other medical professionals but also for consumers. This site has a good search function and provides a full range of easily accessed data on mushroom (and plant) poisoning events as well as complete files on current treatments and supporting references. http://www.emedicine.com.

Another Web site to consult is that of the International Programme on Chemical Safety, http://www.inchem.org/documents/pims/fungi/fungi.htm.

An excellent chemical structure database for toxins of all kinds is the Comparative Toxicogenomics Database, http://www.ctd.mdibl.org/.

For spectacular color photographs and authoritative descriptions of over 500 species of amanitas, the reader is referred to the Web site developed and edited by Rodham E. Tulloss and Zhu-liang Yang (2007); many descriptions are based on the personal research of the two editors, authorities on the genus, and their colleagues. http://eticomm.net/~ret/amanita/mainaman.html.

Check out, also, MushroomExpert.Com (Kuo 2006a, b), and Michael Beug's extremely informative works (Beug 2000, 2004).

TYPES OF POISONOUS MUSHROOMS

Poisonous mushrooms are often classified by the poisons they contain. Eight types of toxins are generally recognized, and the most important poisonous species are included here within these eight types. Although it is not possible to deal here with all known poisonous species, selected examples from these eight groups of poisonous mushrooms are discussed in this book. A classification of 14 distinct syndromes of mushroom toxicity has been proposed (Diaz 2005), but this classification system has yet to be widely adopted.

Type 1

Poisonous substance(s). Amatoxins and phallotoxins (cyclopeptides).
Species. *Amanita phalloides* (death cap); *A. bisporigera* and several related *Amanita* species in the destroying angel complex; *Galerina marginata* (autumn galerina) and several other *Galerina* species; several small *Lepiota* species, including *L. subincarnata*, *L. castanea*, and *L. helveola* (deadly parasols, or deadly lepiotas); *Conocybe filaris* (deadly conocybe), *C. rugosa*. Ninety-five percent of mushroom fatalities in North America are associated with amatoxins; that said, the death rate from amanitas in section *Phalloideae* is under

10% in North America, with prompt medical treatment (otherwise, the death rate is about 60%).

Symptoms. Delayed six to 24 hours after ingestion; abdominal pains, nausea, vomiting, diarrhea lasting a day or more, often followed by short remission; then recurring pain, liver and kidney dysfunction, convulsions, coma, and often death; recovery, with proper treatment, can occur in one to two weeks, but victim can have permanent liver and kidney damage.

Type 2

Poisonous substance(s). Orellanins (bipyridine alkaloids).

Species. Various *Cortinarius* species, including *C. rubellus*, *C. gentilis* (deadly cortinarius), and *C. orellanus* (Poznan cortinarius).

Symptoms. Delayed three to 14 days after ingestion; acute or chronic kidney failure, which can result in death; recovery with treatment can take as long as six months.

Type 3

Poisonous substance(s). Gyromitrin (monomethyl hydrazine, or MMH).

Species. *Gyromitra esculenta* (false morel) and other *Gyromitra* species.

Symptoms. Delayed usually six to 12 hours after ingestion; bloated feeling, nausea, vomiting, water or bloody diarrhea, abdominal pains, muscle cramps, faintness, loss of coordination, and sometimes convulsions and coma. Death in North America is "exceedingly rare" (http://www.emedicine.com/emerg/topic459.htm); recovery with treatment can occur within hours.

Type 4

Poisonous substance(s). Muscarine.

Species. *Clitocybe dealbata* (sweat-causing clitocybe) and other *Clitocybe* species; *Inocybe geophylla* (white inocybe) and most other *Inocybe* species; also present, but not the dominant toxin, in *Omphalotus* species (jack-o'-lantern) and *Amanita muscaria* (fly agaric) and its relatives.

Symptoms. Profuse perspiration, salivation, tears, blurred vision, abdominal cramps, watery diarrhea, constriction of pupils, drop in blood pressure, slow pulse; deaths from *Inocybe* species, fortunately, rare; occasional death from other species in people with preexisting illness (e.g., children with heart conditions), and of particular risk to the young and elderly; *Inocybe* can be deadly with dogs; recovery usually occurs within six to 24 hours.

Type 5

Poisonous substance(s). Ibotenic acid and muscimol (isoxazole-derived alkaloids).

Species. *Amanita pantherina* (panther agaric) complex, *A. muscaria* (fly agaric) complex, and other *Amanita* species.

Symptoms. Occur 30 minutes to two hours after ingestion; dizziness, lack of coordination, delusions, staggering, delirium, hallucinations, muscular cramps, hyperactivity, followed by deep sleep; recovery usually within four to 24 hours; there are cases on record of only one bite causing a victim to exhibit symptoms of delirium.

Type 6

Poisonous substance(s). Psilocin, psilocybin (tryptamine-derived alkaloids).

Species. *Psilocybe semilanceata* (liberty cap), *P. cubensis* (common large psilocybe), and other *Psilocybe* species (magic mushrooms); *Conocybe smithii* (bog conocybe), *Gymnopilus spectabilis* (big laughing gym) and other *Gymnopilus* species, *Panaeolus subbalteatus* (girdled panaeolus) and other *Panaeolus* species.

Symptoms. Usually occur ten to 30 minutes after ingestion; mood changes, laughter, compulsive movements, weakness of muscles, drowsiness, visions, sleep; recovery usually within six hours.

Type 7

Poisonous substance(s). Coprine (antabuse-like amino acid compounds).

Species. *Coprinopsis atramentaria* (alcohol inky-cap) and some *Coprinus* species, *Clitocybe clavipes* (fat-footed clitocybe).

Symptoms. Occur 30 minutes or so after drinking alcohol, as long as five days after eating mushrooms; flushed face, distension of neck veins, swelling and tingling of hands, metallic taste in mouth, palpitations, low blood pressure, nausea, vomiting, perspiration; recovery usually within two to four hours. Symptoms also occur if alcohol is ingested just prior to eating the mushrooms.

Type 8

Poisonous substance(s). Diverse, often unknown but ranging from potentially deadly to gastrointestinal irritants that may cause discomfort but without lasting harm.

Species. *Agaricus meleagris* (western flat-topped agaricus) and other *Agaricus* species; *Amanita rubescens* (blusher) complex and related species (contain the hemolytic amanita toxin, though some are edible after cooking, including one sold in markets in Mexico, called *mantecosa* ["lardy"] because it gets slimy after cooking); *Armillaria mellea* complex (honey mushroom); *Boletus subvelutipes* (red-mouth bolete); *Chlorophyllum molybdites* (green-spored lepiota); *Entoloma sinuatum* (lead poisoner) and some other *Entoloma* species; *Hebeloma crustuliniforme* (poison pie); *Lactarius torminosus* (pink-fringed lactarius) and some other *Lactarius* species; some smaller *Lepiota* species; *Omphalotus* spp. (jack-o'-lantern); *Russula emetica* (emetic russula); *Scleroderma* spp. (poison puffball); *Tricholoma pardinum* (dirty tricholoma); *T. pessundatum* (red-brown tricholoma).

Symptoms. Usually occur within 30 minutes to three hours after ingestion; mild to severe nausea, vomiting, diarrhea, abdominal pain; recovery is normally complete and fairly rapid, usually within one to 48 hours. Sometimes (as in the case of *Chlorophyllum molybdites*) poisoning is more serious, and recovery may take several weeks. *Amanita smithiana* (Smith's lepidella), which has been traditionally grouped with these mushrooms, can cause more than stomach upset; it is known to contain norleucine, a compound proven to damage kidney cells in culture.

Much remains to be learned about mushroom poisoning, and many dangerous mushroom toxins are still to be isolated and analyzed.

THE GENUS *AMANITA*

The mushrooms described in this book are listed in alphabetical order of their scientific names, since the common names are often quite variable and are frequently derived from the scientific names. But first, a closer look at *Amanita*, the most important genus of toxic mushrooms. Three species in the genus are responsible for most mushroom fatalities, and others cause serious illness or occasionally death if not treated. Most of the amanitas of concern are conspicuous, large, and even strikingly beautiful. Field guides usually don't list a full set of characters, nor do they include important microscopic characters that separate amanitas from other genera. People who collect based on family or folk traditions (especially such traditions brought from other lands) are operating in an environment of even less information. Amanitas containing amatoxins are often mistaken for edible *Agaricus* or *Volvariella* species. *Amanita smithiana*, which contains norleucine, has been mistaken for American matsutake.

Amanitas share the following macroscopic features that, taken in a group, will help to identify members of the genus.

1. All amanitas start to develop as spherical or ovoid structures known as buttons (primordia).
2. Both a universal and partial veil are present in the button stage of many species (see illustration) and can usually be seen (at least in faint outline) if a button large enough to be of culinary interest is cut lengthwise. The universal veil is often termed the volva. When a partial veil is present, it is called an annulus, ring, or skirt.
3. As the stem of the button elongates and the cap expands, both veils break. Remnants of the universal veil can often be seen on the cap as warty patches of tissue and at or near the base of the stem as one or more of the following: a) similar warts (*Amanita smithiana*); b) rings of wart-like material (e.g., *A. muscaria*); c) a nearly free membranous or submembranous bag or sack (e.g., *A. sinicoflava*); or d) a membranous flap attached to a roughly globose bulb (e.g., *A. bisporigera*). When a partial veil breaks, it may remain on the stem as an annulus. The annulus is absent in some; in other taxa it may be poorly formed or very delicate and may disappear altogether. In some species (e.g., fly agaric, *A. muscaria*), the volva is not free from the stem but remains as a series of ridges running around the base of the stem.
4. Most North American amanitas have white, yellow, or pale cream gills, which are free from the stem or just reach it. A small number of our amanitas may have pinkish or very pale orange gills.
5. All amanitas have white or whitish spores and spore prints. (However, if the gill edges touch the paper during the making of a spore print, colored cells from gill edges may become mixed with spores, giving the print a false coloring.)

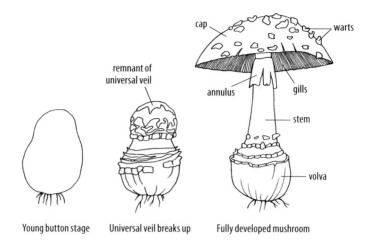

Young button stage   Universal veil breaks up   Fully developed mushroom

Development and typical parts of an amanita mushroom.

While it is not within the scope of this book to present the taxonomy of *Amanita*, a few factors are relevant to toxins and determination of specimens, to which we devote the following paragraphs.

The definition of the genus *Amanita* is simplest when expressed by three characters that are not so often observed but are critical when microscopy is necessary. *Amanita* is the only gilled mushroom genus defined by three characters: 1) mushroom development occurs in a solid mass of tissue and requires surfaces in that mass to die and collapse in order for the final product of development to expand and release spores (e.g., the gills must separate from each other and from the stem and/or the partial veil); 2) the tissue of the stem (even after cooking) will be seen to contain plentiful, club-shaped cells that are longitudinally oriented; and 3) a cross-section of a gill will reveal a strip of tissue running from top to bottom with cells on both sides of the strip curving downward and outward toward the gill's opposing surfaces. Technical names for the three items are schizohymenial (gill splitting) development; longitudinally acrophysalidic stipe context; and bilateral (or divergent) gill trama.

In addition to its distinctive macroscopic, microscopic, and developmental characters, *Amanita* is both large enough and old enough to have had at least four different sets of toxins develop within its species. On morphological and molecular grounds, the genus is divided into seven sections. One of these, section *Phalloideae*, contains those species possessing deadly amatoxins and phallotoxins; one (section *Amanita*), psychoactive isoxazoles; one (section *Lepidella*), deadly toxins that are complex amino acids including norleucine destructive to the liver and kidneys; and one (section *Validae*), hemolytic compounds that will cause gastrointestinal upset if ingested without being destroyed by cooking. For more information about these sections and the species assigned to them, see Tulloss and Yang (2007).

The toxin content of some amanitas, for no known reason, may vary widely from fruiting body to fruiting body, even when the individual mushrooms are found in very close proximity to each other. For example, according to mycologist Rodham E. Tulloss (pers. comm. 2008), some fruiting bodies of *Amanita bisporigera* may have no amanitin at all, whereas others nearby may have enough to fatally poison an adult.

There are actually a number of edible *Amanita* species in North America, and some have been eaten in Europe for centuries. However, there are more species in North America, and (despite the common field guides) they are almost *entirely* different from those found in Europe; furthermore, many of these New World species are still poorly known. Given that some very toxic amanita mushrooms have been repeatedly mistaken for edible amanitas, eating *any* amanita is strongly discouraged.

MUSHROOM SPECIES AND GROUPS

Amanita bisporigera and related spp.
destroying angel, or death angel complex
amanita family (Amanitaceae)

Quick check. Pure white mushrooms of forests or clearings; cap smooth, sticky when wet; membranous volva flap ensheathing stem base; large skirt-like ring on upper stem and attached to stem's bulb. Highly toxic, often fatal. First symptoms appear in six to 24 hours, followed by period of apparent improvement, then by symptoms of liver and kidney failure after four days or more.

Description. CAP pure white, 3–10 cm (1–4 in.) across, rounded, initially egg-shaped, becoming flat; smooth, sticky when wet; FLESH firm, white, sometimes with potato-like scent, often sickeningly sweet (odor of carrion or decaying honey) with age; GILLS white, crowded, free from stem; STEM up to 25 cm (10 in.) long and 2.5 cm (1 in.) thick, smooth to cottony or shaggy (depending on environmental factors), white, having a basal bulb as in *Amanita phalloides*; ANNULUS large, white, skirt-like, flaring downward and outward; VOLVA white, persistent, membranous, free from stem above its attachment to the basal bulb; SPORE PRINT white.

Occurrence. On ground, solitary or in small groups, in hardwood, mixed, or occasionally coniferous forests, in clearings, and sometimes in lawns, in spring, summer, and fall. *Amanita bisporigera* is widely distributed in North America; *A. elliptosperma* is less common but rather widely distributed in the southeastern United States. The only known substantiated species on the West Coast is *A. ocreata*. A very unusual species with a felted annulus, *A. magnivelaris*, is known from the northeastern United States and southern Canada (Tulloss and Yang 2007).

Toxicity. The toxins of destroying angel are similar to those of death cap (*Amanita phalloides*), and the symptoms of poisoning are the same.

Notes. This species and the related *Amanita elliptosperma*, *A. magnivelaris*, and *A. ocreata* have often been grouped under *A. virosa* or *A. verna*, but with the exception of one possible importation with a European tree, *A. virosa* is not known in North America. The name is widely misapplied to our native *A. bisporigera*. No proven case is known of *A. verna* occurring in North America (Rodham E. Tulloss, pers. comm. 2008). Related research in eastern and southern Asia shows that neither of the cited taxa occurs there either, despite plentiful reports in the literature (Tulloss and Yang 2007). The most up-to-

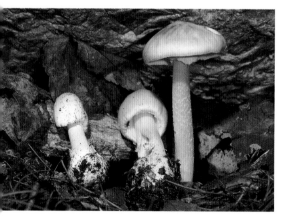

Destroying angel (*Amanita bisporigera*). Michael Beug

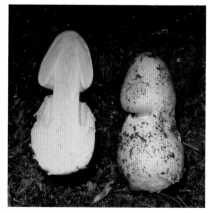

Destroying angel (*Amanita bisporigera*), button stage. Michael Beug

date key to the North American destroying angels is provided by Tulloss (2000). These mushrooms are all strikingly beautiful, but deadly. In fact, mushrooms of the *Amanita phalloides* and *A. verna-virosa* complex (including *A. bisporigera* and *A. ocreata*) are the most poisonous species known.

Amanita muscaria and related spp.
fly agaric, or fly mushroom complex
amanita family (Amanitaceae)

Quick check. Scarlet-red, orange, or yellowish, often fading in sunlight, medium to large-sized mushroom of forests, clearings, or lawns near trees or shrubs; cap covered with whitish, warty spots; stem and gills white; several rings or ridges around the base of the stem and the top of the stem's bulb. Hallucinogenic, with symptoms resembling alcohol intoxication; may cause temporary coma; seldom fatal. First symptoms appear within an hour or so after consuming. Associated with a wide variety of woody symbionts, very easily exported with trees of multiple families, both broad-leaved and coniferous.

Description. CAP 5–30 cm (2–12 in.) across, scarlet-red to orange and yellow, fading to creamy yellow, white; sticky when wet; usually covered with whitish, creamy, or yellow warts or patches (remnants of the universal veil, which may disappear with age or weathering); semispherical when young, becoming flat or saucer-like with age; FLESH firm, white or creamy, without distinctive odor; GILLS whitish, crowded, extending to stem but free from it; STEM whitish, smooth or covered with silky hairs; up to 20 cm (8 in.) long and 2.5 cm (1 in.) thick, enlarged at base, often bulbous there; ANNULUS white, membranous, hanging, and conspicuous; VOLVA white, in the form of one or several concentric rings around the stem base and the upper part of the stem's bulb; occasionally also with single ring *and* with shallow rim on bulb; SPORE PRINT white.

Occurrence. Singly, or sometimes in large groups, in rings or arcs on the ground in hardwood, coniferous, or mixed forests, as well as forest openings, grassy areas, and lawns under a variety of trees. Exported throughout temperate zones of both hemispheres; common in North America from spring through fall. Yellow and orange variants predominate in northern and eastern North America, with two red variants west of the central prairies and along the Pacific Coast from Alaska southward. Peach-colored variants (often with reduced volva remains on their stipes) occur in the southeastern United States and in very restricted habitats in California. One or more red variants are encountered in natural environments southward through Central America to the Colombian Andes. South of the southern limit of naturally occurring conifers in Central America, members of the complex occur with oak.

Toxicity. Deaths directly due to fly agaric poisoning are rare in the northern hemisphere, and its reputation as a deadly poisonous mushroom is probably overrated, but the toxins and their effects on individuals can be serious, especially if their health is already compromised or they are taking drugs, prescribed or otherwise. Furthermore, the disoriented state induced by fly agarics can lead to accidental injury and death, such as from exposure. Fly agaric contains the hallucinogens ibotenic acid and muscimol. The toxin muscarine if present is usually in insignificant amounts (estimated at 0.0025% dry weight basis), varying somewhat from one location to another. Contrary to some reports, fly agaric does not contain atropine.

The mushroom is variable in its effects; eating just one mouthful can cause very violent reactions in some people. The first symptoms, occurring in 30 to 60 minutes, resemble those of alcohol intoxication, with drowsiness and dizziness—a condition sometimes characterized as the pantherine syndrome, after fly agaric's relative, panther agaric (*Amanita pantherina*). This stage is usually followed by confusion, muscular spasms, delirium, and visual disturbances lasting a few hours and generally succeeded by drowsiness and deep sleep. Sometimes the victim becomes comatose. Recovery is usually quite rapid, within six to 24 hours, depending on the amount ingested and the state of health of the patient. Some researchers have characterized the action of ibotenic acid and muscimol on neural transmission as resembling that of the drug LSD. A homeless New Jersey man who apparently ingested several mushrooms of a species (*A. crenulata*) containing the same toxins as fly agaric had to be restrained for several days because of his repeated attempts to attack hospital staff (Tulloss 1990; Tulloss and Yang 2007).

Notes. In North America, members of this complex include *Amanita muscaria* var. *muscaria*; *A. muscaria* ssp. *flavivolvata*; *A. muscaria* var. *persicina*; yellow variants of the first two taxa; *A. breckonii*; and at least two undescribed taxa. A major problem with fly agaric is that it can easily be misidentified as it is so variable in form. Individual mushrooms vary greatly in relative toxicity, and there are many look-alikes, some of which, such as panther agaric (*A. pantherina*), are seriously poisonous. However, neither fly agaric nor panther agaric has been known to cause human deaths in North America in recent years.

Red variants of *Amanita muscaria* (taken together) probably comprise the best-known "single" mushroom in the world. It is strikingly attractive and is illustrated in many children's books, as well as being used in a variety of graphic designs. Its common name, fly agaric, comes from its longstanding use as an insecticide against houseflies; Adam Szczawinski recalled this use from his childhood days in Poland and remembered that many of the flies were not actually killed from eating it but only intoxicated for a few hours. Fly agaric has a long history of use as an intoxicant and hallucinogen by peoples of Europe and Asia, particularly in northern Siberia and the Kamchatka Peninsula. People in these last regions were known to drink the urine of individuals intoxicated by the mushroom, becoming similarly intoxicated thereby (apparently, most of the hallucinogenic compounds pass through the body intact). Fly agaric is the subject of several interesting books (in particular, Wasson 1968), and Benjamin (1995) offers an excellent compilation of information on fly agaric and its use as an inebriant, as well as the toxins involved and the treatment.

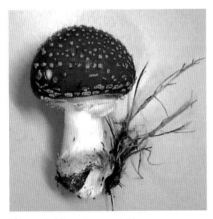

Fly agaric (*Amanita muscaria*).

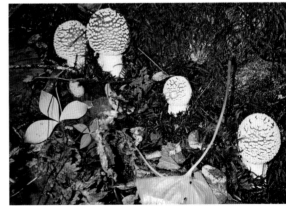

Fly agaric (*Amanita muscaria*) in the duff.

Amanita pantherina and related spp.

panther agaric, panther amanita, or panther cap complex
amanita family (Amanitaceae)

Quick check. Medium-sized to large mushrooms of open woods or wooded lawns; cap pallid to various shades of yellow or dark brown, usually with warty white spots; stem and gills white; annulus membranous, skirt-like, persistent, on upper stem, funnel-shaped at first in some species (e.g., *Amanita velatipes*); often with raised rim of volval tissue around top of roughly globose bulb at base of stem. Highly poisonous, but not generally considered deadly. Symptoms usually appear within an hour after consuming.

Description. CAP 5–15 cm (2–6 in.) across, occasionally larger (most often in *Amanita velatipes*), rounded at first, becoming flat in age, sticky when moist, very pallid to pale tan to a shade of yellow to chocolate-brown, covered with whitish, pointed warts; FLESH firm, whitish without distinctive odor or taste; GILLS white, closely spaced, free from stem; STEM up to 12 cm (5 in.) long and 2.5 cm (1 in.) thick (often larger in *A. velatipes*), white, silky, shiny above the annulus and somewhat fibrillose below the annulus, with a bulb at the base, having a rather shallow raised rim of volval material on the bulb encircling the base of the stem; ANNULUS single, membranous, somewhat cottony above and fibrillose (finely stringy) below; VOLVA adhering to bulb forming a narrow, free roll or collar around the stem; SPORE PRINT white.

Occurrence. Throughout temperate northern hemisphere; common in North America and Rocky Mountains. Grows singly or in groups, occasionally in rings or arcs, on the ground in open coniferous or mixed woods; also on lawns and in gardens and parks in the vicinity of mature coniferous or broadleaved trees. Found from early spring to late fall, occasionally even in winter when weather is mild.

Toxicity. Panther agarics are seriously toxic but generally not considered deadly. The main poisonous compounds are ibotenic acid and muscimol (formerly known as pantherin), both of which may vary in concentration. There are clinically insignificant amounts of muscarine (0.0025% dry weight basis) and related compounds. Pantherine syndrome, the state of inebriation caused by members of this mushroom complex, is similar to but distinguishable from alcohol intoxication. Another species associated with pantherine syndrome is fly agaric (*A. muscaria*), described pre-viously. The toxins responsible are isoxazole derivatives, mainly ibotenic acid, which interfere with nerve transmission in the brain.

Symptoms appear 15 minutes to one hour after eating. A feeling of drowsiness is followed by a state resembling alcohol intoxication. Then a state of confusion sets in, accompanied by muscular spasms, delirium, and disturbance of vision lasting a few hours. Vomiting seldom occurs. Drowsi-ness and sleep follow, and recovery is quite rapid, usually within 24 hours, with little or no memory of the event. Poisoning is potentially fatal for young children or those with kidney or other medical problems, but deaths are rare, or rarely reported. Puppies and other young pets may also be at risk from this mushroom complex.

Notes. In North America, this complex includes *Amanita multisquamosa*, *A. pantherina* in the sense of western U.S. authors (but, so far as is known, not the true *A. pantherina* of Europe), *A. velatipes*, and other undescribed spe-cies of diverse cap colors. Mushrooms of this common, highly toxic *Ama-nita* complex frequently occur on lawns and in woods in populated areas, making the danger of poisoning great. The true (European) *A. pantherina* is named from its dark pigment and leopard-like spots, or warts, on the cap. In the Pacific Northwest, there are several taxa that may be poorly under-stood, named species or undescribed species. This has led to the false belief that the Pacific Northwest "pantherina" intergrades with the usually less poisonous *A. gemmata* in the sense of western U.S. authors (another name

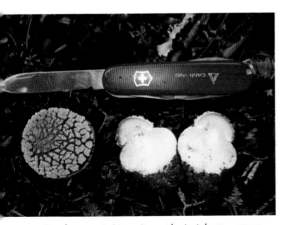

Panther agaric (*Amanita pantherina*), button stage.

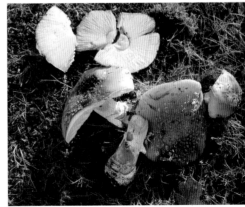

Panther agaric (*Amanita pantherina*), mature.

misapplied in the same region to as many as three yellow taxa.). A taxon formerly called "gemmata" (and identified as causing pantherine syndrome) has been recently described and is now named *A. aprica* (Tulloss and Lindgren 2005, 2007).

Amanita phalloides
death cap
amanita family (Amanitaceae)

Quick check. Attractive, medium-sized mushroom of oak, beech, pine, nut trees, or mixed woods and plantings; cap smooth, yellowish green to greenish brown or (uncommonly) white, with pigment often appearing in streaks; stem and gills white; stem bulbous-based, with membranous flap of volva attached to stem's basal bulb (often below level of soil), and large, skirt-like annulus. Highly toxic, often fatal. First symptoms appear in six to 24 hours; initial symptoms often followed by period of apparent improvement, then by symptoms of liver failure in one or more days.

Description. CAP 5–15 cm (2–6 in.) across, yellowish green to greenish brown, rarely very pale or nearly white, and usually appearing to be streaked radially with darker fibrils near the center (however, examination with a hand lens shows that the pigment is distributed in dots, not lines); convex or flat when fully expanded; slightly sticky; easily peeled; without warty spots, or occasionally with only a few dried traces of membranous white universal veil; FLESH firm, white to light green just below cap; odor becomes foul (described as sickeningly sweet, an odor of death or carrion); GILLS white, close together but well separated and free from stem; STEM up to 15 cm (6 in.) long and nearly 2 cm (0.8 in.) thick, having a roughly globose bulb at the base, white, smooth, solid when young but hollow when mature; ANNULUS thin, membranous, persisting and hanging skirt-like on stem; VOLVA whitish, membranous, in irregular lobe(s) attached to the stem's bulb, persistent, often buried in ground; SPORE PRINT white. In Mexico and Central America south to Andean Colombia, *Amanita arocheae* is a similar, grayer species (Tulloss et al. 1992).

Occurrence. On ground in oak, beech, pine, or mixed woods. Infrequent in North America, sometimes occurring under plantations of European trees. Known from Maine to Virginia and west to Ohio in the East, and from Washington to California in the West, where it has been found with increasing frequency in recent years. Common in Central Europe, and less abundant where introduced in Africa, Australia, South America, Japan, China, and New Zealand. Several Asian reports of *Amanita phalloides* have been found to be erroneous and actually refer to closely related species such as *A. subjunquillea* (Tulloss and Yang 2007).

Toxicity. This mushroom is responsible for more deaths than any of the other species. It has the additional disadvantage of being as easily transported with woody symbionts as *Amanita muscaria*. Hence, it has been introduced to many places that have been former European colonies and to which European trees were introduced. Eating a single mushroom can be fatal. In the United States, it is estimated that amatoxins, found in this and related species, account for as much as 95% of all mushroom-related deaths, with estimated mortality rates of 10 to 60%. The death cap contains two closely related groups of toxins, the amatoxins, which are cyclic octapeptides, and the phallotoxins, which are cyclic heptapeptides. The latter are said to be destroyed by heat and do not survive cooking. There are six known amatoxins, including amanitin, and five phallotoxins, including phalloidin. The

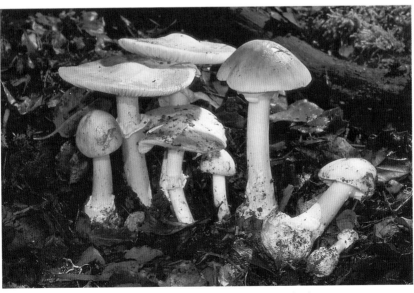

Death cap (*Amanita phalloides*). Kit Scates Barnhart, courtesy Michael Beug

relative toxicity of amatoxins and phallotoxins is still unclear, but it is generally accepted that the amatoxins (mainly alpha-amanitin), and not phallotoxins, are responsible for the lethality of *A. phalloides* and related species.

Poisoning symptoms occur in three distinct stages. The first, developing within six to 24 (usually ten to 14) hours, include dry mouth, nausea, vomiting, sharp abdominal pains, diarrhea (often with blood and mucus), and shock. The longer these initial symptoms are delayed, the better an individual's chances for survival. After about 24 hours, these symptoms may be followed by a period of false recovery lasting up to four days. Then comes the most serious stage of intoxication, with recurrence of abdominal pain and symptoms of liver and kidney failure frequently leading to death in seven to ten days due mainly to liver deterioration and subsequent failure, blood coagulation deficiency, and ultimately, hepatic coma and heart and kidney failure.

About 30 g (half a fresh mushroom) can be fatal to an adult. The larger the quantity consumed, the greater the risk of fatality. The general mortality rate in North America for death cap poisoning is about 10%, including for children; in other parts of the world, mortality can be much higher, in some cases as much as 50% or more. Children generally tend to be more vulnerable to mushroom poisoning, possibly due to the fact that they often eat quantities of mushrooms similar to those simultaneously ingested by adults, but because of their smaller size, absorb a larger dose of the toxins in proportion to their body weight.

Amanita phalloides is also toxic to dogs and some other animals, but cases of poisoning are rare. Certain animals, including rabbits and gray squirrels, are reportedly not affected by oral ingestion of this mushroom.

Notes. On New Year's Day in 2007, six family members ate tacos they made from wild mushrooms they had collected in a park in Santa Cruz, California. They were all admitted to the hospital suffering from amatoxin poisoning, with symptoms of eating death cap. The doctor treating them discovered references to milk thistle and to the effectiveness of an intravenous preparation of silibinin, one of the flavonolignans in milk thistle extract (made from the fruits of milk thistle, *Silybum marianum*) in treating amatoxin poisoning. He had to get special approval to import this standardized preparation, Legalon-Sil, into the United States. He then used it along with penicillin, activated charcoal, and an antidote for Tylenol overdose. Five of the patients recovered, but unfortunately, the oldest victim, an 83-year-old woman, who (characteristically) seemed to be recovering, succumbed to kidney failure (Cavaliere 2007).

In the fall of 1989, a family of Korean immigrants were seriously poisoned after they confused *Amanita phalloides* buttons growing in a park in Vancouver, Washington, with paddy straw mushroom (*Volvariella volvacea*), a popular mushroom widely cultivated and sold in Korea and over much of Southeast Asia. They each ate ten to 12 caps, and ten hours later symptoms of mushroom poisoning were evident. Within 72 hours, four of the five experienced severe liver dysfunction and required liver transplants. The fifth patient recovered after suffering from moderate liver and kidney failure (Benjamin 1995).

Amanita phalloides has also been confused with *A. brunnescens* (which does *not* contain the deadly toxins of *A. phalloides*), a species common in hardwood and mixed forests of eastern North America. Its basal bulb is cleft, or split, and its cap is sticky and pale citrine to deep brown with white, cottony warts. *Amanita brunnescens* also, as implied by its epithet, has a strong tendency to slowly turn brown, a trait absent in *A. phalloides*. Other eastern North American taxa that could be mistaken for *A. phalloides* include *A. aestivalis* (very similar to *A. brunnescens* except for a white cap with a yellow center) and *A. citrina* f. *lavendula* (a citrine-colored taxon with a tendency for its volval remnants to become rusty and with the unique property of becoming lavender after experiencing near freezing temperatures) (Tulloss and Yang 2007). Species of *Russula* with greenish caps might be mistaken for *A. phalloides*, but russulas lack both universal and partial veils, lack a basal bulb on the stem, and have flesh with a uniquely crumbly consistency.

Amanita smithiana
Smith's lepidella
amanita family (Amanitaceae)

Quick check. Medium to large-sized mushroom with white to ivory (sometimes tan, pink, or yellowish tones) rounded cap and white flesh; cap covered with irregularly shaped warty or felty patches; remnants of ring near top of stem and some wartlike remnants of the volva usually found at the base of the stem and on top of the bulb, but often missing in specimens cut off at ground level; often mistaken for American matsutake, or pine mushroom (*Tricholoma magnivelare*); highly toxic, and potentially deadly; first symptoms usually delayed several hours, with eventual kidney damage requiring dialysis.

Description. CAP 5–15 cm (2–6 in.) across, white to ivory (with tan, pink, or yellowish overtones), rounded to convex or flat when fully expanded; covered with irregularly shaped warty spots (remnants of volva), reduced to a few tufts or felty patches in older mushrooms; FLESH white, unchanging and up to 2 cm (0.8 in.) thick over the stem, with unpleasant odor, which is mild and faintly pungent at first, becoming "truly obnoxious" with age; GILLS white, bruising slowly to buff or pinkish when handled, crowded, free from stem or slightly attached, some short gills interspersed among the longer ones; STEM (excluding the deeply rooting bulb) up to 15 cm (6 in.) or more long and 1–3 cm (0.4–1.2 in.) thick, often covered with soft felty or scaly patches; ANNULUS a poorly defined ring of tufted remnants near the top of the stem; VOLVA vague, felted or warty remnants at the base of the stem and on the top of the bulb; BULB thick and rounded at the top, with narrow basal radical that is inevitably cut off in collecting; SPORE

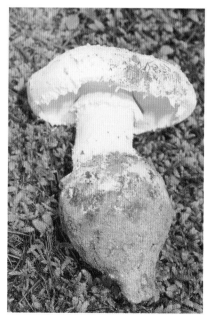

PRINT white. A complete description of this northwestern North American species, including microscopic details, is provided by Tulloss and Lindgren (1992) and on the Amanita Studies Web site (http://pluto.njcc.com/~ret/amanita/species/smithian.html).

Occurrence. In conifer and mixed woods (including alder, oak, Douglas-fir, fir, hemlock, larch, and pine), from southern British Columbia through the United States west of the Great Plains and south to central Mexico; infrequently collected south of Santa Cruz, California.

Toxicity. This species (along with some other amanitas of section *Lepidella*) is known to contain at least one kidney toxin, which is

Smith's lepidella (*Amanita smithiana*). Michael Beug

evidently not dispelled by cooking. The symptoms are similar to those of amatoxin poisoning. There may be a delay of five to eight hours or more before symptoms—nausea, vomiting, abdominal pains, and diarrhea—show. The patient may seem to recover after a day or so, but this may be followed by a recurrence of pain and symptoms of kidney and liver failure, potentially leading to death. There have been several cases reported when kidneys, or both liver and kidneys, ceased to function at least for a time. Other amanitas causing similar symptoms include *Amanita nauseosa* (U.S. Southeast, Caribbean islands, eastern Mexico), *A. proxima* (Europe), *A. sphaerobulbosa* (China, Japan), and *A. thiersii* (central and southern United States, central Mexico). All species taxonomically related to these taxa should be considered suspect.

Notes. The identification and characterization of this species is relatively recent (Tulloss and Lindgren 1992; Pelizzari et al. 1994). *Amanita smithiana* has often been called "*Amanita solitaria*" in mushroom guides printed for western North America, but it is quite distinct from the European species of that name. The greatest risk for Smith's lepidella seems to be its frequent confusion with the choice edible species *Tricholoma magnivelare* (American matsutake, or pine mushroom). Harvesters' practice of cutting off the stems of collected mushrooms at ground level (above the bulb of *A. smithiana*) increases the potential for misidentification.

Clitocybe dealbata and related spp.

sweat-causing clitocybe
tricholoma family (Tricholomataceae)

Quick check. Small to medium-sized mushroom of open, grassy areas and lawns; cap dry, grayish white, smooth, slightly depressed at center when mature, with irregular, incurved margins; gills slightly running down stem, which is short and tough. Very poisonous; sometimes fatal. Symptoms appear within two hours.

Description. CAP grayish white when dry, to grayish tan when moist; 2–5 cm (0.8–2 in.) broad, at first convex, then flat and depressed at center at maturity; margin irregular, indented, and incurved or inrolled; FLESH thin, whitish, with mild taste; GILLS white, close and narrow, attached or running down the stem slightly; STEM 1–7 cm (0.4–2.8 in.) long and up to 8 mm (0.3 in.) thick; solid, tough, same color as cap; sometimes curved, and often off-center; ANNULUS none; SPORE PRINT white.

Occurrence. Single to numerous on ground in open, grassy areas and sometimes woods; often on lawns, where it frequently forms rings. Found throughout North America from summer through fall.

Toxicity. This mushroom, also known as sweating mushroom, contains significant, and potentially fatal, amounts of the toxin muscarine (0.15% dry weight), the same compound present in white inocybe (*Inocybe geophylla*), as well as other members of *Clitocybe* and *Inocybe*. For symptoms of muscarine poisoning, see *Inocybe geophylla*.

Notes. Sweat-causing clitocybe is occasionally abundant on lawns, growing together with other lawn-inhabiting mushrooms such as fairy ring mushroom (*Marasmius oreades*) and meadow mushroom (*Agaricus campestris*). Therefore, it is very important to be aware of and able to recognize this very toxic mushroom. Other North American *Clitocybe* species known to contain muscarine and capable of causing poisoning include *C. dilatata*, *C. morbifera*, and *C. rivulosa*. Benjamin (1995) provides a good review of the *Clitocybe* species and other muscarine-containing mushrooms and the clinical aspects of muscarine poisoning.

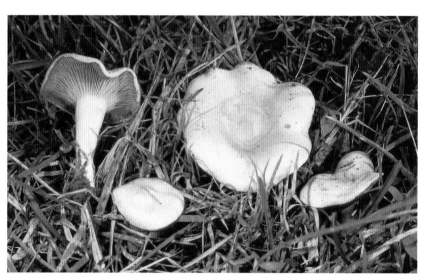

Sweat-causing clitocybe (*Clitocybe dealbata*). Michael Beug

Conocybe filaris (syn. *Pholiotina filaris*)
deadly conocybe, or ringed conocybe
bolbitius family (Bolbitiaceae)

Quick check. Small, brown, gilled mushroom with long, thin stem; conspicuous ring halfway down stem. Deadly.

Description. CAP smooth and tawny brown, up to 2.5 cm (1 in.) across, cone-like to convex or flat, often with central knob; GILLS broad and close together, notched, whitish to rust-colored; STEM up to about 4 cm (1.5 in.) long, thin, and yellow-brown to orange-brown; ANNULUS membranous and movable, central on stalk; SPORE PRINT cinnamon-brown.

Occurrence. Widely distributed in North America; scattered in lawns and grassy areas on rich, humus soils.

Toxicity. This species contains the same lethal amatoxins and phallotoxins as the death cap (*Amanita phalloides*) and is very poisonous.

Notes. This mushroom is a good example of an LBM ("little brown mushroom") that is highly toxic. People should refrain from eating all LBMs unless positive they are edible.

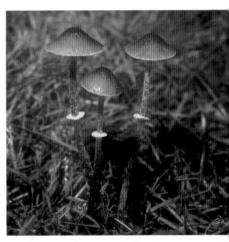

Deadly conocybe (*Conocybe filaris*).
Stan Czolowski, courtesy Trudy Greif

Coprinopsis atramentaria (syn. *Coprinus atramentarius*)
inky-cap, or alcohol inky-cap
inky-cap family (Coprinaceae)

Quick check. Small to medium, grayish mushroom with rounded, cone-shaped to bell-shaped cap, changing into an inky black fluid as the mushroom matures. Often causes unpleasant (but not fatal) toxic reaction if consumed with alcohol. Symptoms appear within 30 minutes after drinking alcoholic beverages and eating the mushroom.

Description. CAP rounded, conical or bell-shaped, dull gray to grayish brown, smooth or mealy, ribbed radially, often splitting at the edges; up to

8 cm (3 in.) long; FLESH thin, grayish white, with no distinctive odor; GILLS crowded, free from stem, grayish white when young, becoming dark gray, then black and dissolving into an inky black fluid; STEM up to 12 cm (5 in.) long and 2 cm (0.8 in.) thick; covered with tiny, flattened hairs; hollow and splitting easily; ANNULUS membrane-like, faint or sometimes conspicuous, located near the base of the stem; SPORE PRINT black.

Occurrence. On ground, in clusters; common in wastelands, grassy areas, gardens, on road shoulders, and on debris. Common throughout North America from late summer to late fall.

Toxicity. Inky-cap contains varying amounts of an amino acid derivative, coprine, which interferes with the body's alcohol metabolism and may cause sterility and testicular damage, as it has done in studies involving dogs and rats (Michael Beug, pers. comm. 2008). The toxic effect of coprine takes place only in the presence of alcohol (ethanol); when no alcoholic beverage has been drunk, the mushroom is not toxic and is in fact considered edible.

A toxic reaction normally takes place within 30 minutes after ingesting inky-cap and drinking alcohol, and lasts about two hours. A recurrence may be experienced if alcohol is taken again within the next few days.

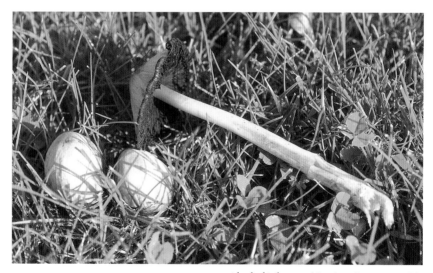

Alcohol inky-cap (*Coprinopsis atramentaria*).

Major symptoms are flushed face and neck, chest pains, palpitations, rapid heartbeat, low blood pressure, feeling of swelling in hands and feet, profuse sweating, metallic taste in the mouth, nausea, vomiting, visual disturbances, weakness, dizziness, and rarely, difficulty in breathing or coma. Poisoning is not fatal, and recovery is usually fairly rapid and complete within a few hours. There is a considerable variation in the reaction of different individuals; some are totally unaffected by the toxin.

Notes. Some species in the related genus *Coprinus* are known to contain coprine, but the well-known edible shaggy mane (*C. comatus*) apparently does not. Like inky-cap, it dissolves into a black fluid when old, but when young it is a choice edible species. However, Michael Beug warns that some people cannot eat shaggy mane and drink alcohol because this causes gastrointestinal upset.

A toxic reaction with alcohol, similar to that of inky-cap, has been reported from Japan for an unrelated mushroom, *Clitocybe clavipes* (fatfooted, or club-footed clitocybe), a species considered edible except when consumed with alcohol.

Coprine may become a useful drug in alcoholism therapy. Its action is similar to that induced by the drug disulfiram, currently used for treatment of alcoholics, but coprine has fewer side effects.

Cortinarius spp.

corts
cortinarius family (Cortinariaceae)

Quick check. Fleshy, often colorful mushrooms with rounded cap, young specimens with cobweb-like partial veil (cortina) extending from edge of cap to stem. Some species highly toxic; potentially fatal, causing kidney failure. Symptoms may be delayed two to 17 days. For safety, do not eat any *Cortinarius* species.

Description. There are hundreds of different species in this genus, with many variations in size, shape, and color, making *Cortinarius* species extremely difficult to identify. CAP fleshy, variable in color (some bright orange, violet, or cinnamon), rounded; a universal veil is often present, adhering to the surface with thin, silky fibrils, becoming slimy or glutinous when wet; spiderweb-like, partial veil (cortina) composed of delicate strands extends from the edge of the cap to the stem, in young specimens usually covering the gills; veil disappearing at maturity; FLESH variable in color; GILLS usually rusty brown in mature specimens; STEM variable in size, color; ANNULUS often reduced to ring or series of partial rings on the lower part of the stem in older specimens; SPORE PRINT rusty brown to cinnamon-brown.

Occurrence. On ground; over 800 species occurring in North America. The thread-like mycelium forms a special symbiotic relationship (mycorrhizal association) with the roots of trees, shrubs, and other plants. In fact, *Cortinarius* is the largest genus of mycorrhizal mushrooms in North America. *Cortinarius gentilis*, a common toxic species, occurs abundantly under conifers and is widespread in North America.

Toxicity. Although some *Cortinarius* species are identifiable and a few are known to be edible, the facts that many are not well known or even described, and that some are highly toxic, make it advisable not to eat any specimen until more is known about them. Several orange-colored species are included in the highly toxic group, including *C. gentilis* (deadly cortinar-

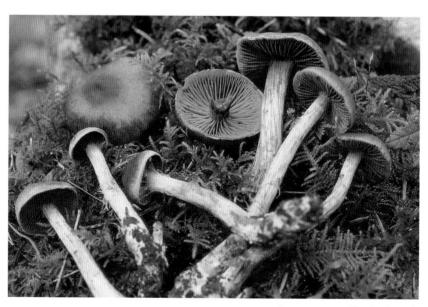

An orange cort (*Cortinarius* sp.).

ius), *C. orellanus* (Poznan cortinarius), and *C. rubellus* (which has been called *C. orellanoides* in Europe, *C. speciosissimus* in eastern North America, and *C. rainierensis* in the Northwest). This last species is particularly deadly. *Cortinarius rubellus* and some other toxic cort species fluoresce under UV light. One series of compounds has been identified; these cortinarins are closely allied to the amatoxin cyclopeptides of *Amanita phalloides*. One of these, cortinarin B, is suggested as the main toxic agent of *Cortinarius*. The toxin from *C. rubellus* differs, as it was found to be a bipyridine alkaloid. Much is still to be learned about these colorful but potentially deadly species.

Cortinarius (orellanine) poisoning can cause liver and kidney damage. The nervous system may also be affected. Symptoms may be delayed three to 14 days after ingesting the mushrooms, with an average of about eight days between ingestion and onset of symptoms. Nausea, vomiting, dry mouth, and loss of appetite, followed by sweating, shivering, and stiffness; pain in the limbs, abdomen, and lumbar region; constipation or diarrhea; severe thirst; reduction and then increase in urine production; sleepiness; and convulsions are all symptoms. Many of these indicate kidney involvement.

Notes. Several fatalities caused by eating cortinarius mushrooms have been reported, mainly from Great Britain and Europe; in the 1950s, in Poland, for example, there were 132 reported orellanine poisonings, with 11% mortality (Benjamin 1995). But mycologist Michael Beug (pers. comm. 2008), who has reviewed cases of mushroom poisoning for nearly four decades, is stunned to note that in this time he has not encountered "a single significant poisoning from the over 800 *Cortinarius* species in North America." Cortinarius toxins are all the more insidious because of the long delay in appearance of symptoms. Because of this, it is quite possible that cortinarius poisoning has occurred from time to time in North America but simply not been diagnosed. In North America, corts are seldom eaten, although *C. violaceus*, a brilliant purple species, is considered edible and occasionally sought by mushroom gatherers. At least one *Cortinarius* species has caused fatal poisoning in sheep. As a final word, all corts should be considered toxic to animals as well as humans.

Galerina marginata (syn. *G. autumnalis*)
autumn galerina
cortinarius family (Cortinariaceae)

Quick check. Small to medium-sized mushroom on decayed wood in forests (or lawns if growing over buried wood); smooth, brownish, broadly bell-shaped cap; hairy, band-like ring around stem. Highly toxic, potentially fatal. First symptoms appear in six to 24 hours, followed by period of apparent improvement, then by symptoms of liver and kidney failure after four days or more.

Description. CAP 2–6 cm (0.8–2.5 in.) across, bell-shaped, becoming rounded with a small, central knob, or umbo; surface smooth, sticky when wet, light tan (when dry) to dark brown (when wet), with distinct lines, or striations, on the margin when wet; FLESH light brown, watery, without distinctive odor; GILLS rusty, attached to stem; STEM up to 8 cm (3 in.) long and 6 mm (0.2 in.) thick, slightly enlarged at the base and tapering upward; brown, covered with whitish hairs; ANNULUS band-like, narrow, white-hairy, sometimes inconspicuous; SPORE PRINT rusty brown.

Occurrence. Common in woods from spring to late fall, sometimes early winter; scattered or in dense clusters, growing on well-decayed wood, both

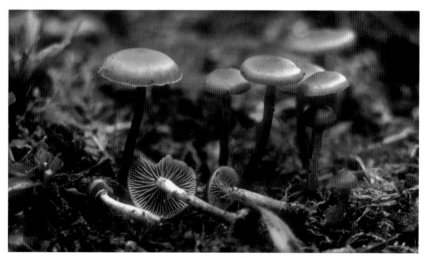

Autumn galerina (*Galerina marginata*). Paul Kroeger

conifer and hardwood, or sometimes on buried wood (even in lawns), chips, or sawdust. Particularly abundant after a heavy rain.

Toxicity. This mushroom contains the same groups of toxins, the fatally poisonous amatoxins and phallotoxins, as death cap (*Amanita phalloides*). The first symptoms appear in six to 24 hours. Nausea, vomiting, diarrhea, and severe abdominal cramps are followed by a period of improvement lasting up to four days. Then liver and kidney failure ensue, sometimes leading to coma and death in seven to ten days.

Notes. The genus *Galerina* includes about 200 species of small, hard-to-identify mushrooms, some deadly poisonous, others with unknown edibility. All should be strictly avoided. The closely related North American species *G. venenata* is similar in appearance and habitat to autumn galerina and just as deadly; it is known only from the Pacific Northwest and grows on lawns. Fortunately, because these mushrooms are smaller than the amanita mushrooms, the relative quantity of toxins consumed is generally less. Nevertheless, the death rate is close to that of *Amanita phalloides*—in the order of 10%. even with prompt treatment (Michael Beug, pers. comm. 2008).

Parents of small children and pets should watch for galerinas on lawns, especially if there is wood buried beneath. In northwestern North America galerinas are sometimes confused with honey mushrooms (*Armillaria mellea* complex) (Michael Beug, pers. comm. 2008). Furthermore, both genera can easily be confused by inexperienced collectors for the hallucinogenic magic mushrooms of *Psilocybe* (Stamets 1996). People who collect the latter should make themselves completely familiar with toxic look-alikes.

Gyromitra esculenta and related spp.
false morel, brain mushroom, or turban fungus
cup fungi family (Helvellaceae)

Quick check. Brownish mushroom of woods and gardens, and recently logged and burned areas, with pale, whitish stem and irregularly folded, convoluted cap; very variable in shape and color. Some strains are highly toxic, especially if eaten raw; potentially fatal, causing liver damage. Symptoms appear in six to 12 hours. Do not confuse with the true, or edible, morel.

Description. CAP tan to reddish brown or chocolate-brown; up to 10 cm (4 in.) high and 15 cm (6 in.) wide; irregular in shape, contorted, folded, and wrinkled, with brain-like ridges (but not pitted, as in true morels); FLESH brittle, pale; STEM up to 6 cm (2.5 in.) high, smooth, fragile, thick and solid at the base, becoming somewhat grooved, hollow, or with open chambers above; pale flesh-colored; ANNULUS none; SPORE PRINT yellowish. (Gills are not present in this mushroom, which is an ascomycete.)

Occurrence. Grows from early spring to early summer, singly or in small groups on the ground in open, moist, wooded areas under coniferous trees, and in gardens and compost heaps. It sometimes fruits "in stupendous abundance" in recently logged or burned-over areas (Michael Beug, pers. comm. 2008). Widely distributed throughout North America and in the temperate zone of the northern hemisphere.

Toxicity. False morel is potentially fatal, especially if eaten raw. Even vapors from cooking these mushrooms can cause poisoning. The main toxic component is gyromytrin. This compound, a hydrazine, is very unstable and is easily converted at moderate cooking temperatures to toxic monomethyl-hydrazine (MMH), a water-soluble toxin that causes the symptoms of poisoning mentioned here. MMH is employed in rocket fuel and causes similar

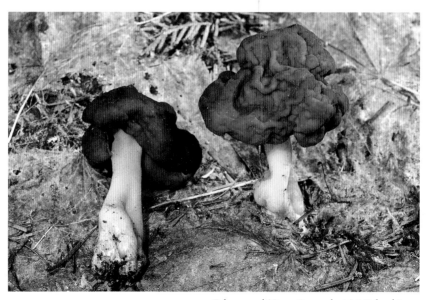

False morel (*Gyromitra esculenta*). Michael Beug

toxic symptoms in aerospace industry workers. Symptoms usually appear six to 12 hours after eating, but cases with symptoms occurring after only two hours are known. Symptoms may include bloated feeling, nausea, vomiting, severe diarrhea, abdominal cramps, headache, dizziness, fever, difficulty breathing, possible rapid heartbeat and low blood sugar, and coma. Death, due to kidney and liver damage, may occur within a few days, but this is relatively rare; in 2003 in the United States, for example, of 71 reports of poisoning from gyromitrin-containing mushrooms, there was only one fatality. The toxin accumulates in the body and until a certain threshold is reached few or no symptoms appear. Consumption of the mushroom once may not induce symptoms, but a second or third meal may produce a severe poisoning. Since the toxin is volatile, it may be removed by parboiling, but this is not guaranteed. False morel is often eaten after such treatment. We strongly recommend, however, that it not be eaten under any circumstances.

Notes. This mushroom is named from its similarity to the true, or edible, morel (*Morchella* spp.), a well-known edible mushroom of springtime, whose stem is hollow, not chambered, and whose dark grayish, elongated cap is pitted with vertically aligned, honeycomb-like cavities. Some species of closely related genera, including *Helvella* (elf's saddle), *Sarcosphaera*, *Peziza*, *Disciotis*, and *Verpa*, may also be toxic, and these, along with edible morels, *should never be eaten raw.*

The toxicity of false morel in North America has caused some confusion, and it appears that the mushroom is variable in its poison content and also causes different reactions in different individuals. Some consider the mushroom more likely to be edible in western North America, but this may well be a myth. It has caused a number of poisonings in North America, with several fatalities. It has been proposed that different chemical strains of these species exist, a theory that would explain its variable toxicity.

False morel is said to be safe to eat if dried or

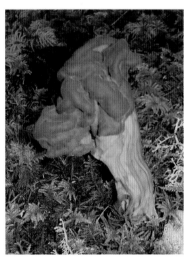

Elf's saddle (*Helvella* sp.).

boiled for ten minutes (discard the water). Mycologist Adam Szczawinski ate young, firm specimens of *Gyromitra esculenta* in both eastern Europe and western North America without any toxic reaction. Until more is known about this mushroom, however, the recommendation is to leave it strictly alone, since its ingestion is definitely a form of "gastronomic roulette," as described by John Trestrail (1993).

Inocybe geophylla and related spp.
white inocybe, or white fiber head
cortinarius family (Cortinariaceae)

Quick check. Small, silvery white to light tan or lilac mushroom of coniferous woods and nearby clearings; small knob at center of cap. Very poisonous; sometimes fatal. Symptoms appear within two hours.

Description. CAP silvery white or occasionally light tan or lilac, dry, with a silvery sheen; 1.5–3.5 cm (0.6–1.4 in.) broad, conical to bell-shaped when young, expanding to nearly flat, with a prominent central knob, or umbo; splitting at the margin at maturity; usually a web-like partial veil (cortina)

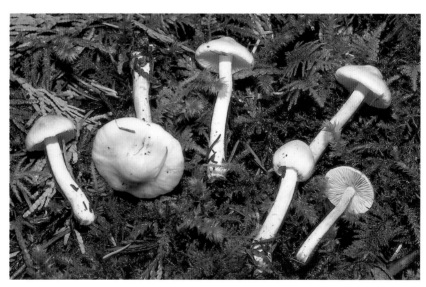

White inocybe (*Inocybe geophylla*).

extends from the edge of the cap to the stem; FLESH thin, white, of no distinctive odor or taste; GILLS close, joined to the stem, white when young, becoming gray, then brown; STEM up to 6 cm (2.5 in.) long and 5 mm (0.2 in.) thick; cylindrical, covered at the top with tiny white hairs; ANNULUS hairy, band-like, often inconspicuous; SPORE PRINT rusty brown.

Occurrence. On damp soil, singly or in small groups, in coniferous or mixed forest; sometimes on open ground or lawns under coniferous trees. Found throughout North America and Europe from fall to early winter.

Toxicity. This mushroom contains muscarine, a toxic alkaloid compound, which may cause serious illness or death, particularly in the young and elderly, and for those with existing health problems. It can be deadly for children with heart conditions. It inhibits the conduction of impulses between nerve cells. Symptoms, which occur from 15 minutes to two hours after ingestion, include copious salivation, profuse sweating, tears, nausea, chest spasms, abdominal pain, and slowed pulse. Vomiting, watery diarrhea, reduced blood pressure, slow heartbeat, asthmatic wheezing, and blurred vision may also occur. A mortality rate of about 5% has been estimated.

Notes. This is one of the most common *Inocybe* species in North America, as well as in Europe. The genus includes about 300 small or medium-sized mushrooms, many very similar in appearance. They are characterized by a convex cap with a central knob. The upper surface of the cap is often covered with radiating fibrils or scales; these are brown in many species. Gills are clay-colored, and spores yellowish to light brown. Identification to species is difficult, and many require microscopy. Many species of this genus contain muscarine and can cause serious illness. Besides *I. geophylla*, another widely distributed toxic North American species is *I. rimosa* (syn. *I. fastigiata*). Some mushroom experts grant the lilac-colored form of *I. geophylla* specific status, as *I. lilacina*. Mushroom collectors should avoid the entire group. These and other mushrooms containing muscarine are very deadly for dogs.

Muscarine was first isolated from fly agaric (*Amanita muscaria*), which contains insignificant amounts. It is found in much higher concentrations in species of *Inocybe* and *Clitocybe*.

Lepiota subincarnata (syn. *L. josserandii*) **and related spp.**
deadly lepiota
lepiota family (Lepiotaceae)

Quick check. Small mushroom of woods and lawns; cap white, with fibrous reddish scales; gills free, white; spore print white; very poisonous; toxins similar to those of death cap (*Amanita phalloides*), with a delay in symptoms of six hours or more.

Description. CAP pale, covered with pointed, reddish scales; 1–3 cm (0.4–1.2 in.) across, elliptical with a central knob, flattening with maturity; margin with veil remnants, sometimes with small flattened scales; FLESH white, turning slightly red when cut, with somewhat fragrant odor; GILLS free from stem, white aging to cream, close and broad, in two or three tiers; STEM 3–6 cm (1.2–2.4 in.) long and up to 4 mm (0.2 in.) thick; solid, pale colored, aging brownish, covered with pale shaggy fibrous patches below and silky above when young; ANNULUS not persistent; SPORE PRINT white.

Occurrence. Single to numerous on ground in woods or on lawns.

Toxicity. This mushroom and its close relatives (including *Lepiota castanea*) contain amatoxins, the same compounds found in death cap (*Amanita phalloides*) and destroying angel (*A. bisporigera* and related spp.), with simi-

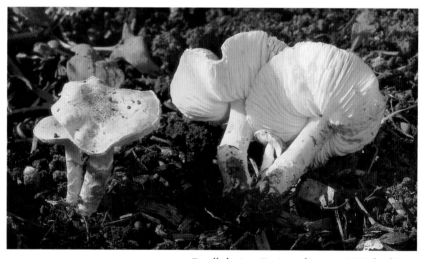

Deadly lepiota (*Lepiota subincarnata*). Michael Beug

lar symptoms of poisoning. Symptoms may be delayed for six to 24 hours, with a period of apparent improvement following the onset of symptoms, but then, one or more days after, liver failure may occur.

Notes. Mycologist Michael Beug (pers. comm. 2008) believes that *Lepiota subincarnata* may be the deadliest mushroom in North America. It was responsible for the death of a man in Vancouver, B.C., who collected a few from a lawn (Seiger 2003). Fortunately, its small size makes it less sought-after by mushroom pickers.

Omphalotus illudens and related spp.
jack-o'-lantern, copper trumpet, or false chanterelle
tricholoma family (Tricholomataceae)

Quick check. Medium-sized, orange to yellowish orange, luminescent mushroom on decaying wood with dry cap, and sharp-edged gills that extend down the stem and glow in the dark. Very poisonous; occasionally fatal. Symptoms appear within two hours. Do not confuse with edible chanterelle.

Description. CAP 5–20 cm (2–8 in.) across, rounded to flat and usually depressed in the middle, with a shallow, central knob; deep orange to yellowish, fading with age; upper surface smooth and dry (not sticky); margin enrolled at first, then upturned and wavy; FLESH whitish and firm, with no distinctive odor; GILLS yellow-orange, sharp-edged, luminescent, running down the stem; STEM light orange, 7–20 cm (3–8 in.) high and 0.5–2.5 cm (0.2–1 in.) thick, tapering at the base; ANNULUS none; SPORE PRINT white to pale cream or pale yellow.

Occurrence. Growing in clusters on decaying wood, including standing trunks, fallen logs, or buried wood, sometimes fruiting in lawns by trees with heart rot; most commonly associated with oak (*Quercus* spp.). Occurs in Canada from the Great Lakes region eastward but is not common. Found throughout the eastern United States and into the South. *Omphalotus illudens* is often mistakenly referred to as *O. olearius*, its European counterpart. Two other species, also toxic, occur in North America: *O. olivascens* occurs in California, and *O. subilludens* in the southeastern United States.

Toxicity. The toxins of this mushroom and its relatives, though potentially deadly, have not yet been fully identified. Some species in the genus *Ompha-lotus* may contain significant amounts of muscarine and the sesquiterpe-noids illudin-s and illudin-m; however, Michael Beug (pers. comm. 2008) suggests that there is probably little or no muscarine in the North American strains. Symptoms of poisoning occur from 15 minutes to two hours after ingestion: salivation, sweating, tears, nausea, chest spasms, abdominal pain, slowed pulse, reduced blood pressure, vomiting, watery diarrhea, asthmatic wheezing, and blurred vision all may occur in severe cases. Additionally, tin-gling fingertips and an unpleasant, metallic taste in the mouth have been

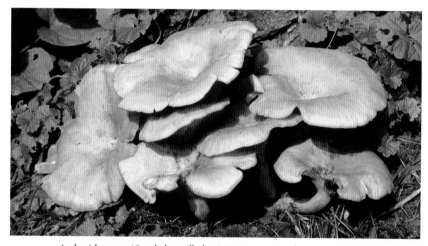

Jack-o'-lantern (*Omphalotus illudens*). Kit Scates Barnhart, courtesy Michael Beug

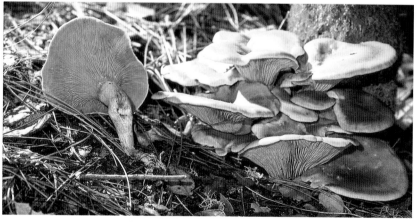

Olive-green jack-o'-lantern (*Omphalotus olivascens*). Michael Beug

noted. Fortunately despite the "exceptionally nasty" character of *Omphalotus* poisoning, the recovery is generally quick, and Michael Beug (pers. comm. 2008) is not aware of any deaths from this mushroom in North America. He notes, however, that the European strains are more toxic.

Notes. *Omphalotus illudens* is sometimes included in the genus *Clitocybe*, as *C. illudens*. A notable case of poisoning by jack-o'-lantern mushroom was in Quebec in 2003, when six women cooked and ate some of these mushrooms. Within 15 minutes all experienced symptoms of drowsiness, dizziness, headache, intestinal cramps, nausea, salivation, sweating, and vomiting. All were given rehydration therapy and recovered (Beug 2004). This mushroom is sometimes confused with the edible chanterelle mushroom (*Cantharellus cibarius*), which is close to it in color but is easily distinguished by its gills, which are shallow ridges and branched (they are sharp-edged and not branched in *Omphalotus illudens*). Furthermore, unlike jack-o'-lantern, chanterelle does not grow on wood. The eerie, greenish luminescence of jack-o'-lantern's gills in the dark often lasts up to two days after it is collected, but old specimens may not show luminescence. In Japan a close relative, *Lampteromyces japonicus*, sometimes causes deaths.

Psilocybe cubensis
common large psilocybe
stropharia family (Strophariaceae)

Quick check. Medium-sized mushroom of well-manured fields, with bell-shaped cap that is chestnut-brown when young, lighter at maturity; ring white, membranous and persisting, and stem staining bluish when bruised. Hallucinogenic, causing confusion, delirium, and visual disturbances within an hour, with recovery in six to 18 hours; no fatalities known, but do not confuse with highly toxic *Galerina marginata* or its relatives.

Description. CAP 2–8 cm (0.8–3 in.) across, conical to bell-shaped, with small knob, or umbo, at tip; expanding to flat-topped with age; chestnut-brown, becoming light brown at maturity; staining bluish when bruised or injured; smooth and sticky when wet; FLESH white at first, bruises blue; GILLS narrow, close, gray, becoming purplish gray to almost black, with distinct, white edges; attached to the stem, and notched at point of attachment;

STEM 5–15 cm (2–6 in.) long, 5–15 mm (0.2–0.6 in.) thick, smooth, whitish, enlarged at the base, and bruising bluish green; ANNULUS white, membranous, persistent; SPORE PRINT purplish brown to blackish.

Occurrence. Scattered or in groups in grassy meadows, mostly on cow or horse manure, or on well-manured ground. Found throughout the southern United States and Mexico, from spring to late fall.

Toxicity. This species contains psilocin and psilocybin, the same hallucinogenic compounds found in the next species described, *Psilocybe semilanceata*. Symptoms of intoxication are the same.

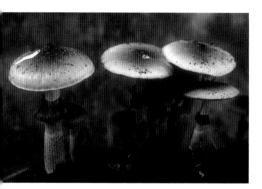

Common large psilocybe (*Psilocybe cubensis*). Paul Kroeger

Notes. *Psilocybe cubensis* is widely used as a hallucinogen and is said to be the most widely cultivated native mushroom in North America. As with *Omphalotus illudens*, the main danger of its use is in misidentification: it closely resembles other, much more toxic species. *Psilocybe* species are commonly referred to as "magic mushrooms," because of their hallucinogenic effects. See Stamets (1996) for a complete treatment of the psilocybin mushrooms.

Psilocybe semilanceata
liberty cap
stropharia family (Strophariaceae)

Quick check. Small, conical-capped, brownish mushroom of wet grasslands, especially on cow dung; cap with distinct knob at tip; a brown, cobweb-like ring around the stem is evident in young specimens but quickly deteriorates with age. Purplish brown to black spores; flesh bruises bluish. Hallucinogenic, causing confusion, delirium, and visual disturbances within an hour, with recovery in six to 18 hours; no fatalities known, but do not confuse with highly toxic *Galerina marginata* or its relatives.

Description. CAP up to 2.5 cm (1 in.) across, sharply conical with prominent knob, or umbo, at tip; semitransparent, usually dark chestnut-brown when moist, drying to light tan or yellowish, occasionally olive-tinted or with a bluish cast; curved under at edges when young; surface sticky and gelatinous when wet; FLESH thin, watery, pale tan to brown; GILLS narrow, close, attached to stem, and not notched at point of attachment; pale tan at first, becoming brown, then purplish brown with pale edges; STEM up to 10 cm (4 in.) long and 2.5 mm (0.1 in.) thick, smooth, flexible, light brown, tending to dark brown at base; injured or bruised spots may turn blue; ANNULUS delicate, brown, cobweb-like, quickly disappearing, leaving a sticky zone darkened by the color of the spores; SPORE PRINT purplish brown to black.

Occurrence. Scattered or in groups on wet meadows and grasslands, often on cow dung. Common throughout the Pacific Northwest, west of the Cascades, from British Columbia to California, also known from the eastern Maritime provinces in Canada. Found in the fall and early winter, occasionally in spring in Oregon and Washington. It also occurs commonly in Europe and in the United Kingdom.

Toxicity. This mushroom contains hallucinogenic alkaloids, psilocin and psilocybin, which are tryptamine derivatives. Concentrations of these active compounds vary from species to species. Their effects on people are similar to those of LSD (lysergic acid diethylamide). Hallucinations and intoxication can occur from eating the mushrooms raw or cooked, or from drinking broth made by boiling them.

Symptoms of intoxication, becoming evident after ten to 30 minutes, include initial sense of exhilaration and euphoria, hallucinations, and visual disturbances with exaggerated and distorted colors, then often confusion, dizziness, muscular weakness, tremors, palpitations, respiratory difficulties, and feelings of anxiety and paranoia. Varying degrees of delirium, laughter, and visual aberration of speed, light, and color may also occur. Recovery normally takes place in six to 18 hours,

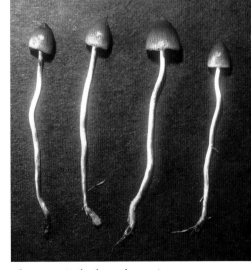

Liberty cap (*Psilocybe semilanceata*). Stan Czolowski, courtesy Trudy Greif

depending on the individual, his or her condition, and the quantity of mushrooms ingested. *Psilocybe semilanceata* is not known to be fatal but can be mistaken for other, more deadly mushrooms.

Notes. Hallucinogenic mushrooms containing psilocin and psilocybin were used since at least 2000 years ago by the Aztecs of Mexico in their religious rituals and were considered "flesh of the Gods." In the 1960s, these "magic mushrooms" became popular among some groups of people, particularly teenagers and young adults, as recreational drugs and symbols of the counterculture; they continue to be sold on streets in North American cities. The species most frequently used are *Psilocybe semilanceata* and *P. cubensis*, as well as *P. cyanescens*, *P. stuntzii*, and *P. baeocystis*. Altogether, of the more than 70 hallucinogenic species in the genus, over 20 occur in North America. Species in a number of other mushroom genera, including *Panaeolus*, *Conocybe*, *Inocybe*, *Gymnopilus*, *Pluteus*, and even a couple of *Lycoperdon* (puffball) species, also contain tryptamine derivatives (and even more deadly toxins). A major problem for anyone purposely seeking magic mushrooms (*Psilocybe* spp.), therefore, is the danger of misidentification. From time to time, highly toxic mushrooms such as *Galerina marginata*, or species of *Panaeolus* or *Stropharia*, have been eaten accidentally, sometimes with fatal results in the case of *Galerina*. The best identification guide to psilocybin mushrooms is by Paul Stamets (1996).

Russula emetica and related spp.

emetic russula
russula family (Russulaceae)

Quick check. Showy, medium-sized mushroom of mossy woods; bright red cap, whitish, brittle stem and gills, and acrid, peppery taste. Causes vomiting and digestive distress within an hour of eating but is not fatal.

Description. CAP up to 10 cm (4 in.) across; rounded at first, becoming flattened, with depressed center and upturned margins; usually bright red, sometimes mottled yellowish and red; smooth, and sticky when wet; margin marked by radiating lines, or striations, which fade with age; FLESH white to off-white, brittle, with a very acrid, peppery taste; GILLS free, or almost free, from the stem; white to yellowish white, and thin; STEM up to

10 cm (4 in.) high and 2.5 cm (1 in.) thick, enlarging toward the base; whitish; smooth and dry, becoming hollow with age; ANNULUS none; SPORE PRINT white to yellowish white.

Occurrence. Grows from late summer to fall singly or in groups on the ground in mossy areas of coniferous or mixed woods; rarely on well-decayed wood or in peat bogs. Common and widely distributed in North America.

Toxicity. The toxins are not yet well known, and not all people are affected to the same degree. Sesquiterpenes have been identified in some *Russula* species, and muscarine has been found but in apparently negligible amounts. Symptoms, which usually occur 30 to 45 minutes after eating the mushroom, are vomiting, nausea, abdominal cramps, and diarrhea. The mushroom is named after the inevitable vomiting and diarrhea it causes. In severe cases, discomfort persists for 24 hours or more, but normally recovery is within a few hours.

Notes. Related russulas are also acrid and should be avoided; these include *Russula sanguinaria* (syns. *R. rosacea*, *R. sanguinea*) and *R. fragilis*. Another, *R. vesicatoria*, causes blistering of the lips and tongue when tasted. Russulas are among the most abundant and conspicuous mushrooms of North American woodlands and forests but are difficult to identify to species and are seldom eaten. According to some, even emetic russula and its relatives become

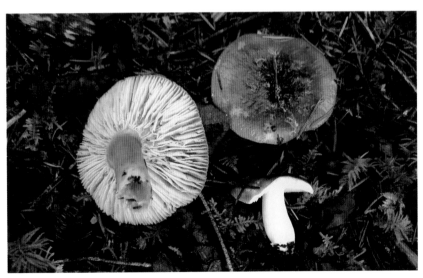

Russula (*Russula* sp.).

edible and palatable after thorough cooking, but until more is known about their toxins, all russulas—especially those with an acrid taste—should be avoided. Sometimes mycologists use a "taste test" to detect the peppery or bitter-tasting qualities of russulas, but repeated "tasting" over a day of mushroom identification has been known to cause gastrointestinal symptoms (Benjamin 1995).

Scleroderma spp.
poison puffballs
fall puffball family (Sclerodermataceae)

Quick check. Thick-skinned, smooth to warty, light brown, puffball-like mushrooms, with purplish black spore mass inside at maturity. Cause nausea and stomach upset, but not fatal. Do not confuse with edible puffballs.

Description. Spherical to flattened puffball-like mushrooms, rooted at the base, without separate cap or stem; up to 10 cm (4 in.) across and 4 cm (1.5 in.) high, sometimes resembling small, rounded potatoes half buried in the ground; covered with smooth to rough and warty, rind-like skin, which is yellowish tan to dark brown; the outer wall breaks irregularly at the top at

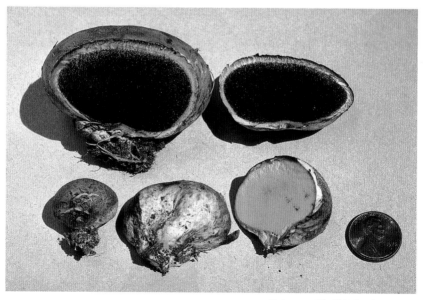

Poison puffball (*Scleroderma* sp.).

maturity to expose the spores; FLESH of skin white; of spore mass, at first white, but soon becoming purplish black to black. Several species occur in North America, and they are often difficult to distinguish.

Occurrence. Poison puffballs are widely distributed in North America, growing from summer through fall on the ground on wood debris, in woods, and sometimes gardens, usually near trees.

Toxicity. *Scleroderma* species are known to cause nausea, vomiting, abdominal cramps, and diarrhea, but their toxins have not been identified. Symptoms appear about 30 minutes after eating. The degree of reaction depends on the individual but can be severe. Recovery is usually fairly rapid. At least one species, *S. citrinum*, can be lethal to dogs and pigs (Michael Beug, pers. comm. 2008).

Notes. Poison puffballs can be confused with true puffballs (*Lycoperdon* spp., *Bovista* spp., and other, related genera), many of which are favorite edibles when young. To distinguish edible puffballs, slice them in half from top to bottom: a true puffball at the edible stage will look and feel like a marshmallow, firm but soft, white, and homogeneous (without gills or discrete stem); puffballs too old for eating will be yellowish or greenish brown and very soft inside, becoming dark brown and powdery when dry. (Some indigenous people consider this puffball spore powder poisonous, and warn against getting it in your eyes or breathing it in.) Poison puffballs at maturity will be firm and purplish black inside, with a thick, rind-like skin. Although some species of *Scleroderma* have been eaten as truffle substitutes, their taste is rather acrid, and all should be avoided because of their potential harmful properties.

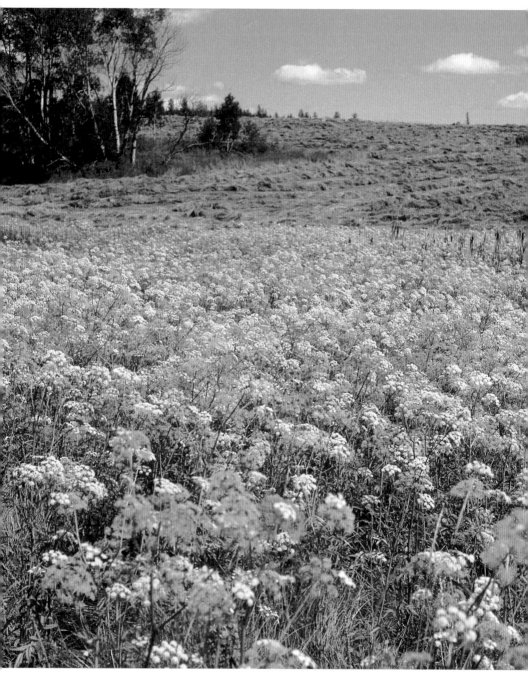

Western water hemlock in wet meadow, Cariboo district, British Columbia.

CHAPTER 3
Poisonous Plants of Wild Areas

ALGAE AND CYANOBACTERIA

Quick check. Shellfish poisoning from microscope algae can be fatal. Almost all the larger seaweeds are harmless. Algae and bacteria can contaminate fresh water: do not drink any water not known to be safe.

Never harvest shellfish for eating without checking with those who know local water conditions, such as fisheries or health authorities. If shellfish poisoning is suspected, contact physician immediately. Keep samples of water and shellfish for identification.

What are algae?

Algae are members of several large groups of simple, mainly aquatic protistans. They include the so-called seaweeds, which are large, easily visible marine or freshwater algae, as well as many microscopic types that in large numbers produce greenish or brownish scum or slime in ponds and tidepools. Many algae, particularly seaweeds, are edible and are an important part of the human diet in many areas of the world, including Japan, China, Hawaii, and the South Pacific. Indigenous and local peoples of coastal North America also eat seaweeds, and some species, such as dulse (*Palmaria palmata*), are widely marketed in Canada and the United States.

Poisonous freshwater algae and cyanobacteria

Some algae and cyanobacteria can be toxic to humans and animals. Among freshwater types, only a few belonging to the cyanobacteria (formerly bluegreen algae) are known to cause poisoning. Cyanobacteria are common in almost any body of water. Although they are mostly microscopic, under some conditions they can grow rapidly and accumulate in large masses in the upper layers of water, forming a "bloom" or scum. Only a few species of the cyanobacteria that form these blooms are poisonous, and since several or many types often grow together, the actual toxic species are difficult to isolate. Furthermore, toxicity varies greatly over time spans as short as a few hours. Slight changes in environmental conditions may dissipate concentrations of the harmful cyanobacteria quite suddenly. Several species have been implicated, but of these, only three are well-substantiated toxic organisms: *Anabaena flos-aquae*, *Aphanizomenon flos-aquae*, and *Microcystis aeruginosa*. These three species are found in quiet, warm, nutrient-rich waters in North America and throughout the world. Surprisingly, the toxin from *Anabaena flos-aquae* has been identified as the same as that from "red tide."

Extensive loss of life and severe sickness of humans and many kinds of animals have been associated with drinking water contaminated with algal blooms in the northern United States and Texas and in southern Canada. One moderately poisonous algal toxin that has been isolated is a cyclic polypeptide containing seven amino acids. Others have not been identified and may be products of decomposition or of other bacteria associated with the cyanobacteria. Symptoms of algae poisoning appear rapidly, within 15 to 45 minutes of drinking contaminated water, and include nausea, vomiting, abdominal pain, diarrhea, prostration, muscular tremors, difficulty in breathing, discoloration of the skin due to lack of oxygen, general paralysis, convulsions, and, occasionally death within one to 24 hours. Other types of bacteria and other organisms in fresh water may also cause illness. The best policy is not to drink stagnant water, or any water not known to be safe.

Paralytic shellfish poisoning: "red tide"

For marine algae, the most serious cause of poisoning is through eating filter-feeding mollusks such as mussels, clams, and oysters, and sometimes their predators that have accumulated the toxin from a large quantity of tiny microscopic algae of the dinoflagellate group. Under conditions difficult to predict, populations of these minute organisms multiply to concentrations of several million cells per liter of seawater. In these quantities, they may color the water brownish or reddish, giving rise to the term "red tide." It should be noted, however, that there are many organisms that cause a reddish coloration in the water that are not poisonous, and dinoflagellate algae in concentrations enough to be toxic do not always produce a visible coloration.

"Red tides" have over recorded history caused hundreds of cases of severe poisoning and death on the West Coast of North America, from Alaska to California, and to a lesser degree on the East Coast as well. Two species, *Alexandrium catenella* on the West Coast and *A. fundyense* on the East Coast, are the main culprits. Saxitoxin is the principal toxin in about a dozen structurally related paralytic shellfish toxins based on a complex perhydropurine skeleton. These water-soluble, extremely stable toxins act on the neuromuscular system in a manner similar to that of curare, the South American arrow poison. Eating only a very few contaminated clams or other bivalves may be lethal for a person. Numbness, nausea, difficulty in walking, thick speech, headache, and increasing general paralysis are typical symptoms. Death is from respiratory failure. If the patient survives the first 24 hours, however, the prognosis is good.

In the winter of 1987 a new form of shellfish poisoning originating on the East Coast was attributed to accumulation in the water of a diatom, *Pseudo-nitzschia multiseries*, and the concentration of its deadly toxin, domoic acid, in mussels. Over 150 people became sick after eating mussels from the Canadian Maritimes region, and there were at least three deaths.

The best prevention for shellfish poisoning is to inquire about local tidewater conditions before harvesting shellfish. The summer months are particularly suspect. Removal of the viscera of the shellfish reduces, but does not eliminate, the level of toxicity. Many clams concentrate the toxin in the pigments at their siphon tips, possibly as a defense against predators that often nip them off. Commercially marketed shellfish are vigorously and effectively inspected through governmental agencies. The main victims of shellfish poisoning are uninformed individuals harvesting their own shellfish. For more information on shellfish and other types of seafood poisoning, see Woods Hole Oceanographic Institutions's "Harmful Algae Page," http://www.whoi.edu/redtide/.

Seaweeds: most are harmless

Of the larger, more easily visible marine algae, or seaweeds, only a few are toxic if eaten in quantity, and members of only one genus, *Lyngbya*, are potentially lethal. *Lyngbya* is actually a genus of hair-like filamentous cyanobacteria (bluegreen algae) forming dense irregular floating mats or growths around atolls and in salt marshes, as well as in fresh water. Many types of

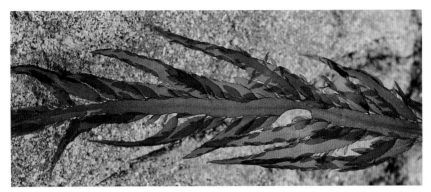

Desmarestia (*Desmarestia herbacea*).

fish feeding on *Lyngbya* species or on other fish that feed on them become poisonous to humans. This type of poisoning, ciguatura poisoning, is prevalent in the Caribbean, the South Pacific, and other tropical regions; studies aimed at detecting and controlling it are ongoing.

Another genus of seaweeds that could cause problems if ingested is *Desmarestia*. Members of this genus are brown algae that have a very high acidity and contain esters of sulfuric acid; they can cause severe digestive upset, but since they taste very sour they are unlikely to be eaten in any quantity.

FUNGI

Quick check. Ergot, a small, hard, black, elongated structure that grows on and contaminates grains, is highly toxic to humans and animals when eaten in quantity or in small doses over a long period of time; rarely a problem for humans in North America, but animal poisoning occasionally severe. Some molds are poisonous and potentially carcinogenic.

If home-grown grains are eaten, check for ergot contamination. If poisoning from ergot-contaminated feed is suspected, have a sample checked by local agricultural authorities. Never eat rotting or moldy food, or feed moldy fodder to animals. Do not breathe in dust from moldy hay or foods. Avoid old or improperly stored grains and nuts.

Ergot

Not just poisonous mushrooms but many other types of fungi cause poisoning to humans and animals. One of the most notorious is ergot (*Claviceps* spp.), including several species of ascomycete fungi with complex life

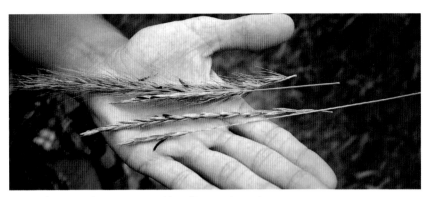

Ergot (*Claviceps* sp.) growing on wildrye (*Leymus cinereus*).

cycles that parasitize the grains of various cultivated and wild grasses. Most prominent is *C. purpurea*, which grows on rye, wheat, and barley. The resting phase of ergot is as a sclerotium, a hard, blackish, elongated structure. It is occasionally found as a contaminant in grain, causing crop loss by reducing the yield and quality of grain. (Grain containing more than 0.3% ergot by weight is prohibited from sale due to potential toxicity.)

Ergot poisoning was known for many centuries as St. Anthony's fire, after the saint who is said to have suffered from it. Russian peasants often developed a chronic form of ergot poisoning, and people who ate bread made from infected grain suffered from ergotism. There are still occasional outbreaks of the disease in some parts of the world, but in North America human poisoning has virtually ceased. Animal poisoning, especially of cattle, however, has occasionally been severe.

Over 40 alkaloids, many toxic, have been isolated from ergot. All are related chemically, being derivatives of lysergic acid. They are present in varying amounts depending on the strain and geographic location of the ergot sclerotia. Some are useful medically in stimulating uterine contractions during labor and in controlling uterine hemorrhage, but used incorrectly they can cause hallucinations and insanity.

Symptoms of ergot poisoning include irritation of the digestive tract (abdominal pain, with nausea, vomiting, diarrhea, and thirst), headache, loss of balance, lack of coordination, muscle tremors, and convulsions. These symptoms are followed by drowsiness and temporary paralysis. Large amounts of ergot ingested per day produce convulsive ergotism: hyperexcitability, belligerency, trembling, and convulsions. Ingesting small amounts of ergot over a period of weeks may cause chronic poisoning characterized by dry gangrene of the extremities. Irregular heartbeat, variable blood pressure, and kidney failure sometimes occur. Humans and animals are affected similarly. For affected animals, care should be taken to avoid undue excitement in moving them away from infected vegetation.

Mold poisons, or mycotoxins

Another type of poisoning results from consuming mycotoxins found in certain molds. Molds are microscopic fungi that sometime contaminate food and can cause poisoning in people and animals. They have been recognized for centuries; some are used in the production of roquefort, camembert, and other cheeses, and of penicillin and other antibiotics. (Even camembert and other cheeses can be harmful when eaten together with certain tranquilizers and antidepressants.) However, it has been shown that many molds produce toxins as secondary metabolites.

A major impact of mold poisons arises from contaminated animal forage. So-called forage poisoning has caused the illness and death of tens of thousands of cattle, horses, pigs, poultry, and other domesticated animals in North America. Several toxic mold species, especially in the genera *Penicillium*, *Aspergillus*, and *Monascus*, have been incriminated through poisoning investigations and experimental feeding. The main losses have been associated with moldy corn.

Originally, many mycotoxicoses (diseases caused by mycotoxins) were blamed on the feed plants themselves rather than on their mold contaminants. Mycotoxins vary considerably in chemical structure and belong to several different chemical groups. In 1961 researchers isolated a common mold, *Aspergillus flavus*, from peanut meal that had been responsible for the deaths of thousands of turkeys in Britain. Subsequently, it was found that this species and another, *A. parasiticus*, produced aflatoxin, a mycotoxin that causes tumors of the liver. Since that time, investigations on mycotoxins and mycotoxicoses have been numerous, and are ongoing.

The tumor-causing properties and other toxic effects of aflatoxin and some other mold poisons certainly have implications for human health. Differences in geographical distribution of liver cancer in humans have been attributed to different levels of occurrence of mycotoxins in food in various parts of the world, although this has not been actually proven. Improved harvesting and storage procedures for crops such as peanuts and grains have significantly reduced the risks of mycotoxicosis in humans.

Food may contain mycotoxins even when not visibly moldy. Furthermore, the presence of mold on stored food does not necessarily indicate the presence of mycotoxins, which are produced only by some mold species. Many mycotoxins have been identified from mold species on a wide variety of grains, cereal, and nuts, and also from the milk and meat of animals that have eaten contaminated feed. Inhaling the spores of many molds is another potential danger; these can produce an allergic respiratory condition in humans and animals. Several species in the genus *Fusarium* are known to cause this problem.

A new danger from the fungus world was identified on eastern Vancouver Island in 1999. A pathogenic yeast relative, *Cryptococcus gattii*, previously found only in tropical and subtropical regions, had by February 2008 caused over 175 diagnosed infections and at least eight deaths in the region, mostly of elderly people with previous respiratory conditions.

LICHENS

Quick check. Lichens—small, moss-like or flattened organisms of various colors growing on rock, bark, soil, or wood—are mostly indigestible and can be acrid and irritating to the digestive tract, but few are seriously poisonous in small quantities. Some lichens can cause allergic skin reactions in some people.

What are lichens?

Lichens are complex structures consisting of two or more separate organisms, one or more algae and a fungus, growing together in a close, mutually beneficial relationship, or symbiosis. They have several different growth forms. Some are crustose, adhering tightly to rock or bark. Others are thallose, with flattened, almost leaflike surfaces. Still others are fruticose, with stiff upright or hanging, branching structures. Some lichens are edible— including black tree hair, or Fremont's horsehair lichen (*Bryoria fremontii*) and rock tripes (*Umbilicaria* spp.)—after leaching, neutralizing with ash, or prolonged cooking. Most cannot be eaten, because they contain bitter acids; furthermore, their complex carbohydrates are not easily broken down by the human digestive system. Eating raw, unprocessed lichens, even edible species, can cause stomach cramps and discomfort. (Deer, caribou, reindeer, and other ungulates are much better able to digest lichens than humans are.)

Poisonous lichens

Some lichens are quite toxic, due to the presence of usnic or vulpinic acid or other lichen substances. One example is wolf lichen (*Letharia vulpina* and related spp.), a bright greenish yellow, finely branched fruticose type growing on trunks and dead branches of coniferous trees in dry areas of northwestern North America. In Scandinavia, wolf lichen was powdered, mixed with ground glass, and sprinkled on meat, as a wolf poison. Another notably poisonous species is ground lichen (*Parmelia molliuscula*), a gray-green irregularly dissected, flattened type. It grows from Nebraska to North Dakota and west to the Rocky Mountains and has been responsible for range poisoning of sheep and cattle, sometimes causing severe paralysis and death. Poisoning usually occurs in winter when other forage is scarce. Some relatives of black tree hair lichen, including *Bryoria tortuosa*, contain much higher concentrations of poisonous vulpinic acid and are potentially toxic; usually, however, their bitter taste precludes people consuming them.

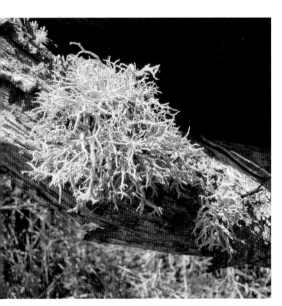

Wolf lichen (*Letharia vulpina*).

Lichens and skin irritation

Some lichens occasionally cause a dermatitis known as woodcutter's eczema. This ailment has been traced to allergic reactions of people coming in contact with lichens containing usnic acid and other substances.

Cautionary note on eating lichens

Because of the difficulty in identifying and distinguishing various lichens, their doubtful digestibility except with special preparation, and their potential toxicity, lichens should not be consumed by the uninformed. Their nutritive value is rather low, although they have been known to sustain life in emergency situations.

FERNS AND THEIR RELATIVES

Quick check. Brackenfern is potentially toxic and carcinogenic; horsetails may be toxic to livestock; some other ferns (male fern, cloakfern, sensitive fern) are poisonous to livestock if consumed in quantity; most ferns are harmless.

Some harmful ferns

Several species of ferns and their relatives are poisonous to humans and animals. Prominent among these are brackenfern and horsetails (both of which are treated here in detail). Others include male fern (*Dryopteris filix-mas*), cloakfern (*Astrolepis sinuata*), and sensitive fern (*Onoclea sensibilis*).

The widely distributed male fern, used medicinally as a deworming agent, is known to contain thiaminase (as do brackenfern and horsetails) and filicin, another potentially harmful substance. Cloakfern, or jimmy fern, an erect, evergreen perennial of dry rocky hills in the southcentral United States and Mexico, contains an unknown toxin that affects range stock, especially sheep. Sensitive fern, a perennial with green, broadly triangular vegetative fronds and deep brown spore-bearing fronds, grows in open woods and thickets throughout eastern North America; it is a suspected cause of nervous disorder in horses.

brackenfern

Pteridium aquilinum
hay-scented fern family (Dennstaedtiaceae)

Quick check. Large, coarse fern of open fields and woodlands, with long-stemmed fronds of broadly triangular outline arising singly from perennial rhizomes. Poisonous to livestock; potentially carcinogenic. Eating bracken fiddleheads not recommended.

Description. Brackenfern, or brake, is a common fern, usually 1–2 m (3–6 ft.) high, growing from long, blackish, branching horizontal rhizomes. The young shoots (fiddleheads) are brownish and scaly, rolled tightly inward from the tip, and bent over at the top like a shepherd's crook. The frond stalks are tall, stiff, and light brown, and the blades (leafy part) are coarse, broadly triangular, and usually three times divided, the ultimate segments oblong. The leaflet margins are inrolled, and spore-bearing structures, when present, are inconspicuous and borne on the undersides of the margins. Fronds are deciduous, turning light brown and dying back in the fall.

Occurrence. This fern grows worldwide in open fields, meadows, and woods, and is often present in abundance. Many varieties are distinguished, including several in North America.

Toxicity. Brackenfern contains a number of toxic constituents, which are apparently present throughout the plant. These include prunasin, a cyanogenic glycoside; thiaminase, an enzyme that results in a thiamine deficiency; and ptaquiloside, a carcinogenic, mutagenic sesquiterpene glycoside.

Not all brackenfern populations contain prunasin; it can be detected in the shoots by the presence of a strong, bitter almond odor. Thiaminase in bracken, highest in the rhizomes and fiddleheads, can induce fatal thiamine deficiency in horses and occasionally in livestock by destroying thiamine (vitamin B_1) reserves, and could be harmful to humans eating large quantities of the fiddleheads.

These toxins, especially the carcinogen ptaquiloside, have serious implications for humans, particularly because young bracken fiddleheads have

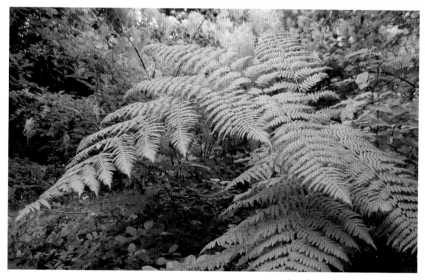

Brackenfern (*Pteridium aquilinum*).

been used as a vegetable in some parts of the world, especially Japan, and are still occasionally recommended as a "wild food" in North America. Human consumption of bracken has been suggested as a cause of the high incidence of stomach cancer in Japan. The fiddleheads contain high concentrations of carcinogenic agents. Furthermore, humans can be exposed to the carcinogens indirectly, through drinking milk from cows grazing in bracken-covered pastures.

Notes. The risks to humans of eating bracken fiddleheads are potentially serious but have not yet been fully established. However, because the plant's toxicity to livestock has been well documented, its safety for humans is at best questionable, and it should no longer be used. Indigenous North Americans of the western United States and Canada traditionally ate the starchy tissue from roasted bracken rhizomes, but this use is now largely unknown.

Bracken fiddleheads should not be confused with the fiddleheads of ostrich fern (*Matteuccia struthiopteris*), which are commonly gathered from the wild in parts of Canada and the eastern United States and are commercially harvested in the Maritimes. These are not carcinogenic and are generally safe for human consumption. There are some records of people eating fiddleheads in restaurant meals and developing severe gastrointestinal cramps, vomiting, and diarrhea (Frohne and Pfänder 2005), but these situations are no doubt due to bacterial contamination, not from the fiddleheads themselves.

horsetail, field

Equisetum arvense and related spp.
horsetail family (Equisetaceae)

Quick check. Herbaceous nonflowering perennials with rush-like, jointed, green, ridged stalks (and branches if present), scratchy to the touch, usually 30–60 cm (1–2 ft.) tall; leaves reduced to papery sheathing rings at the joints. Potentially cause of thiamine deficiency when consumed in quantity or over prolonged periods.

Description. One of the most prevalent of the many species of horsetail in North America is the field horsetail (*Equisetum arvense*), a branching, bright green plant, up to 60 cm (2 ft.) high with stems produced annually from underground rhizomes. The stems are jointed, hollow, and rough-textured, with longitudinal ridges. The branches are slender and numerous, in whorls from the joints. The leaves are small and papery, forming a sheathing ring at each joint. A spore-bearing "cone" is produced at the end of a separate, whitish, nonbranching stalk in early spring. Other species, such as scour-ingrush horsetail (*E. hyemale*), are unbranched, and some have dark green, perennial stems. In some, the spore-bearing structure grows at the tip of the green vegetative shoot.

Occurrence. Field horsetail is widespread in North America, growing in a variety of habitats, from damp, swampy areas to dry, sandy locations in woodlands, pastures, and cultivated land. Other species occur in different regions, mostly in damp soil.

Toxicity. The main toxic compound in horsetails is thiaminase, the same enzyme found in brackenfern, which destroys thiamine (vitamin B_1) in the body. The plants also contain a saponin (equisitonin) and several flavone glycosides. Some *Equisetum* species (e.g., *E. palustre*, marsh horsetail) contain an alkaloid, palustrine. Horsetail is sometimes used in herbal medicine as a diuretic and astringent, but its effectiveness is limited, and it should be used sparingly (Tyler 1987). The young shoots of some species are considered edible but should not be eaten in quantity.

Notes. The silica in horsetails makes them scratchy to the touch and useful as abrasives and pot scrubbers. The young shoots of field horsetail (*Equisetum*

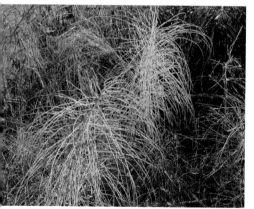

Field horsetail (*Equisetum arvense*), mature plants.

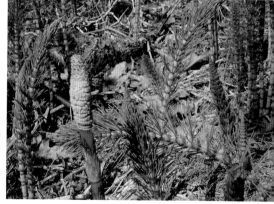

Giant horsetail (*Equisetum telmateia*), young shoots and spore-bearing shoot.

arvense) and giant horsetail (*E. telmateia*) are sometimes eaten as a spring-time vegetable by indigenous peoples of western North America, with no reported detrimental effects, but the mature plants should not be eaten.

CONIFERS

Evergreen (needled or scaled) trees, mostly cone-bearing, are known to contain a wide variety of complex chemical substances in their foliage, bark, and pitch. The "Christmas tree" aroma of pines and firs and the characteristic scent of junipers and their relatives indicate the presence of these compounds. Resins found in resin canals in conifers are suspended in a solvent of many essential oils, collectively referred to as turpentine, which is poisonous in its own right. Most of these trees would be too strong-tasting and unpalatable to eat, but many can be used safely as flavorings or to make beverage and medicinal teas, as long as these are taken in moderation and in low concentrations. Exceptions are the yews (*Taxus* spp.), which are highly toxic (see Chapter 4), and ponderosa pine (*Pinus ponderosa*), a tree of dry western forests, with long needles usually in clusters of three. Some indigenous people ate the inner bark and seeds of this pine, but they knew that pregnant women should not chew on the buds or needles because it would cause a miscarriage (Turner et al. 1980). Eating the foliage of this pine is known to cause abortion in late-term pregnant cattle and other livestock, due to the presence of isocupressic acid, which has also been found in lodgepole pine (*P. contorta*) and Jeffrey pine (*P. jeffreyi*). Other pines, such as loblolly pine (*P. taeda*) of the southeastern United States, should also be regarded with caution.

Additionally, some trees of the cypress family (Cupressaceae)—"cedars," cypresses, and junipers (including *Thuja* spp., *Cupressus* spp., *Chamaecyparis* spp., and *Juniperus* spp.)—have been implicated in cases of illness and poisoning. Juniper "berries," widely used as a flavoring and herbal medicine, are known to cause kidney irritation, uterine contractions, and possible miscarriage in pregnant women if taken in quantity (Tyler 1987). Significant concentrations of isocupressic acid have been found in junipers (*Juniperus scopulorum, J. communis*) and in the aforementioned pines (Gardner and James 1999).

TREES AND TALL SHRUBS

buckeyes: California buckeye, Ohio buckeye, yellow buckeye

Aesculus californica, A. glabra, A. flava, and related spp.
horse chestnut family (Hippocastanaceae)

Quick check. Trees or shrubs with palmately compound leaves, erect flower clusters, and large, glossy brown seeds with a spiny capsule. Entire plants poisonous; children sometimes seriously poisoned from eating the seeds or drinking tea made from the leaves.

Description. Buckeyes are relatives of horse chestnuts and are similar to those ornamental trees. They are deciduous shrubs or small trees, with leaves opposite and palmately compound, with five to seven toothed leaflets. The flowers are red to yellowish, and numerous, in large, erect clusters. The fruits are three-parted capsules with spiny, leathery, greenish to brownish husks splitting open at maturity to reveal one to six large, glossy brown seeds, each bearing a large, pale scar or "buckeye."

Occurrence. Several species of buckeye are native to North America. California buckeye (*Aesculus californica*) grows in the dry hills and canyons of the southern Pacific Coast. Ohio buckeye (*A. glabra*) grows in rich woods from southern Ontario to Nebraska, and south to Texas and Georgia. Yellow buckeye (*A. flava*) is native to the Ohio Valley and Appalachian Mountains of the eastern states.

Toxicity. The main toxin in buckeyes is aescin, a saponin found in the leaves, shoots, bark, flowers, and seeds. The three species listed are toxic to humans and animals. Buckeye honey can also be poisonous.

Children are sometimes poisoned from eating the nuts or making tea from the leaves or twigs. Poisoning symptoms include weakness, loss of coordination, vomiting, twitching, dilated pupils, sluggishness, excitability, and paralysis.

Notes. The nuts of some buckeye species were a traditional food of indigenous peoples but had to be specially prepared to reduce the toxic effects. Buckeye fruits have been used as fish poisons by several Native American groups (Moerman 2003).

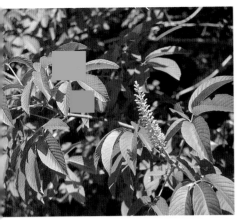

California buckeye (*Aesculus californica*).

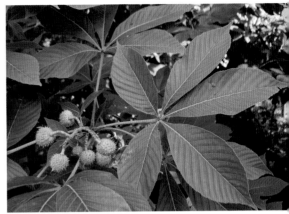

Ohio buckeye (*Aesculus glabra*).

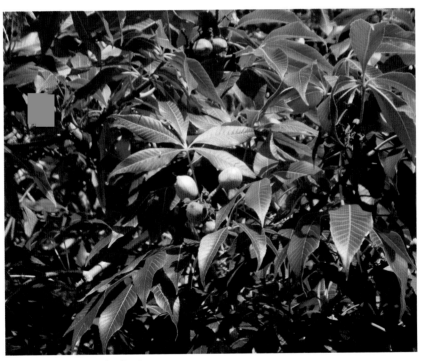

Yellow buckeye (*Aesculus flava*).

cherries, wild: chokecherry, black cherry, bitter cherry, pin cherry

Prunus virginiana, P. serotina, P. emarginata, P. pensylvanica, and related spp.
rose family (Rosaceae)

Quick check. Trees or shrubs (occasionally low) with simple, usually deciduous leaves, clustered white or pinkish flowers, small cherry-like fruits. Leaves, roots, bark, and seed kernels contain cyanide-producing compound; potentially fatal to children swallowing large numbers of seeds when they eat the fruit.

Description. There are several kinds of wild cherries in North America, including some garden escapes. The bark is rough and dark, to smooth and gray or reddish, often peeling off in horizontal strips, with conspicuous horizontal lenticels or eyelets. The leaves, deciduous in most species, are simple and alternate, often with toothed edges. The flowers are whitish or pinkish and five-petalled, in elongated or umbrella-like clusters. The cherry-like fruits are red to blackish, with a fleshy, usually edible, layer covering a single, hard stone.

Chokecherry is a shrub or small tree with small flowers in elongated clusters (racemes), and red, purplish, or blackish fruit. Black cherry is a tree, 15 m (50 ft.) or more tall and 1 m (3 ft.) across at maturity, with flowers in elongated clusters, and black fruit. Bitter cherry and pin cherry are similar; both are shrubs or small to medium trees with flowers in small, umbrella-like clusters (umbels) and small, red fruit.

Occurrence. Wild cherries are found in woods and thickets, often near water, throughout North America except in the far north. Chokecherry (*Prunus virginiana*) is widespread, with varieties occurring from coast to coast in temperate areas. Black cherry (*P. serotina*) occurs in eastern Canada and the United States south to Florida and west to Texas. Bitter cherry (*P. emarginata*) is found along the Pacific Coast east to the Rocky Mountains, and pin cherry (*P. pensylvanica*) from eastern British Columbia to the Atlantic Coast, ranging into the central and northeastern United States.

Toxicity. Although most wild cherries have fruit that is palatable and pleasant to eat when ripe, several species are known to contain dangerous levels of the cyanide-producing compound amygdalin, a cyanogenic glycoside, in their leaves, twigs, bark, and seeds (stones). Another related compound, prunasin, has been isolated from black cherry (*Prunus serotina*). These compounds have been responsible for much livestock loss, as well as occasional illness and fatalities in humans. There is considerable variation in level of cyanide production among species and in different parts or growth stages. The highest concentrations of cyanide are produced in the largest, most succulent leaves on vigorous shoots. Wilting leaves usually produce larger amounts than fresh leaves.

Symptoms of cyanide poisoning include anxiety, confusion, dizziness, headache, and vomiting, with an odor of bitter almonds on the breath or vomit. Difficulty in breathing, fluctuations of blood pressure and heart rate, and possible kidney failure may also occur. Convulsions, coma, and death may occur very suddenly, within a matter of minutes following very large doses.

Children are sometimes fatally poisoned by eating wild cherries and swallowing the cyanide-producing stones; these should always be discarded before the fruits are eaten.

Notes. Domesticated cherries, plums, apples, pears, peaches, apricots, and almonds contain the same cyanide-producing compound in their seeds, leaves, and bark as the wild cherries. Other wild plants in the rose family known to be cyanide-producing and hence toxic are mountain mahoganies (*Cercocarpus* spp.) and Carolina laurelcherry (*Prunus caroliniana*). Wild plums are also toxic but less likely to cause poisoning in humans because their stones are larger and are seldom swallowed. Saskatoon serviceberry

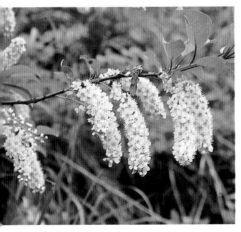

Chokecherry (*Prunus virginiana*).

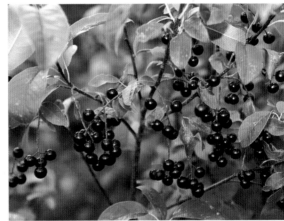

Chokecherry fruits.

(*Amelanchier alnifolia*) and its relatives in the genus have edible fruit, but their leaves and twigs may produce toxic amounts of cyanide, and their seeds, though small, also contain cyanide-producing compounds.

coyotillo
Karwinskia humboldtiana
buckthorn family (Rhamnaceae)

Quick check. Simple-leaved shrub or small tree of dry hills, canyons, and valleys of the far Southwest; small brownish black "berries." Eating these fruits causes delayed paralysis, and potentially death, in humans and animals; foliage also poisonous.

Description. Coyotillo, or tullidora, is a shrub or small tree 1–6 m (3–20 ft.) tall. The leaves, mostly opposite, are stalked and elliptical to oval, with smooth or wavy, slightly recurving margins and distinct straight veins. The small, greenish flowers are borne in clusters at the leaf axils. The fruit is an ovoid, berry-like drupe (fleshy outer covering, with single stone) about 1.2 cm (0.5 in.) across.

Occurrence. Dry, gravelly hills, canyons, and valleys in southwestern Texas, New Mexico, Arizona, southern California, and Mexico.

Toxicity. The fleshy fruits have long been known to be poisonous to humans and livestock, including goats, sheep, cattle, pigs, and poultry. The foliage is also toxic and may be fatal to browsing livestock. Eating the fruits can cause severe paralysis, which may be delayed for a few days to several weeks without any visible signs of poisoning in the lag period. Then weakness, lack of coordination, and finally complete prostration may ensue. Recovery may take many weeks. A number of neurotoxic substances have been isolated from the fruits, including anthra-

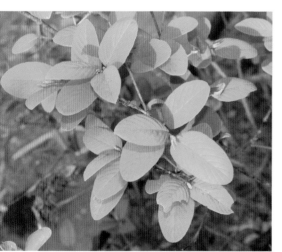

Karwinskia humboldtiana. Jan Dauphin

cenes, which are linked with a naphthalene derivative (Frohne and Pfänder 2005).

Notes. The seeds are the most toxic part of the plant. Children have been fatally poisoned from eating the fruits, and should be kept away from them. The delayed onset of the paralysis caused by ingesting the fruits can make detection of the poisoning source very difficult.

elderberries: red elderberry, black elderberry, blue elderberry

Sambucus racemosa, *S. nigra* ssp. *canadensis*, *S. nigra* ssp. *cerulea*, and related spp. honeysuckle family (Caprifoliaceae)

Quick check. Tall deciduous shrubs, with opposite, pinnately compound leaves, and small red, bluish, or purple-black berries in flat-topped or pyramidal clusters. Leaves, stems, bark, and roots strongly purgative and cyanide-producing; uncooked berries may cause nausea in humans.

Description. These are coarse shrubs, up to 4 m (12 ft.) high, with stout, pithy, grayish-barked stems. The leaves are opposite and pinnately compound, with lance-shaped, toothed leaflets. The small, numerous flowers are whitish or creamy, in dense flat-topped or pyramidal clusters. The berries are small but produced in large, conspicuous masses. Depending on the species, the fruits range in color from bright red to grayish blue to purple-black.

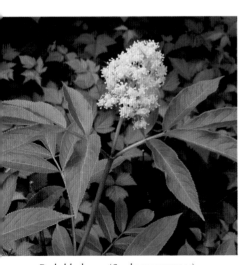

Red elderberry (*Sambucus racemosa*).

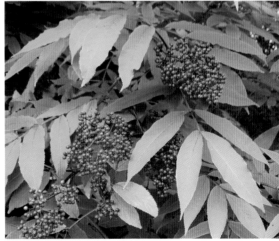

Red elderberry fruits.

Young growths may be distinguished by their opposite leaves and absence of tuberous roots.

Occurrence. Moist, rich soils in woodlands throughout much of North America. Red elderberry (*Sambucus racemosa*) occurs from Alaska south to California and New Mexico, and east to the Maritimes in Canada. Blue elderberry (*S. nigra* ssp. *cerulea*) is found from British Columbia east to Montana and south to New Mexico. Black elderberry (*S. nigra* ssp. *canadensis*) grows in eastern North America from Manitoba to the Maritimes and south to Georgia and Louisiana. Other species occur in the wild and increasingly in gardens throughout much of North America.

Toxicity. The roots, stems, bark, and leaves (and to a much lesser extent, the flowers and unripe fruits) contain a poisonous alkaloid and cyanogenic glycoside causing nausea, vomiting, and diarrhea. In addition, a lectin is present. People are sometimes poisoned by drinking medicinal tea, especially if it is made from the leaves or branches. Children have been poisoned by using hollowed elder stems for popguns and peashooters.

Notes. Elderberry stems, bark, and roots are used medicinally as an emetic and purgative by several North American indigenous groups. Elder flowers and fruits are edible, and the latter are commonly used to make wine and jelly; however, there have been reports of the raw fruits of red elderberry causing nausea.

A number of other plants in the honeysuckle family (snowberry, for example, which see) are considered to be poisonous to some extent. Many indigenous peoples maintain that the fruits and entire plant of twinberry honeysuckle, or black twinberry (*Lonicera involucrata*) are poisonous, and that eating them will cause one to lose his voice; these berries are variously called raven's berries, crow's berries, or monster's food in different languages (Moerman 2003; Turner 1995).

Kentucky coffeetree

Gymnocladus dioicus
pea family (Fabaceae)

Quick check. Large, much-branched tree of the eastern United States, with large, divided leaves and large, brown, hard "bean" pods. Seeds poisonous to humans but seldom fatal; foliage and shoots highly toxic.

Description. A large, rough-barked forest tree up to 30 m (80 ft.) or more tall, with short trunk and many major branches. The leaves are alternate, twice pinnately divided, and up to 1 m (3 ft.) long, with oval-shaped, smooth-margined leaflets. The flowers, produced in May, are whitish, in elongated terminal clusters. The fruit is a hard, flat, reddish brown "bean" pod up to 15 cm (6 in.) long and about 2.5 cm (1 in.) broad, containing four to seven hard, flat seeds with sticky pulp between them. The fresh pods exude yellow resin when broken.

Occurrence. Rich, moist woods from southern Ontario to Alabama and Oklahoma; occasionally planted elsewhere as a lawn or street tree.

Toxicity. The main toxic substance in this tree is cytisine, a quinolizidine alkaloid with action similar to nicotine. Humans may be poisoned by eating the seeds or pulp between the seeds, although the roasted seeds were used by early settlers as a coffee substitute. Livestock have been fatally poisoned from eating the foliage or young shoots. Symptoms of poisoning include intense irritation of the digestive tract, diarrhea, vomiting, congestion of mucous membranes, irregular pulse, and coma. Death may occur within a day after appearance of symptoms.

Notes. The fruits of this tree may be confused with those of the more common honeylocust (*Gleditsia triacanthos*), whose seed pulp is sweet and edible; honeylocust is usually thorny, and its pod is much longer (20–30 cm, 8–15 in.), often twisted or curved, with thinner walls. Do not confuse honeylocust with black locust (*Robinia pseudoacacia*), another poisonous-fruited tree of the pea family, which is also sometimes called honeylocust.

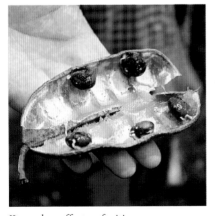

Kentucky coffeetree fruiting pod with seeds.

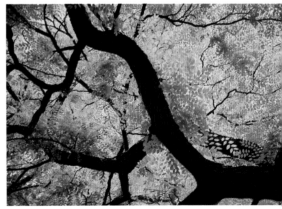

Kentucky coffeetree (*Gymnocladus dioicus*).

Keep children away from the pods of Kentucky coffeetree. Livestock should be kept away from the felled trees, cut branches, and sprouts from cut stumps.

laurels: sheep laurel, mountain laurel, alpine laurel

Kalmia angustifolia, K. latifolia, and *K. microphylla*
heather family (Ericaceae)

Quick check. Small trees to occasionally low shrubs of rocky or sandy acidic soils or peat bogs, with dark green, evergreen leaves and whitish to pink or deep red, clustered bell-shaped to urn-shaped flowers. Leaves and flowers highly toxic, sometimes fatal, to humans and browsing animals. Flower nectar and honey also toxic.

Description. The laurels all have smooth, evergreen leaves and showy, clustered, five-pointed, ornate flowers with the petals fused together, and dry, capsulate, many-seeded fruits.

Sheep laurel (*Kalmia angustifolia*), also known as lambkill, is an open, woody shrub, 0.3–1.3 m (1–4 ft.) tall. The leaves are opposite, or whorled in threes, and elongated, 2.5–6.5 cm (1–2.5 in.) long. The branches are upright, and the flowers rose or crimson, widely bell-shaped, and produced in lateral clusters.

Mountain laurel (*Kalmia latifolia*) is a shrub or small tree 2–10 m (6–30 ft.) high, with alternate leaves up to 10 cm (4 in.) long. The flowers are white to rose with purple markings and borne in terminal clusters.

Alpine laurel (*Kalmia microphylla*), also known as bog laurel, is a small shrub usually under 60 cm (2 ft.) high. The leaves are opposite and shiny, whitish beneath, and usually less than 2.5 cm (1 in.) long. The flowers, rose to purple, are similar to those of sheep laurel but smaller, and in terminal clusters.

Occurrence. Sheep laurel is found in old pastures and meadows throughout northeastern North America. Mountain laurel grows in moist woods and clearings and along streams from eastern Canada southward in the Appalachian Mountains and Piedmont, and infrequently in the eastern coastal plain of the United States. Alpine laurel occurs in peat bogs and wet meadows at low to high elevations from northern California to Alaska.

Toxicity. Mountain laurel has caused human deaths. All three species have caused livestock deaths, especially of sheep and cattle. Poisoning is due primarily to a poisonous diterpene, acetylandromedol. This compound varies in its concentration across and within species. There is an initial burning of the lips, mouth, and throat with ingestion of the plants, followed up to six hours later by salivation, nausea, severe vomiting, abdominal pain, watering of the mouth, eyes, and nose, loss of appetite, repeated swallowing, headache, low blood pressure, and drowsiness with convulsions, weakness, difficulty in breathing, and progressive paralysis of the limbs, followed by coma and death in the most severe cases.

Notes. Children have been poisoned by sucking the flowers of mountain laurel and making tea from the leaves. Even honey from the flowers is poisonous, and people have been affected, especially from honey of laurels in central Europe and Turkey. Laurels are usually avoided by livestock, but poisoning can occur, especially in late spring and fall, when no other green foliage is available. At the Washington Zoo, a valuable monkey and angora goats were poisoned at different times by being fed laurel flowers and leaves by visitors.

Several other plants in the heather family contain the same poisonous compounds as laurels. These include rhododendrons, pieris, false azalea, and Labrador tea. Laurels are sometimes grown as garden ornamentals.

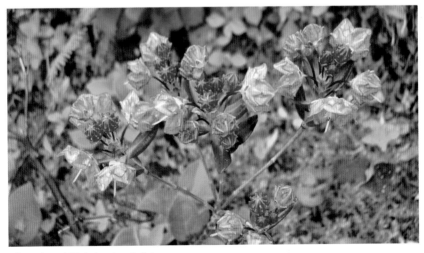

Alpine laurel (*Kalmia microphylla*).

mescal bean

Sophora secundiflora
pea family (Fabaceae)

Quick check. Evergreen shrub of dry areas of the far Southwest; pinnately compound, often hairy leaves; purplish, pea-like, clustered flowers; large, jointed, cylindrical fruiting pods. Seeds hallucinogenic and highly toxic; potentially fatal in small quantities to children; entire plant toxic to livestock but rarely fatal.

Description. Mescal bean, also known as frijolito or Texas mountain laurel, is an evergreen shrub or small tree, to 10 m (30 ft.) tall, with leaves that are stalked and alternate, 10–15 cm (4–6 in.) long, and pinnately compound with seven to 13 leathery, smooth-edged, oblong leaflets. The leaves may be covered with dense, whitish hairs. The pea-like flowers are violet-blue and very fragrant, produced in large, one-sided terminal clusters. The fruits are woody, jointed, cylindrical pods, each 2.5–18 cm (1–7 in.) long, containing one to eight bright red, hard seeds, on average about 13 mm (0.5 in.) long.

Occurrence. Mescal bean grows naturally on dry limestone hills and canyons of southwestern Texas and New Mexico into Mexico. Widely grown in the southern United States as an ornamental.

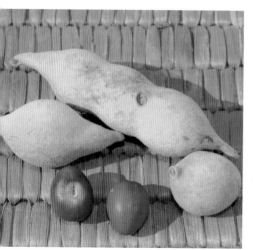

Mescal bean (*Sophora secundiflora*), pods and seeds.

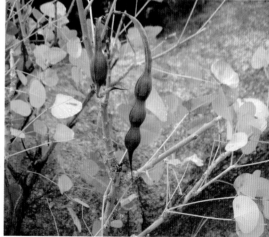

Coralbean (*Erythrina flabelliformis*).

Toxicity. This plant, like other species of the genus *Sophora*, contains poisonous quinolizidine alkaloids including cytisine, which is also present in *Laburnum*. The seeds are most commonly implicated in human poisoning. Symptoms include nausea, vomiting, diarrhea, excitability, delirium, convulsions, coma, and occasionally death through respiratory failure. One seed, thoroughly chewed, is said to be enough to kill a child.

Notes. Mescal bean is hallucinogenic and has long been used medicinally and ritually by Southwest Native Americans. Another native leguminous shrub, coralbean (*Erythrina flabelliformis*), also has showy red beans containing toxic alkaloids, borne in hanging pods. The seeds of both mescal bean and coralbean are sometimes used to make jewelry.

oaks

Quercus spp.
beech family (Fagaceae)

Quick check. Usually deciduous trees or shrubs with alternate, simple, often lobed or toothed leaves, and capped nut-like fruits (acorns). Young shoots, foliage, and some acorns poisonous. Acorns of some species are eaten by humans but only after special treatment to remove toxins and bitter compounds.

Description. Oaks are very common and probably recognized by most people. They are a large, variable group with some 60 native tree-size species in North America. There are also many hybrids and varieties, shrubby species, and introduced ornamentals. Oak leaves are alternate, simple, pinnately veined, and variable in size and shape. The flowers are greenish or yellowish, solitary or clustered, often appearing before the leaves. The fruits are spherical or elongated acorns partially enclosed by a scaly cup. Native oaks can be subdivided into three main groups: the white oaks, with deciduous leaves that are usually deeply lobed with rounded edges; the red oaks, with deciduous, usually sharply lobed, often bristle-tipped leaves; and the live oaks, with leaves that are thick, leathery, often spiny-margined, and evergreen.

Occurrence. Open, dry to moist deciduous woods throughout North America.

Toxicity. The acorns, leaves, and young shoots of many different oak species are toxic, reportedly due to the presence of various classes of tannins, including ellagitannin, condensed tannin (proanthocyanidin), and gallotannins. There are, fortunately, no reported human fatalities from oaks. Acorns, especially of the white oak group, were an important traditional food for indigenous peoples of North America and are still eaten by some; however, the kernels have to be carefully processed to remove the astringent, toxic principles. Since taste has everything to do with palatability, poisoning was probably avoided in the past by the bad taste of those having high tannin content. Nevertheless, we know of several people who consumed raw, untreated acorns on an experimental basis, resulting in painful and lingering irritation of the mouth and throat. There is also a danger of young children being poisoned from acorns, but fortunately there is little likelihood of a child chewing more than one acorn because the tannins are so bitter. In severe cases, oak tannins can cause inflammation, irritation, and hemorrhaging of the intestinal walls and degeneration of the liver and kidneys.

Notes. There are innumerable records in North America and Europe of livestock loss from oak shoots, leaves, and acorns. Cattle are particularly susceptible to oak poisoning, and sheep and goats are also affected. Poisoning usually occurs in spring, when new foliage is eaten; in the fall of heavy acorn crop years; and during drought years, when other forage is scarce. Squirrels and many types of birds, such as jays, rely on acorns as a food.

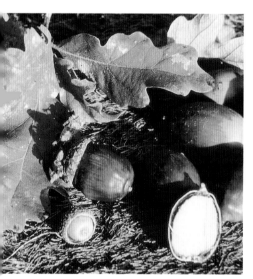

Garry oak acorns.

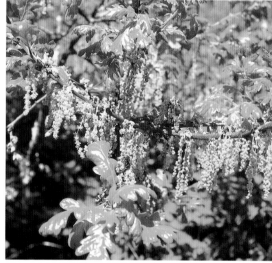

Garry oak, or Oregon white oak (*Quercus garryana*).

poison sumac

Toxicodendron vernix (syn. *Rhus vernix*)
cashew family (Anacardiaceae)

Quick check. Small tree to occasionally low shrub of bogs and swamps, with deciduous, alternate, pinnately compound leaves. Entire plant causes severe allergenic skin irritation.

Description. A much-branched low to tall shrub, or, in crowded stands, a single-trunked tree up to 8 m (25 ft.) tall. The bark is smooth and grayish. The leaves are deciduous, alternate, and pinnately divided into seven to 13 leaflets, each short-stalked, pointed, and smooth-edged. The leaf stalks are reddish. The flowers are tiny, greenish yellow, and inconspicuous; the fruits are small, dry, whitish to creamy yellow berry-like drupes, in hanging clusters that may persist over the winter.

Occurrence. Swamps, wet woods, and around boggy ponds from southern Ontario and Quebec south to eastern Texas and Florida; predominantly east of the Mississippi River.

Toxicity. The sap of the roots, stems, leaves, flowers, fruits, and the pollen contain a potent skin irritant, released by contact with the plant (especially with bruised portions) and affecting many people who have an allergic sen-

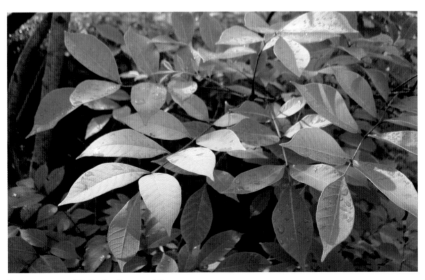

Poison sumac (*Toxicodendron vernix*).

sitivity to it. The toxic components, urushiols, are similar to those found in its relatives, poison ivy and poison oak. Danger of poisoning is greatest in spring and summer when the sap is produced abundantly. Symptoms are the same as for poison ivy.

Notes. Other, nonirritant shrubby sumacs (*Rhus* spp.) can be distinguished from poison sumac, also known as swamp sumac, or poison elder, by having toothed leaflets and flowers and fruits in dense, terminal, erect clusters. They also grow in drier habitats. (Some of these, such as staghorn sumac, *R. typhina* of eastern North America, however, have a high tannin content in their fruits and leaves that can produce stomach upset if eaten.) Elderberries (*Sambucus* spp.) and ashes (*Fraxinus* spp.) may also be confused with poison sumac due to their pinnately compound leaves, but their leaves are opposite, not alternate.

Florida poisontree (*Metopium toxiferum*), another irritant plant of the same family, is a tall shrub or small tree found in Monroe and Dade counties in Florida. It has compound, five- to seven-parted leaves and fleshy fruits about 2.5 cm (1 in.) long. It is presumed to contain the same poisonous compounds as poison sumac and poison ivy.

MEDIUM TO LOW SHRUBS

broom, Scotch
Cytisus scoparius
pea family (Fabaceae)

Quick check. Upright, bushy shrub of open areas; twigs green and angled; flowers pea-like, bright yellow (or variegated); fruits flat pea-like pods. Potentially poisonous to humans and livestock, but no fatalities reported.

Description. Scotch broom is a stiffly upright, much-branching shrub, 2 m (6 ft.) or more high, with angled, evergreen twigs. The leaves are small and deciduous, usually three-parted. The flowers are numerous, bright yellow and pea-like (sometimes whitish or marked with dark red); often more or less covering the plant. The fruit is a flat pod, green with whitish, silky hairs along the margins when young, turning blackish at maturity and snapping open explosively, the two halves twisting backward to release the small, flattened, brownish seeds.

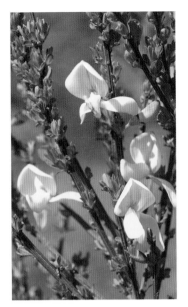

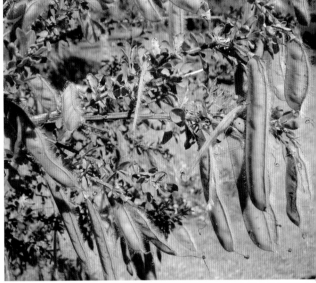

Scotch broom (*Cytisus scoparius*).

Scotch broom, green fruiting pods.

Occurrence. This noxious weedy shrub was introduced from Europe and is now widely naturalized in North America. It is common on dry hillsides, roadsides, wastelands, and shorelines on both the Atlantic and Pacific coasts.

Toxicity. Scotch broom contains several toxic quinolizidine alkaloids, including sparteine, isosparteine, and cytisine. These compounds can depress the heart and nervous system, sometimes paralyzing the motor nerve endings. Fortunately, the alkaloids are present in relatively small amounts, and only a few cases of livestock poisoning from Scotch broom have been reported. Still, it should be regarded as potentially dangerous to humans as well as animals. Symptoms would be expected to be similar to those of lupine poisoning: nausea, vomiting, dizziness, headache, and abdominal pain.

Notes. Broom seeds have been used as a coffee substitute, and broom flowers have been pickled, and used to make wine. However, extreme caution is advised. There is a potential for children to be poisoned from eating the pods and seeds, which resemble small peas. Related plants that contain similar quinolizidine alkaloids include Spanish broom (*Spartium junceum*) and greenweeds (*Genista* spp.).

poison ivy, eastern, and western poison ivy

Toxicodendron radicans and *T. rydbergii*
cashew family (Anacardiaceae)

Quick check. Low shrub (western poison ivy) or woody vine (eastern poison ivy) with three-parted, pointed leaves, inconspicuous flowers, and whitish, clustered, berry-like fruits. Entire plant is allergenic, causing severe and continuing skin irritation on contact for most people.

Description. Eastern poison ivy (*Toxicodendron radicans*) is typically a trailing or climbing vine, whereas western poison ivy (*T. rydbergii*) is a low, bushy shrub. The leaves are alternate, three-parted, often drooping, with shiny, oval, pointed leaflets having smooth, toothed, or lobed edges. The flowers are small and inconspicuous, in hanging clusters, and the fruit is a smooth, whitish, berry-like drupe. The seeds are white and longitudinally grooved.

Occurrence. Widespread in North America, with several varieties or forms; found in sandy, gravelly, or loamy soil in disturbed places, on floodplains, along lakeshores and streambanks, and in woods throughout the United States and southern Canada.

Toxicity. Eastern and western poison ivy are the best known and most widespread of a group of related species in the genus *Toxicodendron*, including poison oak and poison sumac, all containing the same highly irritating, widely allergenic catechol derivatives, urushiols. These are composed of a mixture of compounds, the worst being a phenolic resin, 3-n-penta-decyl-catechol. All parts of the plant—roots, stems, leaves, flowers, and fruits—

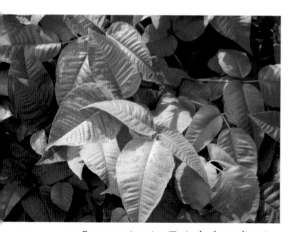
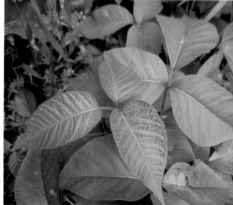

Eastern poison ivy (*Toxicodendron radicans*).   Western poison ivy (*Toxicodendron rydbergii*).

are potentially irritating, and even the pollen, smoke from burning plant material, or clothing and tools coming in contact with the plant, can produce symptoms.

Symptoms of poison ivy allergy include itching, burning, and redness of the skin. Small blisters may appear after a few hours or as long as five days after contact. Severe dermatitis, with large blisters, swelling, headache, and fever, may occur in some individuals, or after prolonged contact, and may require hospitalization. Fluid in blisters contains traces of the irritant, and if the blisters are broken, they can further irritate the surrounding skin or become infected.

Notes. Not everyone is equally sensitive to poison ivy and its relatives, but most people are potentially vulnerable to them sooner or later. Sensitivity is usually acquired in childhood or early adult life and tends to decline in later life. Remove contaminated clothing. Immediately wash all affected areas thoroughly with strong soap and water, then apply rubbing alcohol. Do not break blisters. Apply first aid cream with antihistamine to ease the itching. Keep contaminated clothing separate from other laundry and wash thoroughly several times. In severe cases, see your doctor.

poison oak, Atlantic, and Pacific poison oak

Toxicodendron pubescens and *T. diversilobum*
cashew family (Anacardiaceae)

Quick check. Woody shrubs, or climbing vines (Pacific poison oak only), with three-parted, oak-like leaves; flowers and fruits in hanging clusters; fruits yellowish or whitish and berry-like. Entire plant causes severe allergenic skin irritation on contact.

Description. Atlantic poison oak (*Toxicodendron pubescens*) is a woody shrub, never vine-like, whereas Pacific poison oak (*T. diversilobum*) is sometimes shrubby but is commonly a vine up to 15 m (50 ft.) tall. The leaves are alternate and three-parted (sometimes five-parted), the leaflets deeply toothed or lobed, resembling oak leaves. The small, greenish flowers are borne in loose, hanging clusters. The fruits are small, berry-like drupes, each containing a single seed. Pacific poison oak berries are whitish; those of *T. pubescens* are yellowish and hairy. Pacific poison oak most closely resembles poison ivy, and occasionally these plants hybridize.

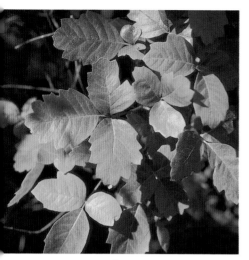

Pacific poison oak (*Toxicodendron diversilobum*).

Occurrence. Atlantic poison oak grows in sandy soil, of the dry barrens and oak-pine and pine woods of the Atlantic and Gulf coastal plains from southern New Jersey to northern Florida and west to eastern Texas and Kansas. Pacific poison oak is mainly confined to thickets and wooded slopes of the Pacific coastal region, from Puget Sound to California and Mexico, west of the Cascades and Sierra Nevada ranges, and inland along the Columbia River.

Toxicity. The sap of all parts of these species contains urushiols, the same irritating oleoresins and their derivatives that are found in poison ivy (*Toxicodendron radicans, T. rydbergii*) and poison sumac (*T. vernix*). Most people are allergic to these substances to some degree, and on contact break out in a burning, itching rash. For details of toxicity, see the previous entry on poison ivy.

Notes. Every year, according to estimates, approximately two million people in the United States experience irritating or painful effects from direct or indirect contact with poison oak, poison ivy, or poison sumac.

snowberry, common
Symphoricarpos albus and related spp.
honeysuckle family (Caprifoliaceae)

Quick check. Medium to low deciduous shrub with rounded, opposite leaves, and white, clustered berries. Berries poisonous, especially for children.

Description. Common snowberry, or waxberry, is an erect, much-branching, deciduous shrub up to 1 m (3 ft.) or more high. The leaves are dull green, 2–5 cm (1–2 in.) long, oval-shaped, and sometimes deeply lobed. The small, pinkish white, clustered flowers are bell-shaped and hairy inside. The berries are waxy white, pea-sized, spherical, and tightly clustered, often persisting over winter.

Occurrence. Dry, open woods throughout most of temperate North America from Alaska and northern Canada south to California and Colorado, and east to Virginia. Sometimes grown as an ornamental in North America and Europe.

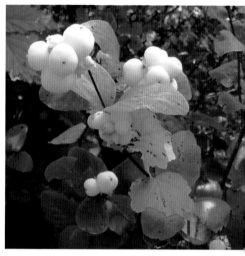

Toxicity. A number of classes of compounds with known toxic properties have been found in the berries, including saponins, tannins, terpenes, triglycerides, and coumarins. Although experimental findings suggest that the berries are generally nontoxic, the fruits do have a longstanding reputation for being poisonous in some areas, especially for children (Frohne and Pfänder 2005). Cases of snowberry poisoning have

Common snowberry (*Symphoricarpos albus*).

been documented in children in the United States, Britain, and Poland. In Britain, a child eating only three berries experienced vomiting, slight dizziness, and mild sedation. Gastrointestinal irritation, blood-stained urine, delirium, and a semi-comatose state are other reported symptoms. On Vancouver Island, an elderly Saanich man told one of us (NT) that his younger sister died at the age of six from eating the berries. Most Native Americans and Canadians regard the berries as inedible and possibly fatally poisonous if many are consumed.

Notes. Several other species of snowberry occur in different parts of North America. All should be regarded as potentially dangerous if the berries are eaten in quantity. Other members of the honeysuckle family, including honeysuckles (*Lonicera* spp.) and highbush cranberries (*Viburnum* spp.), are popularly considered to be poisonous and may contain coumarins, iridoids, diterpenes, and other pharmacologically active compounds. The ripe berries are concluded to be generally safe, at most bringing about a mildly upset stomach if eaten raw or unripe in excess. The ripe fruits of several *Viburnum* species are in fact frequently eaten. For example, *V. edule* fruits, cooked and mixed with fish oil, are a highly prestigious traditional food for indigenous peoples of coastal British Columbia, with productive patches being owned by families and individuals and passed hereditarily from one generation to the next.

Among some indigenous peoples of British Columbia, eating a snow-berry or two is said to be an antidote to discomfort caused by eating too much fatty food. The berries are known in several indigenous languages as ghost-berries, or corpse-berries.

VINES

NOTE. Eastern poison ivy (*Toxicodendron radicans*) and Pacific poison oak (*T. diversilobum*), both of which may grow as vines, are treated in the previous section on medium to low shrubs.

manroot, coastal
Marah oreganus and related spp.
cucumber family (Cucurbitaceae)

Quick check. Trailing or climbing vine with large, woody root, palmately lobed leaves, and oval, usually spiny, green fruits with large, rounded seeds. Entire plant is toxic, potentially fatal.

Description. This cucumber-like plant, also known as bigroot or wild cucumber, is an herbaceous perennial vine with branching tendrils, growing from a much-enlarged, woody root. The leaves are long-stalked and rather irregularly palmately lobed. The plants are monoecious, producing female and male flowers on separate plants. The female flowers are single; the male flowers, borne in elongated clusters. The flowers, small and greenish white, bloom from April to June. The fruits are elliptical to oval, usually 3–8 cm (1–3 in.) long, green, and usually prickly, containing two to eight large, rounded, brown seeds.

Occurrence. Bottomlands, fields, thickets, open hillsides, coastal bluffs, and roadsides from extreme southern British Columbia to northern California, mostly west of the Cascade Mountains.

Toxicity. This plant is fatally toxic under some circumstances. In 1986 an Oregon man went into shock, lost consciousness, and died 24 hours after consuming a homemade potion of the seeds. Within two hours of drinking at least one cup of the tea, he complained of chest pains and tightness of the chest, followed by loss of muscle control and shortness of breath. Restlessness, low blood pressure, and internal bleeding due to loss of the blood clotting function followed. Death was attributed to heart failure and internal bleeding. It is unclear why he took the drink, but possibly it was to obtain some hallucinogenic effect from the seeds. The cucumber-like fruits themselves are very bitter, but because they resemble cucumbers and children sometimes play with them, their potential toxicity is notable. The poisonous principles include cucurbitacins, which are tetracylic triterpenes. Cucurbitacins are said to be the bitterest naturally occurring plant compounds known.

Notes. Indigenous peoples of western North America recognize coastal manroot as toxic, but some used it medicinally. The seeds were eaten for kidney trouble, a decoction of the plant was drunk for venereal diseases, and the crushed roots were used as a poultice for sores of horses. The root, which is very bitter, was crushed and placed in streams to stupefy fish (Moerman 2003). Rich in tannins, in Mexico it has been used for tanning.

Another plant of the cucumber family, reportedly poisonous, is balsampear, balsamapple, or bitter gourd (*Momordica charantia*). It is a cucumber-like vine of sandy soils and wastelands of the coastal plain from Florida to Texas and is often cultivated in the southern Midwest. Its flowers are small

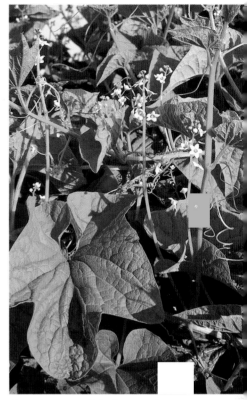

Coastal manroot (*Marah oreganus*).

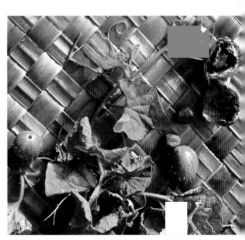

Coastal manroot fruits.

and unisexual, borne singly in the leaf axils. The leaves are deeply dissected, similar to those of watermelon but much smaller. The foliage and the outer coat and seeds of the gourd-like fruits are cathartic, causing diarrhea and vomiting if eaten. Nevertheless, the fruits are eaten in China and South Asia for their "cooling" effect, as well as being used as a major curry ingredient. In China the seeds are removed, and the fruits are soaked in salty water or roasted to reduce the bitterness. *Momordica charantia* contains some potentially harmful compounds, including cucurbitacins, abortifacients, alkaloids, and momordin, a toxic lectin that acts through inhibiting protein synthesis. Recovery from poisoning can be lengthy, and at least one death of a child in India is attributed to this plant.

moonseed, common

Menispermum canadense
moonseed family (Menispermaceae)

Quick check. Woody vine with grape-like leaves and fruit; fruits with single, crescent-shaped seed. Fruits highly toxic, sometimes fatal.

Description. Moonseed is a woody, perennial, twining vine resembling grape. The leaves are alternate and palmately lobed, with three to five shallow smooth-edged lobes (rather than the prominent saw-toothed lobes of grape). The greenish white flowers are borne in small clusters and bloom in June and July. The fruits are globular and purplish black, in grape-like bunches, but each contains a single, large, grooved, crescent-shaped seed, rather than several to many teardrop-shaped seeds, as in grapes.

Occurrence. This vine is found growing on other vegetation in woods, thickets, and fencerows of eastern North America, from Canada south to Georgia and Oklahoma.

Toxicity. Moonseed contains isoquinoline alkaloids, including dauricine, a compound with curare-like action. The fruits, which resemble small purple grapes, are the main cause of poisoning, and when eaten in quantity can be deadly. There are reports of fatalities in children who mistook them for grapes.

Notes. Birds eat moonseed fruits readily, apparently without harm. Again, many berries and plants poisonous to humans are eaten by birds and ani-

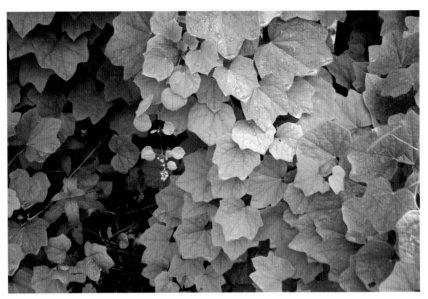

Common moonseed (*Menispermum canadense*).

mals; observing wildlife eating plants is therefore no guarantee that people can safely eat them too.

nightshade, climbing

Solanum dulcamara
nightshade family (Solanaceae)

Quick check. Slender vine with simple leaves often basally lobed, deep purple potato-like flowers, and bright red (when ripe) clustered berries. Entire plant, especially unripe fruit, toxic and potentially fatal.

Description. Slender, woody-based perennial vine up to 2 m (6 ft.) or more high. The leaves are dark green, pointed, and oval to heart-shaped, often with two opposite lobes at the base of the blade. The clustered, deep purple or bluish flowers have recurved petals and bright yellow exserted stamens. They bloom throughout the summer. The berries are oval, hard and green when unripe, maturing to soft, translucent, bright red, and shiny.

Occurrence. This vine, introduced from Europe (hence its other common name, European bittersweet), is commonly found trailing over the ground or twining on other plants in damp woods, thickets, wastelands, and occasionally gardens, throughout North America.

Toxicity. The entire plant contains solanine, a toxic glyco-alkaloid present in other members of the genus *Solanum* (including in green potatoes), and dulcamarine, a glycoside similar in its structure and effects to atropine, which is present in belladonna (*Atropa bella-donna*). Climbing nightshade berries have been implicated in the fatal poisoning of children, and the plants have been responsible for livestock loss in both Europe and North America. The ripe fruits are less toxic than the leaves and unripe berries, but even fully ripe berries should be considered poisonous. The actual quantity of toxins varies with light, soil, climate, and growth stage. Symptoms of poisoning include varying degrees of abdominal pain, headache, flushing and irritation of the skin and mucous membranes, and tiredness. In severe cases, vomiting, thirst, difficulty in breathing, restlessness, subnormal temperature, paralysis, dilated pupils, diarrhea, blood in urine, shock, extreme weakness, loss of sensation, and occasionally death, may occur.

Notes. The highest concentrations of toxic solanine are reported in the unripe fruit of *Solanum* species. In some taxa—some strains of black nightshade (*S. nigrum* and *S. americanum*), for instance—the fully ripe berries are actually edible, but unless edibility is absolutely certain, leave the berries of all species alone. Leaves of climbing nightshade and black nightshade have shown up occasionally among mixed greens in restaurants or groceries, gathered by mistake together with spinach and other edible leaves.

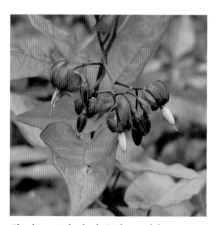

Climbing nightshade (*Solanum dulcamara*).

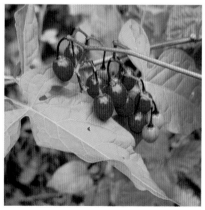

Climbing nightshade fruits.

peas, wild

Lathyrus spp.

pea family (Fabaceae)

Quick check. Herbaceous vines with white, yellowish, or purplish flowers and long, flat pods. Foliage and seeds toxic and potentially fatal when consumed in quantity over an extended period; small quantities not harmful.

Description. Many species of the genus *Lathyrus* are found in North America, some introduced from Europe, some native. All are climbing vines with herbaceous, winged or angular stems. The leaves are alternate and compound, divided into two to many elongated or rounded leaflets and terminating in slender tendrils. The flowers, which consist of five irregularly shaped petals, are whitish or yellowish to shades of pink or purple and often quite showy. The fruits are elongated, flattened pods, usually containing several small seeds.

Occurrence. Wild peas, or vetchlings, are widespread, occurring from seaside to mountains in a variety of habitats, from marshes and open woods to fields and wastelands, throughout North America.

Toxicity. The foliage and especially the seeds of many species in this genus, when consumed in quantity, can be poisonous to humans and livestock, due to the presence of lathyrogens, toxic amino acids, in particular, beta-aminopropionitrile. Small or even moderate amounts have been eaten without apparent harm. Long-term or intensive use of the seeds as food can result in lathyrism, a potentially fatal disease.

Notes. Cooking the seeds does not eliminate their long-term toxicity for humans. However, toxicity is caused only when large quantities are eaten, not when relatively small amounts are consumed as part of a mixed diet. Wild *Lathyrus* species known to have seeds potentially poisonous to humans include Caley pea (*L. hirsutus*), hoary pea (*L. polymorphus* ssp. *incanus*),

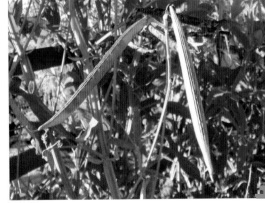

Perennial pea (*Lathyrus latifolius*), pods.

tiny pea (*L. pusillus*), and flat pea (*L. sylvestris*); garden sweetpea (*L. odoratus*) may also cause poisoning.

All species of *Lathyrus* should be regarded with caution. However, a strong case is made for the edible qualities of perennial pea, or wild sweet pea (*L. latifolius*) by wild food expert John Kallas (2004a, b), who considers both the peas and the young shoots, flowers, and green pods of this species to be perfectly edible and delicious, raw or cooked, for most people eating a healthy diet. They would only be harmful if eaten in enormous quantities, for people who are suffering from severe chronic nutrient deficiency, for those whose livers are compromised or with some type of abnormal metabolism, or for fetuses and infants (i.e., for people who are growing very fast). For healthy, well-fed adults, he maintains, there is little or no chance of any negative impact. Cooper and Johnson (2003) concur for white peas, or chick peas (*L. sativus*), noting that when only relatively small quantities are eaten, as part of a mixed diet, they are harmless and nutritious.

vetch, garden
Vicia sativa
pea family (Fabaceae)

Quick check. Small, herbaceous vine with pinnately compound leaves, purple pea-like flowers, and narrow, pointed pods. Foliage and seeds toxic and potentially fatal if large quantities are consumed.

Description. Herbaceous vine usually under 1 m (3 ft.) tall, climbing on other plants, especially grasses, by means of slender tendrils. The leaves are small and pinnately divided, with paired, oval leaflets 1–2 cm (0.5 in.) long, and pointed stipules at the leaf bases. The small, pea-like flowers, pale pink to deep reddish purple, are borne singly or in pairs. The fruits are narrow, beaked pods, usually 2–5 cm (1–2 in.) long, each containing four to ten small "peas."

Occurrence. A widespread weed of gardens, wastelands, meadows, and hillsides throughout North America; sometimes cultivated for animal feed as a hay crop and for silage.

Toxicity. Various species of vetch, and particularly garden vetch, have been reported from time to time to produce disease and loss of life in humans and livestock. The main toxic components are cyanogenic glycosides, such as vicianine, which release hydrocyanic acid in the presence of enzymes in the plant or in the digestive tract. Different species, varieties, populations, and life cycle stages of vetch exhibit differing concentrations of the glycosides and the enzymes that break them down. The seeds of garden vetch have been shown to contain lethal levels of cyanogenic glycosides in some populations, and some strains are known also to contain the toxic amino acids beta-cyanoalanine and beta-aminopropionitrile. Symptoms of vetch poisoning are typical of cyanide poisoning: rapid breathing followed by difficulty in breathing, excitability and restlessness, and in severe cases, prostration, convulsions, coma, and death.

Notes. Because vetch pods and seeds resemble those of vegetable garden peas, there is a danger of children eating them in play. Many *Vicia* species occur in North America, some indigenous and some introduced and naturalized, or grown as forage. One often implicated in fatal cattle poisoning is winter vetch (*V. villosa*); another, *V. faba* (fava bean, broadbean), is not normally poisonous but can cause severe hemolytic anemia in some individuals. All vetches should be considered potentially toxic and should be treated with caution until more is known about individual types.

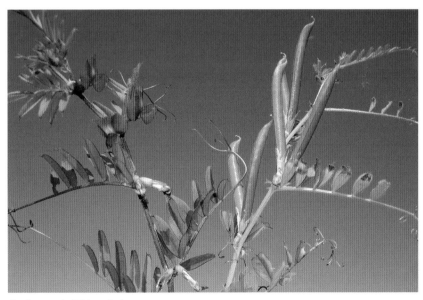

Garden vetch (*Vicia sativa*).

HERBACEOUS PLANTS

baneberry, red, and white baneberry

Actaea rubra and *A. pachypoda*
buttercup family (Ranunculaceae)

Quick check. Bushy, herbaceous plants with compound leaves, small, whitish flowers in dense, elongated clusters, and bright red or white berries. All parts of the plants toxic and potentially fatal.

Description. Herbaceous plants up to 1 m (3 ft.) tall, growing from thick rhizomes. The leaves are large, spreading, and coarsely two or three times divided into six or more pointed, sharply toothed leaflets. The flowers are small and whitish, borne in dense, long-stalked terminal clusters, or racemes. The berries are bright red or white, and very showy. Red baneberry (*Actaea rubra*) usually has red berries, but a white-fruited form sometimes occurs; its berry stalks are very slender. *Actaea pachypoda* (white baneberry, doll's eyes) is usually white-fruited, rarely red-fruited, and its berry stalks are stout, or swollen.

Occurrence. Red baneberry is found from Alaska to central California and east to the central United States. White baneberry occurs from Canada south to Georgia and Louisiana, and west to the northern Rockies. Both species grow in moist, rich woods and along creeks.

Toxicity. All parts of the plants, especially the roots and berries, are toxic; eating only six berries can produce severe symptoms, lasting up to about three hours, including acute stomach cramps, dizziness, vomiting, increased pulse, delirium, circulatory failure, and headache. Baneberries, like some other species in the buttercup family, contain protoanemonin, but their toxicity is apparently mainly due to as yet undetermined toxins, possibly an essential oil or poisonous glycoside. *Actaea spicata* (European baneberry) does not contain protoanemonin (Frohne and Pfänder 2005); nevertheless, there are several documented cases of fatal poisoning in children from eating European baneberry. No deaths have been reported for the North American species.

Notes. The plant is used medicinally by some indigenous peoples, usually in the form of a decoction, which is drunk. The Lillooet (Stl'atl'imx) of British Columbia used red baneberry (*Actaea rubra*) as a general tonic, but their name for the plant translates as "it-makes-you-sick," and they and other indigenous people were very aware of the poisonous qualities of this species (Moerman 2003). Black cohosh, or black baneberry (*A. racemosa*), a close relative, is used as an herbal alternative for hormone replacement therapies in the treatment of menopause (see Appendix 6).

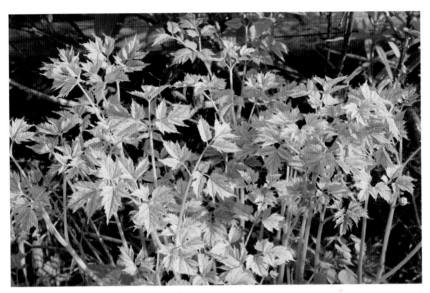

Red baneberry (*Actaea rubra*), young shoots.

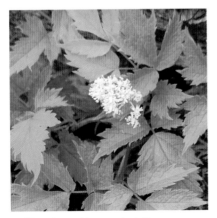

Red baneberry (*Actaea rubra*), flowers.

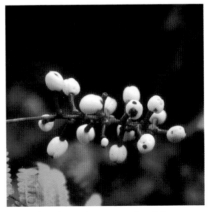

White baneberry (*Actaea pachypoda*), berries. Richard Hebda

bleeding hearts
Dicentra spp.
fumitory family (Fumariaceae)

Quick check. Delicate, herbaceous, early spring-flowering plants with finely divided, fern-like leaves and hanging, clustered, two-sided flowers. Occasional cause of human poisoning but no reported fatalities.

Description. Herbaceous plants up to 60 cm (2 ft.) high, growing from a fleshy, sometimes branching rootstock. The leaves are long-stalked, broadly triangular, and finely dissected, giving the plants a delicate, lacy appearance. The showy flowers are loosely clustered, often hanging, each with four petals fused into two flattened pairs, rounded at the tops, or prolonged backward into two prominent spurs. About a dozen species occur in North America, most potentially poisonous. Most prominent are Dutchman's breeches (*Dicentra cucullaria*), with bulbous rootstock, and white or pinkish, yellow-tipped flowers that resemble baggy pants hanging upside-down; squirrel corn (*D. canadensis*), with tuber-producing rhizomes and greenish white or pinkish heart-shaped flowers; and turkey corn (*D. eximia*) and Pacific bleeding heart (*D. formosa*), both with branching rhizomes and rose-pink to purplish heart-shaped flowers. Showy bleeding heart (*D. spectabilis*), a frequent garden ornamental, is also potentially poisonous.

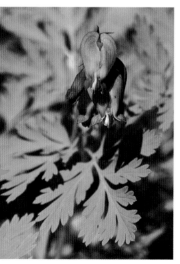

Pacific bleeding heart
(*Dicentra formosa*).

Occurrence. Bleeding hearts and their relatives are found in moist, rich woodlands and meadows throughout North America and are often grown in gardens. Dutchman's-breeches is found in eastern North America from Nova Scotia to Missouri and Alabama. Squirrel corn grows in the East from Nova Scotia to North Carolina and Tennessee. Turkey corn is found in the southern Appalachians, and Pacific bleeding heart in the West from British Columbia to California.

Toxicity. Various species of bleeding hearts have been shown to contain isoquinoline alkaloids, including aporphine, protoberberine, and protopine. They are toxic to both humans and animals. Symptoms of poisoning include trembling, agitation, heavy salivation, vomiting, diarrhea, convulsions, tenseness of muscles, difficulty in breathing, and prostration. Fortunately, human poisoning is rare, and recovery is usually rapid and complete.

Although not reported to have caused human deaths, bleeding hearts are potentially harmful to children, since they are showy and attractive and are often found around meadows, in gardens, or as potted ornamentals. Contact with the plants can cause an allergic skin reaction in some individuals.

Notes. Members of the genus *Corydalis*, related to *Dicentra*, also contain toxic isoquinoline alkaloids. Several *Corydalis* species are native to North America, and they too are increasingly grown as garden flowers. Although not implicated in human poisoning, they have caused poisoning and death in animals. Livestock loss from bleeding hearts and their relatives usually occurs on early spring woodland pasture. Cattle find the plants distasteful and eat them only when other food is scarce. Heavy trampling of the ground when soft may expose the fleshy rootstocks, which may then be eaten, with harmful results.

bloodroot
Sanguinaria canadensis
poppy family (Papaveraceae)

Quick check. White-flowered herbaceous plant with large, palmately lobed leaves; rhizome, leaves, and stems exude a bright red-orange sap when cut. Highly toxic; potential poisoning from herbal medicine preparations.

Description. Herbaceous perennial, growing from a stout, knotted rhizome. The leaves are single, large and long-stalked, and palmately lobed with three to nine rounded lobes. The flowers are white and conspicuous, 2–5 cm (1–2 in.) across, growing singly on a stalk up to 15 cm (6 in.) high. They bear eight to 16 petals, with four usually longer than the others. The fruit is an elongated capsule up to 5 cm (2 in.) long. The rhizome, leaves, and stems all exude a red-orange sap, or latex, when bruised.

Occurrence. Common, well-known spring wildflower of rich woods of eastern and central North America from southern Canada to Florida and Texas.

Toxicity. The red-colored latex found throughout this plant contains several alkaloids, including sanguinarine, chelerythrine, protopine, and homoch-

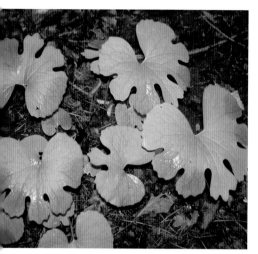

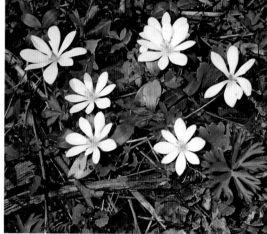

Bloodroot (*Sanguinaria canadensis*).   Bloodroot flowers.

elidonine, as well as resins. These physiologically active compounds can, if consumed, cause vomiting, diarrhea, fainting, shock, coma, and potentially death. They can also cause fluid retention (edema) and glaucoma. However, no cases of human or livestock poisoning by bloodroot under natural conditions are known.

Notes. The red latex was formerly extracted from the rootstock and used as a medicinal drug. It is now also used in research to induce glaucoma in laboratory animals. The alkaloids contained in bloodroot latex are present in other members of the poppy family.

buttercups
Ranunculus spp. and related genera
buttercup family (Ranunculaceae)

Quick check. Low to moderately tall, herbaceous plants with variously lobed or entire leaves, many species with attractive yellow flowers. Fresh plants contain an irritant oil that can cause painful blistering of the skin and irritation of the mouth and digestive tract; human fatalities unknown.

Description. Buttercups (some also known as crowfoot or blisterwort) are a very large group of annual or perennial herbs. The stem leaves are alternate, palmately veined, entire, lobed, or finely divided. Basal leaves are often present, numerous, and variable in shape. The flowers are usually yellow, sometimes cream-colored, and are borne singly or in loose terminal clusters, each with five (or sometimes more) petals. The fruits consist of a group of small, one-seeded achenes on a rounded receptacle.

Occurrence. Buttercups are usually spring-flowering and are found throughout North America in a variety of habitats, from open fields, clearings, and gardens, to moist woods. Some are aquatic; many are common weeds.

Toxicity. Buttercups and other members of the buttercup family, such as anemones (*Anemone* spp., *Pulsatilla* spp.) and marsh marigolds (*Caltha* spp.), contain varying quantities of an acrid, blister-causing juice that yields protoanemonin, a highly irritant yellow oil. This substance is produced in the plant through the enzymatic breakdown of ranunculin, a glycoside. Although it is present through-

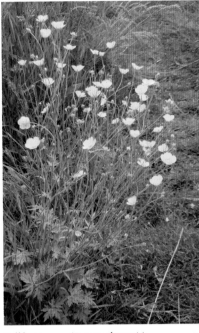

Tall buttercup (*Ranunculus acris*).

out the tissues of fresh plants, especially during flowering, protoanemonin is unstable, and changes, when the plants are dried, into an innocuous form, anemonin. Protoanemonin can cause severe irritation and blistering of the skin, or, if consumed, severe gastrointestinal irritation. It is also irritating to the eyes.

Buttercups and their relatives, especially those with showy flowers, are potentially poisonous to humans, and some species have been known to poison children, causing burning of the mouth, abdominal pain, and diarrhea. However, these plants are mainly known for their toxicity to grazing animals; in severe cases they can be fatal, but since they are strongly distasteful, they are seldom eaten in quantity.

Notes. Buttercup species vary in the amount of protoanemonin they contain. Known poisonous species include tall buttercup (*Ranunculus acris*), bulbous buttercup, or St. Anthony's turnip (*R. bulbosus*), littleleaf buttercup (*R. abortivus*), creeping buttercup (*R. repens*), sagebrush buttercup (*R. glaberrimus*), and cursed buttercup (*R. sceleratus*).

Many North American indigenous groups traditionally used buttercups and their relatives as counter-irritant medicines, applied externally to draw out pain and infection from underlying tissues. They were aware of their potentially poisonous properties, however, and did not usually use them internally (Moerman 2003; Prieto et al. 2003; Turner 1984).

cocklebur, rough
Xanthium strumarium
aster family (Asteraceae)

Quick check. Coarse, weedy annual with palmately lobed leaves and thick, prickly burs along the upper stem of mature plants. Seeds and seedlings toxic to animals and potentially fatal; no human poisonings reported.

Description. Coarse, herbaceous, annual weed up to 1 m (3 ft.) or more high, with erect, stout, branching stems. The leaves are alternate, stalked, and pointed, with toothed or irregularly lobed margins. The flower heads lack colored rays and are separated into small, many-flowered male (pollen-producing) heads near the tops of the stems and two-flowered female (seed-producing) heads clustered at the leaf axils below. The fruits are conspicuous, elongated, two-chambered burs with dense, hooked prickles, which attach easily to clothing and animal fur. This is a highly variable species; several of its varieties are recognized by some authorities as separate species.

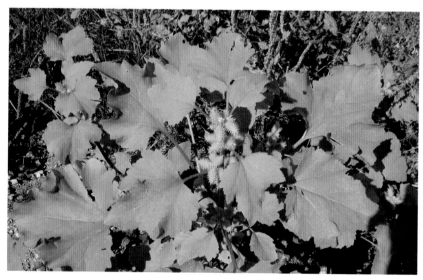

Rough cocklebur (*Xanthium strumarium*).

Occurrence. Introduced from Europe, rough cocklebur is a widespread weed of fields, wastelands, shorelines, and floodplains; it is found throughout North America. The seeds sprout readily when present in soil that has recently been under water.

Toxicity. The main toxic agent of this plant, concentrated in the seeds and seedlings, is carboxyatractyloside, a highly toxic diterpene glycoside. Widely known as a livestock poison, it produces symptoms including loss of appetite, digestive tract inflammation, excitability, weakness, loss of coordination, prostration, and in severe cases, convulsions and death. Human poisoning from rough cocklebur has not been reported, but children should be kept away from it. It is also known to cause allergic skin irritation on contact.

Notes. Another plant in the same family, burdock (*Arctium* spp.), may be confused with rough cocklebur, but it is usually larger, and its burs are more spherical. The burs of both burdock and cocklebur can cause mechanical injury, and burdock causes dermatitis in some people, but it is not considered to be poisonous to eat; in fact, its taproot and peeled stems are a well-known food in Japan and elsewhere.

deathcamas, meadow

Zigadenus venenosus and related spp.
lily family (Liliaceae)

Quick check. Perennial with bulb, basal and grass-like leaves, and showy, cream-colored flowers in a dense, terminal cluster. Entire plant, especially the onion-like bulbs, highly toxic and sometimes fatal for humans; extremely toxic to grazing livestock.

Description. There are about a dozen species of *Zigadenus* in North America, known generically as deathcamas. They vary in toxicity, but all should be considered potentially poisonous. One of the commonest and best known is meadow deathcamas (*Z. venenosus*). It is a perennial lily-like plant, usually 30–60 cm (1–2 ft.) high, growing from a bulb, which resembles a small onion, but lacks any onion odor. The leaves are smooth, grass-like, and V-shaped in cross-section, mostly growing from the base. The six-petalled flowers are creamy white and crowded together in a dense, terminal cluster; the fruits are cylindrical, three-parted capsules. The stalk tends to elon-

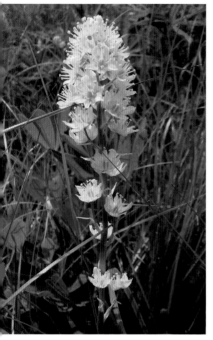

Meadow deathcamas
(*Zigadenus venenosus*).

gate at the fruiting stage, so that the capsules are further spread apart than the flowers. Other species have greenish, white, yellow, or pink flowers, in some cases more loosely clustered; some grow from rhizomes.

Occurrence. *Zigadenus venenosus* is common in moist, grassy meadows in western North America, from southern British Columbia to California, and east to Utah and Nevada. Flowers in May and June. Other species occur throughout North America, from Alaska to Florida.

Toxicity. *Zigadenus* species contain several toxic alkaloids, similar to those found in false hellebores (*Veratrum* spp.). These include zygacine, zygadenine, iso- and neogermidine, and protoveratridine. The entire plant, including the bulb and flowers, is poisonous. Deathcamas species have been responsible for large losses of livestock, especially sheep and cattle. Symptoms in animals are similar to those of humans.

Human poisonings from deathcamas are rare but sometimes occur when people mistake the bulbs for those of edible species such as blue camases (*Camassia* spp.) or wild onions (*Allium* spp.). Symptoms of poisoning include excessive watering of the mouth, burning followed by numbness of the lips and mouth, thirst, headache, dizziness, nausea, stomach pain, persistent vomiting, diarrhea, muscular weakness, confusion, slow and irregular heartbeat, low blood pressure, subnormal temperature, and in severe cases, difficulty in breathing, convulsions, coma, and death. Symptoms may be delayed one to eight hours after eating deathcamas, depending on the species. Recovery usually occurs within 24 hours.

Notes. Most indigenous people who eat bulbs such as blue camases (*Camassia* spp.) and mariposa lilies (*Calochortus* spp.) as part of their traditional diet are well aware of deathcamas and are careful to avoid its "poison onions," as some call them, in their harvesting. Still, accidental poisonings among indigenous peoples have occurred. Aside from *Zigadenus venenosus*, the most toxic species of deathcamas include Z. *paniculatus* (foothill deathcamas), Z.

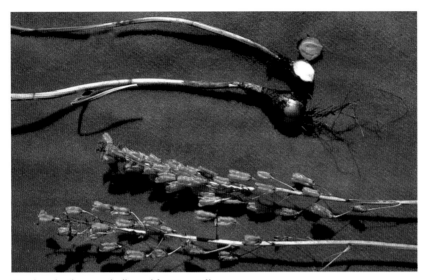

Meadow deathcamas, bulbs and fruiting stalks.

nuttallii (Nuttall's deathcamas), and Z. *leimanthoides* (syn. Z. *densus*, pine barren deathcamas). Several other plants in the lily family are also considered toxic by indigenous peoples: wavyleaf soapplant (*Chlorogalum pomeridianum*), whose bulbs were used as a fish poison by a number of Native Californian groups; western featherbells, or mountainbells (*Stenanthium occidentale*), with purplish flowers on an elongated stalk; and *Trillium* species, with distinctive three-petalled flowers. Another wildflower with reputed toxicity known to indigenous peoples is an orchid, scentbottle (*Platanthera dilatata* var. *dilatata*) (Moerman 2003; Turner 1995).

false hellebore, green
Veratrum viride and related spp.
lily family (Liliaceae)

Quick check. Tall, erect herbaceous perennial with large, alternate, parallel-veined, distinctly pleated leaves and greenish or whitish flowers in dense, terminal clusters. All parts of plant highly toxic, potentially fatal; occasional human poisoning, most from misuse of medicinal preparations.

Description. Green false hellebore is a leafy, unbranched, herbaceous perennial, 1–2.5 m (3–8 ft.) high, growing from a thick rootstock. The leaves are oval, pointed, and densely but finely hairy beneath, up to 30 cm (1 ft.) long and 15 cm (6 in.) wide near the base of the plant, becoming smaller and narrower toward the top. The six-parted flowers, up to 2 cm (0.8 in.) across, are hairy, and greenish white or greenish yellow, often with a dark central blotch. They grow in dense, branching, terminal clusters 30 cm (1 ft.) long or more, the branches spreading and somewhat drooping. The fruits are three-parted capsules, straw-colored to dark brown. Other North American *Veratrum* species, including *V. californicum* (California false hellebore), with whitish flowers and erect flower clusters, and *V. parviflorum* (Appalachian bunchflower), with narrower upper leaves and hairless flowers, are also poisonous, as are European and Asian species.

Occurrence. Rich, moist woods and mountain meadows along streams and wet areas, from Alaska to northern Oregon and eastward to the Atlantic Coast. *Veratrum californicum* occurs in mountain meadows and valleys of the western states from the Pacific Coast to the Rocky Mountains, and *V. parvi-*

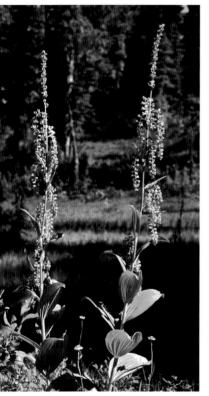

florum in the mountains of the eastern states from West Virginia to Georgia.

Toxicity. Green false hellebore and its relatives contain numerous, complex glyco-alkaloids as well as ester alkaloids. These include jervine, germidine, germitrine, veratroidine, veratrosine, and veratramine. All parts of the plant are toxic, but the highest concentration of toxins is said to be in the inner rhizome.

Most instances of *Veratrum* poisoning in humans have been as a result of misuse of medicinal preparations containing the plant. There are scattered reports of fatalities in humans and various types of livestock from eating the plant itself. Symptoms of poisoning include burning sensation of mouth and throat, and pain in upper abdomen, followed by watering of the mouth, vomiting, diarrhea, sweating, blurred vision, hallucinations, headache, general paralysis, and spasms. In severe cases, shallow breathing, slow or irregular pulse, lower temperature, convulsions, and death

Green false hellebore
(*Veratrum viride*).

may occur. The combined symptoms have been characterized as similar to those of a heart attack. Symptoms usually disappear within 24 hours.

The greatest danger of livestock poisoning by green false hellebore is in early spring, when it produces young, succulent shoots, and when other forage is scarce.

Notes. *Veratrum viride* has been used medicinally for treating high blood pressure; small doses are used to reduce blood pressure with no noticeable effect on respiratory or cardiac rate. Unfortunately, the complexity and relative instability of the alkaloids in this plant make the drug difficult to standardize.

Indigenous people in many areas of the continent, particularly the Pacific Northwest, are well aware of the toxic and medicinal properties of green false hellebore, also known as Indian hellebore. Its rootstock was widely used as an external medicine and local anaesthetic for innumerable ailments, including arthritis and bruises. It was also sometimes taken, with great caution and in very diluted form, as a cleansing purgative during certain rites of hunters, shamans, and others seeking special powers. However, there are several reports of accidental poisoning by this plant. Some British Columbia indigenous people have stressed that the only effective antidote for green false hellebore poisoning is eating large amounts of salmon oil or oulachen grease, rendered from a small oily fish by coastal First Peoples. This treatment is also known for treating poisoning by deathcamas and water hemlock.

Veratrum californicum is the cause of monkey-face, a usually fatal type of

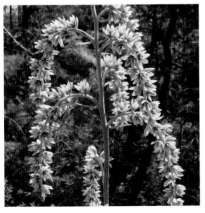
Green false hellebore flowers.

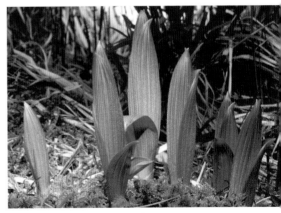
Green false hellebore, young shoots.

birth deformity in lambs traced to ewes feeding on this plant during their early pregnancy in late summer.

Prolonged numbness of the mouth and nausea from drinking water in which false hellebore was growing has been reported.

grasses, wild
various genera
grass family (Poaceae)

Quick check. Grasses are variable in size and flower head shape, but all have jointed stems, long, slender, parallel-veined leaves, petalless flowers in clusters, and seed-like fruits (grains). Some species have potentially toxic grains; all grains can be infested with toxic molds or other fungi; some grass fruits can cause choking if swallowed.

Description. Grasses are well-known and important economic plants, having jointed stems, slender, sheathing, parallel-veined leaves, and usually small, inconspicuous flowers borne in bracted spikelets that are variously clustered into loose or compact heads. Although they include some of the most important edible plants of the world (the cereal grains—wheat, maize, rice, oats, rye, and barley), some grasses are potentially harmful. It is not possible to include here descriptions of individual types, but some are mentioned as potentially dangerous.

Occurrence. Grasses are common and widespread in North America, growing in almost every environment, and recognized by most people as belonging to a distinct group.

Toxicity. Several types of poisoning have been attributed to grasses, mostly related to their widespread use as forage and hay crops for animals. The deadly fungus ergot (*Claviceps purpurea*) commonly infects cereal grains; other fungi, including molds such as species of *Penicillium*, are also known to render toxic grass species that are otherwise edible.

Fungi have been implicated in the toxicity of one well-known poisonous grass genus, *Lolium*, which includes perennial ryegrass (*L. perenne*) and an annual species, darnel ryegrass (*L. temulentum*). Perennial ryegrass is known to cause a nervous disorder, ryegrass staggers, in grazing animals, and there are records dating back to ancient times of people being poisoned by eating flour or bread contaminated with darnel grains. Occasional live-stock poisonings from darnel ryegrass have also been reported.

Some grasses, such as velvetgrass (*Holcus lanatus*) and mannagrasses (*Glyceria* spp.), contain cyanogenic compounds, but these are present in low concentrations and are usually harmless. Many bamboos contain cyano-genic compounds in very high concentrations in their young shoots, but boiling or drying the shoots eliminates virtually all the prussic acid.

Other grass species, such as foxtail barley (*Hordeum jubatum*), brome-grasses (*Bromus* spp.), porcupine grasses, needlegrasses, or needle and threads (*Hesperostipa* and *Stipa* spp.), and bristlegrasses, or foxtails (*Setaria* spp.), have long, sharp, wiry bristles or awns associated with their fruiting heads. These awned fruits are often barbed and can easily become lodged in the ears, noses, and throats of animals and people. Once they penetrate, they can be difficult to remove. In the summer and fall, dogs often must be taken to the veterinarian for removal of grass fruits from deep inside their ears. Berry pick-ers should be careful to remove any awned grass fruits from their harvest, because they can cause choking if swallowed.

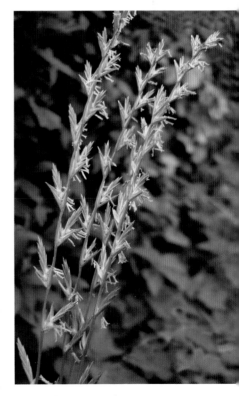

Cutting sharply awned grasses before they go to seed, and not allowing dogs and other animals into areas where these grasses are present during the danger period (early sum-mer to fall) can reduce the hazard of mechan-ical injury from sharp grass fruits. Close inspection of fur and ears after animals have been in a danger area is also recommended.

Notes. One toxic syndrome related to grass pas-turage, variously known as grass tetany, grass staggers, wheat pasture poisoning, protein poisoning, and hypomagnesemia, has caused livestock loss, especially of cattle, in various parts of North America. It is associated with pasturing cattle on the lush young growth of pasture or range grass, or wheat forage, in

Perennial ryegrass (*Lolium perenne*).

early spring or during mild winters in some areas. The exact cause of this disorder is not known but is believed to be related to an inability of the animals to absorb magnesium, resulting in a deficiency of this element.

Large quantities of domesticated cereal grains—wheat, oats, barley, rye, sorghum, and maize, or corn—are used as livestock feed in North America. They sometimes cause digestive disorders and other problems, but, with the exception of rye (which contains some growth-depressing substances and one that produces rickets in chicks), none produces any toxic substances. Most problems with them are caused by fungal contamination due to poor storage, or to poor feeding practices. The best means of preventing grass-related poisoning is to provide animals with good, properly tended pasturage and properly stored feed: estimated losses of $600 million in the beef cattle industry are incurred annually in the United States from myco-toxin-contaminated fodder. For more information on grass genera and animal poisoning, see Frohne and Pfänder (2005).

Indianhemp

Apocynum cannabinum
dogbane family (Apocynaceae)

Quick check. Tall, bushy herb of roadsides and clearings, with opposite, smooth-edged leaves, small, clustered whitish flowers, long thin seedpods, and milky sap. Potentially highly toxic; possible human poisoning from herbal medicine preparations.

Description. Indianhemp, or hemp dogbane, is an erect, bushy herbaceous perennial 1–1.5 m (3–5 ft.) tall, growing from spreading rhizomes. The leaves are simple, opposite, smooth-edged, and oval to elliptical. The flowers are small, whitish, and urn- or bell-shaped, borne in clusters toward the tops of the stems, and the fruits are long, narrow, paired pods containing numerous seeds attached to long, silky, milkweed-like hairs. The stems are very fibrous and exude a milky juice when broken. A shorter, pink-flowered species, spreading dogbane (*Apocynum androsaemifolium*), has similar characteristics and is also considered toxic.

Occurrence. Common summer-flowering patch-forming plant of roadsides, pastures, and clearings, especially in moist areas, widely distributed in

North America. Spreading dogbane is also common in many parts of the continent.

Toxicity. Indianhemp and its relatives contain several resins and glycosides, some cardioactive, including cymarin, apocannoside, and cyanocannoside. Cases of poisoning in humans have not been reported, but their toxicity to animals is known, mainly through laboratory testing. The plants are distasteful to animals and not usually consumed. One glycoside, apocynamarin, is known to increase blood pressure, and some of the resins caused gastric disturbance and death in a dog. The milky sap may cause dermatitis.

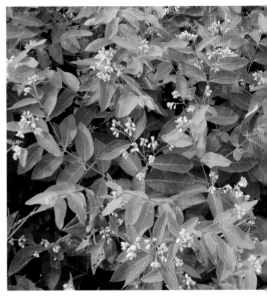

Indianhemp (*Apocynum cannabinum*).

Notes. Indianhemp and spreading dogbane were officially recognized in the 19th century as diaphoretics and expectorants, with emetic, cathartic, and diuretic properties. Indigenous peoples also used them as medicines for kidney problems and other ailments. However, their pharmacological effects are probably due to their toxic cardiotonic activity, and they should be used only with extreme caution. Indianhemp is a primary source of stem fiber for cordage and fishing line and nets for indigenous peoples across its range.

Indian-tobacco

Lobelia inflata
lobelia family (Lobeliaceae)

Quick check. Erect, branching annual weed, with inconspicuous blue flowers, and inflated seedpods. Highly toxic; potentially fatal. Most human poisonings from misuse as herbal medicine.

Description. A branching annual up to 1 m (3 ft.) tall, with simple, alternate, toothed leaves tending to run down the stem. The flowers, clustered at the ends of the stem and branches, are small, pale blue to white, tubular, and

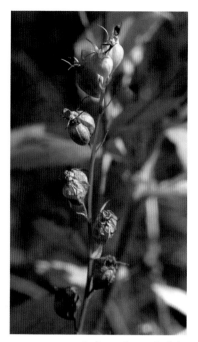

Indian-tobacco (*Lobelia inflata*), inflated fruits.

bilaterally symmetrical, with two lobes above and three below, the tube split nearly to the base along the top. The fruit is a capsule, conspicuously inflated and bladderlike. There are many other species of *Lobelia* in North America, including the showy, red-flowered cardinalflower (*L. cardinalis*), and great blue lobelia (*L. siphilitica*). All should be considered toxic.

Occurrence. Indian-tobacco is a common herbaceous weed of fields, woods, and wastelands throughout eastern North America. Cardinalflower and great blue lobelia occur along water courses and in damp soil in southeastern Canada and the eastern United States and are frequently cultivated as ornamentals.

Toxicity. Several species of *Lobelia*, including Indian-tobacco and cardinalflower, are toxic to both humans and livestock, due to the presence of a variety of pyridine alkaloids, especially lobelamine and lobeline. Over 14 of these alkaloids have been isolated from Indian-tobacco alone. Similar in structure to nicotine, they produce symptoms in humans including nausea, progressive vomiting, sweating, pain, tremors, weakness, paralysis, depressed temperature, rapid but weak pulse, and, in serious cases, convulsions, coma, and death from respiratory failure. Most human poisoning results from inappropriate use of lobelias or their extracts as medicinal preparations. *Lobelia* species can also cause skin irritation in humans.

Livestock poisoning is not common but does occur occasionally, with symptoms appearing after about three days of eating lobelia. The entire plant, including extracts of the leaves or fruits, is potentially poisonous.

Notes. The leaves of Indian-tobacco were dried and smoked by indigenous peoples of eastern North America, and it has been employed as a deterrent to smoking tobacco. The plant was also used in folk medicine and pharmacologically as an emetic, expectorant, and respiratory stimulant.

Jack in the pulpit

Arisaema triphyllum and related spp. and genera
arum family (Araceae)

Quick check. Distinctive herbaceous perennials with three-parted leaves and brownish or greenish "flower" consisting of a central cone-like spike encased within a hood-like spathe. Corm and entire plant contains irritants that cause intense burning and inflammation to mouth and throat; not usually fatal.

Description. Herbaceous perennials growing from a swollen corm. The paired, long-stalked leaves are compound, and usually three-parted, with pointed, smooth-edged leaflets. The flowers are tiny and crowded together in a short, blunt cluster, or spadix, surrounded by an ensheathing spathe, which is purplish, brown, or green, striped with brown or white, and shaped like an old-fashioned pulpit with a long, oval-shaped hood extending over the spadix. The fruits are scarlet berries borne in a dense, egg-shaped cluster about 2.5 cm (1 in.) long. Green dragon (*Arisaema dracontium*) is similar but has a seven- to 13-parted leaf, with a pointed spadix extending well beyond the summit of the greenish spathe.

Occurrence. Jack in the pulpit occurs in rich woods, thickets, swamps, and bogs throughout much of eastern North America.

Toxicity. The entire plant, including the corm, contains numerous microscopic bundles of needle-like crystals of calcium oxalate. When the plants or corms are eaten fresh, these pierce the tender tissues of the mouth, tongue, and throat, and cause intense burning and inflammation. In serious cases, choking may result from swelling of the throat. Salivation, nausea, vomiting, and diarrhea may occur, and, very rarely, irregular heartbeat, dilation of the pupils, fits, coma, and potentially death. Because of the immediate reaction, rarely more than the first mouthful is consumed; hence, the plant is seldom life-threatening. The leaves and roots can cause skin irritation on contact. All *Arisaema* species have similar irritant properties.

Notes. Many species in the arum family have irritating crystals in their leaves and roots, including several grown as houseplants. Three other wild species of this family, eastern skunkcabbage (*Symplocarpus foetidus*), west-

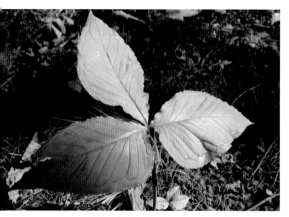

Jack in the pulpit (*Arisaema triphyllum*).

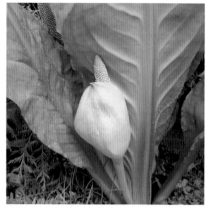

Western skunkcabbage (*Lysichiton americanus*).

ern skunkcabbage (*Lysichiton americanus*), and water arum (*Calla palustris*), are similarly toxic. All are herbaceous perennials of swampy ground. The skunkcabbages have large, fleshy leaves giving off a pungent, skunk-like odor when bruised. Their numerous small flowers form a dense, club-like head surrounded by a large sheath, or spathe. Blooming time is in early spring. In eastern skunkcabbage, the spathe is purplish or brownish mottled; in western skunkcabbage it is bright yellow and showy. Water arum has long-stalked heart-shaped leaves, with a smaller, inconspicuous greenish white flower spathe, and red berries borne in dense clusters.

Despite the irritant properties of Jack in the pulpit corms, they were called Indian turnip, and used as a source of flour by indigenous peoples and early pioneers, after being thoroughly dried and pulverized to break up the calcium oxalate crystals. Boiling alone does not dispel them. The rootstocks and young leaves of skunkcabbages were also sometimes eaten as a famine food after prolonged cooking, but since some residual poison remains, their use is not recommended.

jimsonweed and sacred thorn-apple

Datura stramonium, D. wrightii, and related spp.
nightshade family (Solanaceae)

Quick check. Large, weedy annuals or perennials with big, irregularly toothed leaves, white or purplish tinged funnel-shaped flowers, and prickly, spherical or egg-shaped fruiting capsules. Entire plants highly toxic. Sometimes misused in herbal medicine or as hallucinogens; potentially fatal.

Description. Jimsonweed (*Datura stramonium*) is a large, branching, annual weed 1–1.5 m (3–5 ft.) tall, ill-smelling, and generally lacking hairs. The leaves, 8–20 cm (3–8 in.) long, are alternate, oval, and irregularly toothed or lobed. The showy, funnel-shaped flowers are erect, up to 10 cm (4 in.) long, and white (or purplish in one variety), with a five-pointed rim. The fruit is an ovoid, spiny capsule, splitting regularly into four parts and bearing numerous wrinkled, black seeds. Sacred thorn-apple (*D. wrightii*; syn. *D. meteloides*) is a bushy, branching perennial, up to 1 m (3 ft.) tall and 2 m (6 ft.) across, with a grayish green coloring from a dense covering of hairs. The leaves and flowers are similar to those of jimsonweed, but generally larger. The spherical capsules are nodding or reflexed, with short, hairy spines, splitting open irregularly when ripe.

Several related species are toxic, including desert thorn-apple (*Datura discolor*), of the Colorado Desert area of California, and pricklyburr (*D. inoxia*; syn. *D. metel*), from India but introduced and cultivated widely. Angel's-trumpets (*Brugmansia* spp.) and their relatives have similar toxic properties.

Occurrence. Jimsonweed is widely naturalized around the world and is presumed native to the eastern United States. It is now a common weed of fields, roadsides, and wastelands throughout much of the United States and southern Canada. Sacred thorn-apple is native to southwestern United States and Mexico.

Toxicity. All parts of *Datura* and related *Brugmansia* plants, especially the leaves and seeds, are toxic, containing several indole alkaloids, mainly hyoscyamine (an isomer of atropine that blocks the parasympathetic nervous system) and scopolamine, which is hallucinogenic. Symptoms of poisoning, similar to those of belladonna (*Atropa bella-donna*), may appear from a few minutes to several hours after ingesting the plant. They include intense thirst, dilated pupils, blurred vision, flushing and dryness of the skin and mucous membranes, headache, nausea, rapid but weak pulse, high temperature (occasionally), high blood pressure, urinary retention, hallucinations, delirium, incoherence, amnesia, fever, convulsions, coma, and death. Sometimes people become combative, hyperactive, and paranoid at some stages of intoxication. Intense symptoms may abate after 12 to 48 hours, but disturbance of vision may last up to two weeks. There have been many

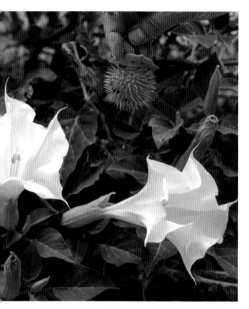

Sacred thorn-apple (*Datura wrightii*).

cases of human poisoning: of children, from sucking the flower nectar or eating the seeds; of those drinking a tea from the leaves as a medicinal preparation for relief of asthma and other ailments; or of people deliberately seeking a hallucinogenic experience from the plant. Eating less than 4–5 gm (⅕ oz.) of the seeds or leaves can be fatal to a child.

Jimsonweed leaves and flowers can cause skin irritation when handled. Jimsonweed, sacred thorn-apple, and their relatives are also toxic to all classes of livestock, and poisoning has occurred when the plants contaminate hay, or the seeds become inadvertently mixed in with grain for poultry. Symptoms in livestock are similar to those in humans. Atropine can often be detected in the stomach contents and body tissues for some time after the death of a poisoned animal.

Notes. An excellent review of jimsonweed and its relatives is provided by Busia and Heckels (2006). The common name for *Datura stramonium* is derived from a 1676 incident at Jamestown, Virginia. British soldiers sent to quell Bacon's Rebellion (a protest led by town resident Nathaniel Bacon against the policies of the governor of that colony) were reportedly given young datura as a "boil'd salad." Some of them, who "ate plentifully of it," exhibited strange and erratic behavior. In one account, "they turned natural fools upon it for several days" and had to be confined "lest they should, in their folly, destroy themselves." "Jimson" is a corruption of Jamestown; the genus name comes from early Sanskrit *dustura* or *dahatura* ("divine inebriation").

Datura species have been used in many parts of the world since ancient times as hallucinogens and folk medicines, valued for their reputed ability to induce visionary dreams foretelling the future and revealing causes of disease and misfortune. In Europe, jimsonweed was used to treat mania, epilepsy, melancholy, rheumatism, convulsions, and madness. Jimsonweed has been an ingredient in powders used to relieve asthma and is recognized for its potential psychotherapeutic applications. The "controlled psychosis" it induces may help to improve clinical management of alcohol intoxication and advance our understanding of schizophrenia and other psychotic disorders.

Botanical gardens have sometimes had to remove this plant because of poaching by those wishing to experience its hallucinogenic properties. The "erratic" behavior alluded to in the Jamestown case is at least as much of a threat to people's safety as the effects of the plant on one's physiology. The drowning of a youth in Skaha Lake in British Columbia's Okanagan Valley in 2006 was attributed to a state of confusion and disorientation from taking datura (Brett 2006).

mayapple
Podophyllum peltatum
barberry family (Berberidaceae)

Quick check. Herbaceous perennial of open woods and meadows with large, lobed, umbrella-shaped leaves, a single white flower, ripening into a large, yellowish berry. Entire plant, except fully ripe berries, violently purgative; large quantities potentially fatal and can cause birth defects; used with extreme caution in pharmaceutical preparations.

Description. Perennial growing from a fleshy, spreading underground rootstock to a height of 30–50 cm (12–18 in.). The leaves are large and umbrella-like, with five to nine prominent lobes spreading out like fingers on a hand, and the stalk joining to the middle of the blade. The leaves are single on flowerless plants, paired on flowering plants. A single large, white, nodding, five- to nine-petalled flower is borne between the leaves in early spring. The fruit is a fleshy, yellowish, blotchy berry, ovoid and up to 5 cm (2 in.) long.

Occurrence. Often found in large patches in open deciduous woods, wet meadows, and along roadsides in southern Ontario and Quebec and throughout the eastern United States west to Minnesota and Texas.

Toxicity. This plant contains over 15 biologically active compounds, particularly within podophyllin, a resinoid component that includes several lignans, notably podophyllotoxin and alpha- and beta-peltatin. The ripe ber-

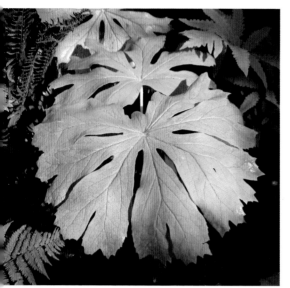

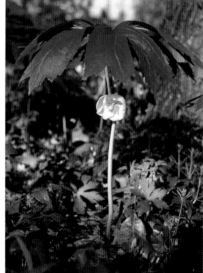

Mayapple (*Podophyllum peltatum*).   Mayapple flower.

ries may be slightly cathartic if eaten in quantity but are well known as an edible wild fruit. Other parts of the plant—rhizome, shoots, leaves, flowers, and unripe fruit—are violently purgative, producing severe digestive upset and diarrhea accompanied by vomiting. They also have a toxic effect on dividing cells, which could potentially lead to birth defects if consumed by women during pregnancy. Children have been poisoned from eating unripe fruit. Poisoning sometimes results from misuse of medicinal preparations of the plant. Eating large quantities of the plant, or repeated application of the resin to the skin may be fatal, producing blood abnormalities, kidney failure, and eventual coma. People handling the powdered rhizomes in commercial drug preparations have experienced eye irritation, keratitis, and ulcerative skin lesions.

Livestock rarely eat this plant, and hence poisoning of them is rare, but deaths do occur occasionally when leaves or shoots are browsed.

Notes. Mayapple has long been a part of both Native American folk medicine and general American materia medica, used to treat cancerous tumors, soft warts, and other growths. Unfortunately, the satisfactory use of mayapple resin against cancer has been complicated by its toxicity.

milkvetches and locoweeds

Astragalus spp. and *Oxytropis* spp.
pea family (Fabaceae)

Quick check. Herbaceous perennials with pinnately compound leaves, pea-like flowers in elongated clusters, and variously shaped pods. Many types fatally poisonous to animals; leaves, pods, and seeds potentially toxic for humans, especially children who might be attracted to pea-like pods.

Description. Milkvetches (*Astragalus* spp.) and locoweeds (*Astragalus* and *Oxytropis* spp.) are a large, diverse group of plants in two closely related genera. Botanists recognize some 400 species of *Astragalus* and more than 25 species of *Oxytropis* in North America alone, and even experts find it difficult to identify them or in some cases to distinguish between members of the two genera. Since both contain toxic species, they are treated here together.

These are perennials, with or without stems, growing in clumps or patches from woody rootstocks. Their leaves are alternate and mostly pinnately compound (with leaflets arranged along a central rib). The flowers, few to many, grow in elongated clusters (racemes) from the leaf axils. They are relatively small and pea-like, varying from white to purple to yellowish, depending on the species. In *Astragalus* the flower stems are leafy, and the keel (lowermost) petal of the flowers is blunt, whereas in *Oxytropis* the flower stems are leafless, and the keel is prolonged into a distinct point (hence, the further common names, point locoweed, or pointvetch). The fruits are pea-like pods varying in size, shape, and texture and containing one or more kidney-shaped seeds.

Occurrence. Milkvetches and locoweeds are found in a wide range of habitats throughout North America, from dry plains, open woods, and hillsides to moist shorelines and alpine meadows.

Toxicity. Some species of milkvetches and locoweeds have low toxicity or are nontoxic, and these are desirable as forage and soil-building plants. However, milkvetches as a group are recognized as among the most poisonous to livestock in North America. They should be considered potentially poisonous to humans too, especially since they have pea-like pods that may attract children. In most cases, however, large quantities have to be consumed to be fatal.

Several species of both *Astragalus* and *Oxytropis* are known to cause a disease of grazing livestock known as *loco* (Spanish for "crazy"), which has been widespread in rangelands of western North America. Typical symptoms of this disease, reflected by its name, include staggering, trembling, and paralysis. Major toxic constituents include toxic amino acids (e.g., selenium-containing) and aliphatic nitro-compounds. In addition, a fungal endophyte (*Embellisia* spp.) produces elevated levels of a toxic indolizidin alkaloid, swainsonine (Ralphs et al. 2008). A second type of poisoning is caused by timber milkvetch (*A. miser*), a small, delicate plant with fine, small leaflets, scanty pinkish mauve blossoms, and slender pods, and by relatives of this species. *Astragalus miser* is common on rangelands of western North America. Symptoms appear relatively quickly after eating the plant and include paralysis with respiratory difficulties—huskiness of voice and coughing, roaring, or wheezing. In this case, poisoning is apparently due to the presence of miserotoxin, the glycoside of nitropropanol, or glycosides of nitropropionic acid.

Notes. At least one species of milkvetch is known to have flower nectar that is poisonous to honeybees, and to have caused serious losses to apiarists in Nevada. Some milkvetches may accumulate toxic amounts of selenium in regions where this element occurs in the soil.

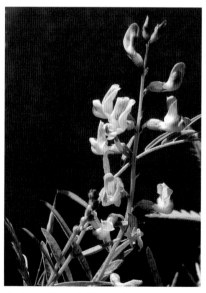

Timber milkvetch (*Astragalus miser*).

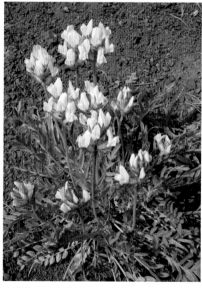

Field locoweed (*Oxytropis campestris*).

Several other wild legumes are toxic. One is prairie thermopsis, or buffalobean (*Thermopsis rhombifolia*), a common, yellow-flowered herbaceous perennial of the prairies, which has seeds that have reputedly caused poisoning in children and foliage toxic to livestock. Another is nineanther prairieclover (*Dalea enneandra*), whose root is considered poisonous by the Dakota (Moerman 2003). The lupines (*Lupinus* spp.) are treated as garden plants; see Chapter 4.

milkweeds

Asclepias spp.
milkweed family (Asclepiadaceae)

Quick check. Large, herbaceous perennials with leaves in opposite pairs or whorls, attractive white, orange, or purplish flowers in umbrella-like clusters, and pointed fruiting pods with silk-tufted seeds; plants exude milky sap when broken. Well known as livestock poisons; potentially toxic to humans when some species are used as wild greens or in herbal preparations.

Description. It is likely that all of the more than 20 species of milkweeds that occur in North America, many of them widespread, have some degree of toxicity. They are upright, herbaceous perennials up to 1 m (3 ft.) or more tall, often branching and growing in large clumps from creeping rhizomes. All parts of the plants exude a milky juice (latex) when broken or injured. The leaves, in opposite pairs or whorls, are broad and elliptical or oblong, or narrow and smooth-edged, and up to 20 cm (8 in.) long, often with a prominent central vein. A dense mat of soft, silky hairs may cover both surfaces of the leaves, or the upper side only. The five-parted flowers are usually fragrant, ranging in color from white to red, orange, or lilac-purple, depending on the species. They are attractive and intricate, with two series of petal parts, the outer whorl strongly curved back, and the inner modified and horned, and arranged in dense, umbrella-like clusters borne on the upper part of the main stem and branches. The fruits are large, greenish, warty pods, splitting along the side when ripe to expose numerous silky-tufted seeds that are very attractive when they become airborne.

Occurrence. Milkweeds are widely distributed in North America, growing from coast to coast, from southern Canada throughout the United States, on dry prairies, pastures, clearings, roadsides, dry streambeds, and lake-shores. Some species grow in wet places, swamps, and bogs.

Toxicity. At least some milkweed species (and probably all, to some extent) contain toxic resinoids in their milky sap, notably galitoxin, as well as several cardioactive cardenolides and bitter-tasting steroidal glycosides with saponin-like properties. The milky latex may cause allergic dermatitis in some individuals.

Although no fatal poisonings of humans by milkweeds are reported, some species are used as edible wild greens and should be selected and prepared with caution. There are many cases of livestock poisoning by milkweed species, the symptoms produced by various species differing only in degree. Initial symptoms are depression, weakness, and staggering, followed by prostration, titanic seizures, labored breathing, high temperature, dilation of the pupils, coma, and death within one to a few days in fatal cases. Fortunately, most milkweeds are distasteful to livestock, and animals eat them only when no other forage is available.

Notes. Although the young shoots, flowers, and green pods of some species are popular as wild vegetables when cooked, the uncooked shoots and the mature plants should never be consumed. Only known edible species of milkweeds, such as showy milkweed (*Asclepias speciosa*) and common milk-

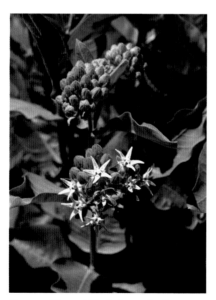 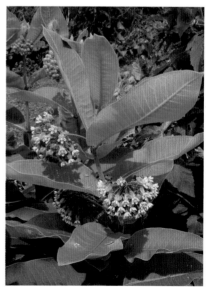

Showy milkweed (*Asclepias speciosa*).   Common milkweed (*Asclepias syriaca*).

weed (*A. syriaca*), should be eaten, and then only after cooking the young shoots or pods in one or more changes of water; this eliminates most of the bitter, poisonous compounds, which leach out in the water.

nightshade, black
Solanum nigrum and *S. americanum*
nightshade family (Solanaceae)

Quick check. Leafy annuals with white, potato-like flowers and clustered berries, green when unripe and shiny black when ripe. Foliage and green berries highly toxic, sometimes fatal. Fully ripe berries of some varieties edible when cooked, but use caution.

Description. Branching annuals, erect or sprawling, 15 cm (6 in.) to 1 m (3 ft.) high. The stems and leaves are smooth or roughly hairy. The leaves are alternate, simple, smooth-edged or with blunt teeth, and oval to triangular or lance-shaped. The star-shaped flowers are small and white, resembling potato flowers, with spreading or reflexed petals and yellow stamens grouped tightly around the stigma at the center. The berries, hanging in small clusters, are green when unripe, black and shiny when ripe. Both native (*Solanum americanum*; American black nightshade) and introduced (*S. nigrum*) populations of black nightshade occur in North America, but the two species are difficult to distinguish, and both are poisonous. Several other species of *Solanum*, also toxic, are found in various parts of North America; all have characteristic potato-like flowers, varying in color from white to blue to violet.

Occurrence. Black nightshades occur as weeds of fields and open woodlands, gardens, pastures, wastelands, and disturbed ground throughout North America.

Toxicity. Black nightshades contain solanine, a toxic glyco-alkaloid. The mature foliage and green berries are especially toxic. The fully ripe fruits of some varieties are edible when cooked, but toxicity varies; unless you are certain the berries are from an edible strain, leave them alone. Both humans and animals of various types have been poisoned by black nightshade, sometimes fatally. Symptoms are similar to those of climbing nightshade (*Solanum dulcamara*), a vine treated earlier in this chapter.

Notes. Another common toxic *Solanum* species is Carolina horsenettle (*S. caro-*

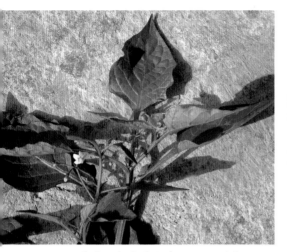

Black nightshade (*Solanum nigrum*), leaves.

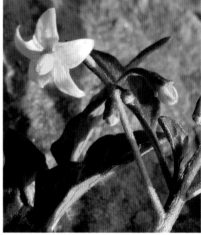

Black nightshade (*Solanum nigrum*), flower.

linense). A tall herbaceous perennial, it is a weed of fields and wastelands, with prickly stems and leaves, and large, yellowish berries, which may remain over the winter and cause poisoning even in spring. It is widespread but especially common in the southeastern United States. The red-berried Jerusalem cherry (*S. pseudocapsicum*) is yet another toxic relative (see Chapter 5).

Solanum nigrum is highly variable, with a complex of subspecies and forms. In some parts of the world, the greens are grown as a potherb, and the ripe berries are often eaten. Most authorities grant specific status to wonderberry, or sunberry (*S. burbankii*) and garden huckleberry (*S. melanocerasum*; syn. *S. intrusum*), both with edible fruit.

peyote cactus
Lophophora williamsii
cactus family (Cactaceae)

Quick check. Small, spineless, rounded cactus with one or more stems having rounded sections around the top, a central pinkish flower, and small, pink fruit. Distributed as small, dried mescal buttons. A potent hallucinogen with potentially dangerous physiological and psychotic effects, but not usually fatal.

Description. Peyote is a small, fleshy cactus with one or more short, rounded

stems growing from a large, branching perennial rootstock. Each stem, 2–5 cm (1–2 in.)
across, is divided around the top into several low, rounded sections, each bearing a tuft
of yellowish white hairs. The flower, white to
rose-pink, grows at the center, and ripens into
a small, pinkish, berry-like fruit. The seeds are
black. The plant is distributed, usually illegally,
as a hallucinogen in the form of small, dried
buttons, which are brownish and have a bitter,
disagreeable taste.

Occurrence. Peyote's natural range is the desert
land of southern Texas to central Mexico; dried
buttons are shipped to other parts of North
America for use as a ceremonial hallucinogen,

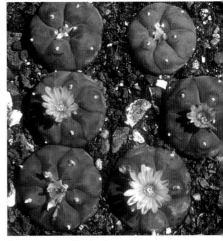

Peyote cactus (*Lophophora
williamsii*). Paul Kroeger

and peyote plants are sometimes cultivated. However, possession of peyote, which is classed as a narcotic, is unlawful in some areas, and there are
legal restrictions against its cultivation or importation from Mexico, despite
conservation concerns in the United States.

Toxicity. Peyote contains many alkaloids, which can be divided into iso-
quinoline-derived compounds (peyotline, pellotine, anhalamine, anhalo-
mineanine, anhalodine, lophophorine) and phenylethylamine derivatives
(mescaline, anhaline). Since the alkaloids act together (and their effects
vary according to their relative concentration, the dosage, and the mental
and physical state of the person eating peyote), it is difficult to characterize the specific actions of each; however, it is known that lophophorine is
the most toxic, having strychnine-like effects, whereas mescaline (or 3,4,5-
trimethoxy-beta-phenylethylamine) is probably the most hallucinogenic,
acting through paralysis of the central nervous system and producing color
visions and awareness of the heaviness of the limbs. Some of the others have
sedative functions. Shortly after ingestion or after a tea from it is drunk, peyote produces nausea, chills, headache, and severe stomach pain and vomiting, often accompanied by terror, anxiety, pupil dilation and visual disturbances, hot, flushed face, muscular relaxation, dizziness, slight decrease in
pulse, loss of sense of time, and wakefulness. As these symptoms subside,
mental stimulation begins, with clarity and intensity of thought, brilliantly

colored, sometimes bizarre, visions, and exaggerated sensitivity to sound and other senses. Peyote apparently does not cause a physiological addiction, but its long-range effects and psychotic reactions are dangerous, and it can be psychologically habit-forming. Peyote intoxication usually occurs among young people experimenting with the plant and trying to experience its psychedelic effects.

Notes. Peyote has long been used by indigenous peoples in religious rites and is still used legally in the communion services of the Native American Church. Mescaline has also been used as a drug in experimental psychiatry.

poison hemlock
Conium maculatum
carrot family (Apiaceae)

Quick check. Young plants carrot-like, with basal rosette of finely dissected leaves; mature plants are tall, much-branched, with numerous tiny white flowers in umbrella-like clusters; stems smooth, hollow, and purplish-speckled; plants with unpleasant "mousy" odor. Highly toxic and potentially fatal, especially for children, who may mistake the leaves for parsley or the roots for carrots.

Description. An erect, branching biennial (sometimes annual or perennial) up to 2 m (6 ft.) or more high when mature, growing from a white, fleshy taproot. The leaves, up to 30 cm (1 ft.) long, are triangular in outline, finely cut, fern-like, and delicate. The young plant closely resembles Queen Anne's lace, or wild carrot (*Daucus carota*), but the latter has distinctly hairy leaves and stems, whereas those of poison hemlock are hairless. The stems are rigid, hollow except at the nodes, smooth, and slightly ridged, with irregular purple blotches or streaks. The flowers are tiny and white, borne in numerous umbrella-like clusters 2–5 cm (1–2 in.) across, distributed from branch tips throughout the upper part of the plant. The fruits are small, grayish brown, and flattened, each with five prominent wavy ridges running lengthwise. When the plant is bruised, crushed, or even touched, a strong, unpleasant odor is emitted, resembling the smell of mice to some people.

Occurrence. Originally introduced from Europe, poison hemlock has become a noxious weed of wastelands, pastures, fields, roadside ditches, and sometimes gardens, throughout southern Canada and the United States, particularly the northern states and adjacent Canada.

Toxicity. Poison hemlock contains a group of closely related piperidine alkaloids, including coniine, gamma-coniceine, N-methyl coniine, conhydrine, and pseudoconhydrine. These alkaloids are structurally related to nicotine and act similarly, producing initial stimulation followed by severe depression of the central nervous systems, resulting in paralysis, slowing of the heart, convulsions, and death from respiratory paralysis. All parts of the plant are toxic, especially the leaves before flowering, and the flowers and

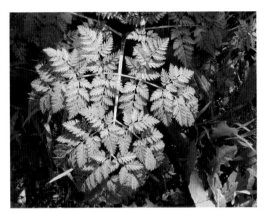

Poison hemlock (*Conium maculatum*).

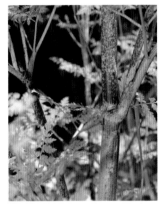

Poison hemlock stalk.

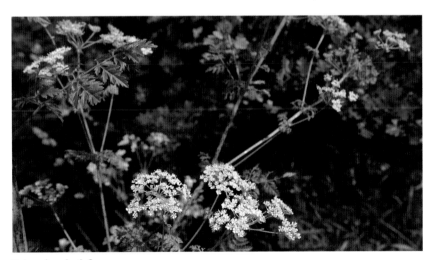

Poison hemlock flowers.

fruits. The concentration of alkaloids varies with climatic conditions; sunny summers produce greater quantities.

The plant is toxic to both humans and animals and has often produced fatalities (see Preface). Sometimes people mistake the finely dissected leaves of the young plants for parsley, or the seeds for anise, with fatal results. Symptoms of human poisoning, appearing one to three hours or more after eating the plant, include nausea, vomiting, salivation, abdominal pain, diarrhea, headache, dilation of the pupils, lack of coordination, confusion, sweating, difficulty in breathing, coldness of the extremities, drowsiness, fluctuations of blood pressure, rapid or irregular heartbeat, convulsions, and coma. Death usually results from stoppage of breathing. Fortunately, the taste of the plant is so unpleasant that seldom is enough eaten to cause death.

Animals are repelled by the unpleasant odor but are sometimes poisoned in the spring, when the leaves of poison hemlock are low and often mixed in with grasses and other forage. Cattle are the most susceptible, but all classes of livestock may be affected. The unpleasant odor of the plant is often detectable in the urine and breath of a poisoned animal. Birth deformities may result when pregnant females eat the plant.

Notes. To prevent the possibility of children and animals being poisoned, eliminate poison hemlock plants from yards, playgrounds, and pasturage before the flowers have a chance to go to seed.

It was this plant that was used in 399 B.C. to kill the Greek philosopher Socrates. The most notorious toxic relatives of poison hemlock are the violently poisonous water hemlocks (*Cicuta* spp.). Several other species in the family have been implicated in poisoning, including wild chervil (*Anthriscus sylvestris*), fool's parsley (*Aethusa cynapium*), some species of *Angelica* (e.g., *A. venenosa*), and some species of *Lomatium* (e.g., fernleaf biscuitroot, *L. dissectum*) and waterparsnips (*Sium* spp.), although most *Lomatium* species and some species of *Sium* are considered edible (Moerman 2003; Turner 2006). Another relative, water parsley (*Oenanthe sarmentosa*), is implicated by the known toxicity of a European species of this genus, hemlock waterdropwort, or dead men's fingers (*O. crocata*), which caused at least ten fatal poisonings in the 20th century. *Oenanthe sarmentosa* is a strong emetic and laxative and has been used—with caution—in Native American medicinal applications (Moerman 2003).

Poison hemlock and water hemlock should not be confused with hemlocks (*Tsuga* spp.), the native coniferous trees, which are not poisonous. However, the shrub called ground hemlock (*Taxus canadensis*), notwithstanding one of its common names, is a yew, and its seeds, foliage, and bark are all poisonous.

pokeweed, American
Phytolacca americana
pokeweed family (Phytolaccaceae)

Quick check. Tall, large-leaved perennial with whitish flowers and round, purple-black berries borne in elongated clusters. Entire plant, especially raw berries, highly toxic and potentially fatal. Even young shoots, considered edible by some, *should not be used* due to the presence of a blood cell altering chemical; poisoning sometimes occurs from misuse of herbal preparations.

Description. American pokeweed, or pokeberry, is a large herbaceous perennial up to 2.5 m (8 ft.) or more tall, growing from a thick, fleshy taproot, with greenish or reddish branching stems. The leaves are alternate, oblong, and smooth-edged, those near the base as much as 30 cm (1 ft.) long. The many small flowers, with greenish white to pink sepals, are borne in an erect or drooping cluster (raceme) up to 20 cm (8 in.) long. The fruits are round, shiny, dark purple, juicy berries. Various related species are similar, and all should be considered toxic.

Occurrence. Common native plant of rich, disturbed soils; found in open fields, moist woods, and wastelands and along fencerows and roadsides

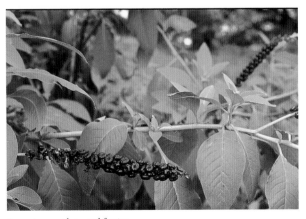

American pokeweed fruits.

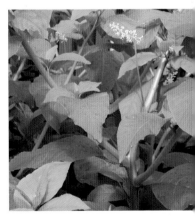

American pokeweed
(*Phytolacca americana*).

throughout eastern United States and southeastern Canada; occasional weed on the West Coast. Sometimes grown in gardens.

Toxicity. The entire plant, especially the roots and seeds, is highly poisonous. Water-soluble triterpenoid saponins, especially phytolaccatoxin and its aglycone phytolaccagenin, are believed to be responsible for this plant's toxicity. Poisoning symptoms, generally developing one to two hours after eating American pokeweed, include abdominal cramps, persistent vomiting, diarrhea, and, in severe cases, convulsions and death. Salivation, heavy perspiration, weakness and drowsiness, slowed pulse, difficulty in breathing, and visual disturbances may also be experienced. An immediate burning sensation in the mouth is the first warning, and fortunately usually stops people from eating a fatal dose. Most fatalities occur in children who eat the berries. Infants and toddlers can be seriously poisoned from eating only a couple of raw berries. One five-year-old died from drinking a quantity of crushed pokeberries added to sugar and water to simulate grape juice. Animals find pokeweed distasteful and do not usually eat it, although pigs are sometimes poisoned from eating the roots, and the plant is a potential hazard to all classes of livestock.

American pokeweed also contains mitogenic lectins that can cause serious and wide-ranging blood cell abnormalities. The pokeweed mitogens affect division of human white blood cells and induce the proliferation of B and T lymphocytes, disturbing the body's immune system. The mitogens can be absorbed through cuts and skin abrasions, as well as through ingesting the plant. Therefore, American pokeweed *should not be* handled except with gloves. Gardeners and others trying to eliminate the plant should be particularly careful.

Notes. The young leafy shoots of American pokeweed are frequently used as a springtime cooked vegetable in eastern North America. The cooked berries have also been eaten. Although thorough cooking (in two waters for the shoots) eliminates most of the toxins, the danger of absorbing the cell-altering mitogens during harvesting and preparation of the shoots and berries is very real. Furthermore, people may be poisoned from improperly cooked leaves or from roots pulled up with the shoots. Because of the potential dangers involved, people should avoid using pokeweed altogether. Folk medicinal preparations from pokeweed roots or other parts are also potentially dangerous.

ragwort, tansy

Senecio jacobaea and related spp.
aster family (Asteraceae)

Quick check. Tall, weedy plant of pastures and roadsides with irregularly lobed leaves, and yellow flowers in conspicuous flat-topped clusters. Toxic and potentially carcinogenic; may produce severe liver damage; seldom immediately fatal in humans, but may be a harmful contaminant of milk and honey. Do not use in herbal preparations or teas.

Description. *Senecio jacobaea*, also known as stinking willie, is a tall, coarse herbaceous biennial, winter annual, or occasional perennial, up to 1 m (3 ft.) or more high, with tough upright stems often red-tinged near the base and branching above the middle. A basal rosette of leaves usually dies before flowering, but the stem leaves persist. They are deeply and irregularly lobed or divided, dark green, and tough. The composite (daisy-like) flowers are small, bright yellow, and numerous, borne in dense, conspicuous, flat-topped clusters. The single-seeded fruits are topped with a downy parachute-like tuft of hair, making them readily dispersible. Over 25 of the many other species of ragwort have proven poisonous. Some, such as common groundsel, or old-man-in-the-spring (*S. vulgaris*), are weedy annuals; others (e.g., lambstongue ragwort, *S. integerrimus*) are native perennials. In cases where ragwort poisoning is suspected, a botanist should be consulted for accurate identification, because the genus *Senecio* is complex and difficult to characterize.

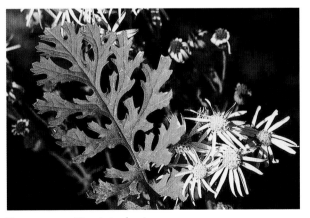

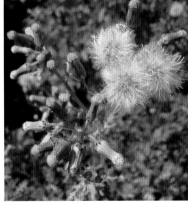

Tansy ragwort (*Senecio jacobaea*).

Groundsel (*Senecio vulgaris*).

Occurrence. Introduced from Europe, tansy ragwort is now a common weed of roadsides, fields, and pastures throughout much of North America, particularly in the Atlantic and Pacific coastal regions of Canada. It has taken over entire fields of previously productive pastureland.

Toxicity. Most ragworts should be considered potentially poisonous, but tansy ragwort (*Senecio jacobaea*) is the most notorious and is considered in Britain to be one of the most important of all poisonous plants. It contains a wide spectrum of pyrrolizidine alkaloids, including senecionine, seneciphylline, jaconine, and jacobine. They are apparently metabolized in the liver to bound pyrrole derivatives, both soluble and insoluble, that are highly toxic and carcinogenic. The toxins are not destroyed by drying or storage. In some parts of the world, such as Africa and the West Indies, humans have suffered from chronic ragwort poisoning caused by eating bread made from flour contaminated with seeds of ragwort species or by drinking medicinal tea from some species. Symptoms of human poisoning include abdominal pain, nausea, vomiting, headache, enlarged liver, apathy, and emaciation. Additionally, people may be harmed indirectly from ragwort-tainted milk or honey. Some ragwort species also cause contact dermatitis.

Grazing livestock are frequently affected by ragwort. Field poisoning of livestock usually occurs only when there is a heavy infestation of the plants and when other forage is scarce. Cattle and horses are the most frequent victims. Symptoms of ragwort poisoning—digestive disturbances, restlessness, lack of coordination, and paralysis—may develop from a few days to several weeks or months after animals have eaten the plants. Once symptoms are obvious, an animal may die within a few days.

Notes. Ragwort poisoning of animals was first identified in 1906 in Nova Scotia; there, a condition known as Pictou disease, after the town of that name, had become common following the introduction of ragwort from Scotland. In Britain, ragwort poisoning causes tremendous economic losses in livestock.

Several plants in the borage family (Boraginaceae), including heliotropes (*Heliotropium* spp.), comfreys (*Symphytum* spp.), gypsyflower (*Cynoglossum officinale*), viper's buglosses (*Echium* spp.), and fiddlenecks (*Amsinckia* spp.), also contain liver-damaging pyrrolizidine alkaloids, and *should not be* used internally as medicinal herbs, even though some have been in the past. The pyrrolizidine alkaloids in these species can also be accumulated and excreted through the milk of cows and other animals that feed on them and, through the milk, can be toxic to infants and young animals.

rattlebox, showy
Crotalaria spectabilis and related spp.
pea family (Fabaceae)

Quick check. *Crotalaria spectabilis* (showy rattlebox) is a dense herbaceous annual up to 2 m (6 ft.) tall, with large, simple leaves, yellow, pea-like flowers in showy clusters, and inflated pods whose seeds rattle inside when dried. Entire plant highly toxic, producing severe liver damage; seeds and medicinal tea from leaves are the usual causes of human poisoning.

Description. Several species of rattlebox occur in North America, most of them coarse, yellow-flowered herbs with distinctive, inflated pods that rattle when shaken. In terms of toxicity, *Crotalaria spectabilis* is the most important and widely distributed. It is a dense, erect annual (sometimes perennial, but never woody), growing up to 2 m (6 ft.) high, with smooth, erect stems. The leaves are simple and oval, up to 18 cm (7 in.) long, hairless above and finely hairy beneath. The flowers are 2.5 cm (1 in.) long and yellow, with purple tinges or veins, borne in large, elongated terminal clusters. The fruiting pods, up to 5 cm (2 in.) long, are inflated, black at maturity, and contain about 20 glossy black seeds, which detach when ripe and rattle when the pod is shaken.

Occurrence. *Crotalaria spectabilis* is a common weed of fields and roadsides from the southern states north to Missouri and Virginia; occasionally cultivated as an ornamental or soil conditioner. Other species of *Crotalaria* occur as garden plants or introduced weeds in parts of the United States. One native species, *C. sagittalis* (arrowhead rattlebox), is found in scattered populations in valley bottoms of the southern and central states.

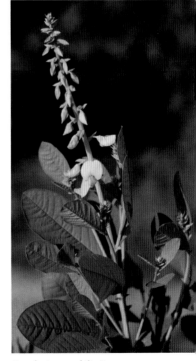

Crotalaria spectabilis. Larry Allain at USGS, National Wetlands Research Center

Toxicity. As with ragworts (*Senecio* spp.) and some members of the borage family, rattlebox species contain a dangerous group of pyrrolizidine alkaloids in their seeds, leaves, and stems. The major compounds include monocrotaline, spectabiline, retusine, retusamine, anacrotine, and nilgirine. Humans have been poisoned through eating the seeds (as a contaminant of grain) or drinking a medicinal tea made from the plants. The main effect is severe liver damage (veno-occlusive liver disease, or Budd-Chiari syndrome, with hepatic vein thrombosis leading to cirrhosis). Symptoms are abdominal pain, enlargement of liver and spleen, loss of appetite, nausea, vomiting, and diarrhea.

Livestock of all types, particularly horses, cattle, poultry, and pigs, are often poisoned by *Crotalaria spectabilis* and other rattlebox species. Animal poisoning generally parallels that of humans, with severe damage to liver and spleen.

Notes. *Crotalaria spectabilis* and several other rattlebox species were originally introduced to the United States in the 1920s by the Bureau of Plant Industry as potential soil builders, hay, and forage crops; it was not until a decade later that their toxicity was discovered.

Another toxic plant in the same family is *Sesbania punicea*, also commonly known as rattlebox, as well as false poinciana and sesbane. Its seeds and flowers contain toxic saponins and are potentially fatal. It is grown as an ornamental shrub and also occurs as a garden escape in the southeastern United States.

St. Johnswort

Hypericum perforatum
St. Johnswort family (Hypericaceae)

Quick check. Erect, opposite-leaved herbaceous perennial; leaves spotted with tiny translucent dots; flowers bright yellow and numerous, in terminal clusters. Entire plant contains a phototoxin that can cause dermatitis and inflammation of the mucous membranes on exposure to direct sunlight; use extreme caution if taking as medicinal herb.

Description. St. Johnswort, or Klamath weed, is a perennial up to 1 m (3 ft.) tall or more, with winged or two-edged stem and branches. The stems are smooth and erect, with a woody base. The leaves are opposite, lacking stalks, elongated and elliptical, with pointed tips, and up to 2.5 cm (1 in.) long; they are spotted with many tiny glandular dots; when held up to the light, these appear translucent. The flowers are five-petalled, yellow, with numerous prominent yellow stamens, and are borne in flat or round-topped clusters toward the top of the plant. The fruiting capsules, brown when mature, contain numerous small pitted seeds.

Occurrence. St. Johnswort was introduced to the eastern United States many years ago and is now an aggressive weed of roadsides, pastures, and ranges throughout most of the United States and southern Canada.

Toxicity. St. Johnswort and most other *Hypericum* species contain naphtho-dianthrone derivatives (especially hypericin, a reddish, fluorescent substance), which have photosensitizing properties that can potentially cause skin irritation when activated by sunlight, specifically ultraviolet rays. They also contain a broad range of flavonoids, phloroglucinols, essential oils (mosly monoterpenes and sesquiterpenes), and xanthones. St. Johnswort is commonly used as an herbal medicine, to treat mild depression and nervous restlessness, as well as in the form of St. Johnswort oil, which is rubbed on wounds for its antibiotic properties. There is little evidence that the photosensitizing or other potentially toxic properties of these plants have been harmful to humans, according to Blumenthal (2000); the usual dosage is far lower than the concentration that would cause problems. Nor is there proof of any carcinogenic effect from St. Johnswort, although the flavonoid-aglycone quercetin occurring in this plant has been shown to have mutagenic effect (Frohne and Pfänder 2005). This herb has excellent benefits but should be used with some caution. A review of St. Johnswort's phytochemistry and therapeutic use is provided by Upton (1997).

For grazing animals, St. Johnswort is much more dangerous. It causes swelling, blistering, and lesions on the unprotected skin of animals consuming the plant, particularly of albinos and others of light coloring. Once sensitivity to hypericin is developed, subsequent reactions to eating the plant or its extracts and exposure to sunlight become more and more serious.

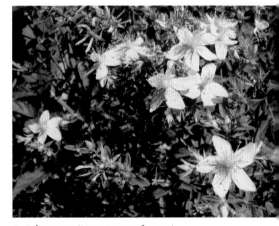

St. Johnswort (*Hypericum perforatum*).

Seriously affected animals may also exhibit thrashing of limbs, loss of appetite, diarrhea, increased respiration and heartbeat, high temperature, blindness, staggering, convulsions, and sometimes coma and death. Depending on conditions, symptoms may appear from two to 14 days after an animal has eaten St. Johnswort. Sometimes an animal may survive the acute stages of poisoning but die eventually from a secondary reaction, such as refusal to eat.

Notes. St. Johnswort is common and widespread, but it was formerly much more noxious. Introduced into California around 1900, Klamath weed, as it was soon named, had spread by the 1950s over an estimated 2⅓ million acres in that state alone and was considered the worst cause of economic loss of pasture and rangelands of California. It caused stock fatalities both directly and indirectly, by reducing the available areas of useful grasses and forage. Fortunately, a biological control program using beetles that feed specifically on it has brought a dramatic decrease in its spread.

There are many other species of *Hypericum* in North America, both native and introduced. Some are grown as garden ornamentals. The same phototoxic compound is known or suspected in some of these, but *H. perforatum* is by far the best known.

St. Johnswort is used worldwide as an herbal treatment for mild to moderate depression, and indications are that, when applied responsibly, it is safe and effective. Furthermore, as reviewed by Mark Blumenthal (2005) and the American Botanical Council, it has significantly fewer side effects than the leading conventional drug used to treat depression of this type. However, there are counter-indications for taking St. Johnswort. There is, for example, a potential for interactions between this herb and tacrolimus, an immunosuppressive drug taken by organ transplant recipients to prevent rejection of a transplanted organ. Therefore, transplant recipients taking tacrolimus should not take St. Johnswort without medical consultation. St. Johnswort may also interfere with other prescription pharmaceuticals: cardiac glycosides (digoxin), other immunosuppressants (cyclosporine), protease inhibitors, anticoagulants, sedatives and antidepressants, oral contraceptives, and active ingredients in cancer drugs (Oliff 2004). It should not be used during pregnancy, and people, especially fair-skinned individuals, should avoid bright sunlight and UV light treatment when taking St. Johnswort preparations.

snakeroot, white

Ageratina altissima (syn. *Eupatorium rugosum*)
aster family (Asteraceae)

Quick check. Tall, herbaceous perennial with long-stalked, toothed leaves, and small, white flower heads in terminal clusters. Entire plant highly toxic; can contaminate milk of cows browsing it and cause milk sickness, or tremetol poisoning, a severe, potentially fatal illness in humans; with modern dairy milk production, milk sickness is almost unknown today, but people owning milk cows should be wary.

Description. Also known as fall poison, this plant is a showy, erect perennial, with branched or unbranched stems, up to 1.2 m (4 ft.) tall. The leaves, 8–15 cm (3–6 in.) long, are paired and opposite, long-stalked, oval to heart-shaped, thin, strongly three-ribbed beneath, sharply toothed at the edges, and pointed. The composite flower heads are white, and borne in open, rounded clusters at the top of the plant. Fruits are small achenes with parachute-like tufts of hair to aid in dispersal. There are many other species of white-flowered *Ageratina* and related *Eupatorium* species, and white snakeroot is itself highly variable. Therefore, if poisoning is suspected, a botanist should be asked to confirm the identification. Only *A. altissima* is implicated as being toxic.

Occurrence. A common plant of rich, open woods and recently cleared areas from eastern Canada to Saskatchewan, and south to eastern Texas, Louisiana, and Georgia. It typically grows in low, moist wooded areas, or along streams, draws, and ravines.

Toxicity. The whole plant contains a highly toxic complex alcohol, tremetol or tremetone. It was responsible, especially in the early 1800s, for many human deaths from North Carolina to the midwestern states. Cows eating large quantities of this plant would develop a disease called "trembles." The milk they produced contained high concentrations of tremetol, and the people drinking the milk developed

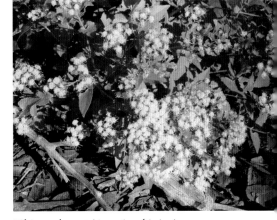

White snakeroot (*Ageratina altissima*).

"milk sickness," the symptoms of which include weakness, nausea, vomiting, tremors, jaundice, constipation, prostration, delirium, and in severe cases, death. Fortunately, with a better understanding of the cause of poisoning, and because most milk is now produced commercially, tremetol poisoning is rare today. White snakeroot, fresh or dried, is also toxic to other animals as well as humans. Symptoms of direct poisoning include sluggishness, difficulty in walking, salivation, loss of appetite, and labored breathing, as well as the characteristic trembling and other symptoms of milk sickness.

Notes. Milk sickness from white snakeroot was said to have been the cause of death of Abraham Lincoln's mother.

Many other plants in the aster family are toxic to livestock and potentially harmful to humans if used as herbal preparations or if they contaminate milk. Some notable poisonous composites are *Anthemis cotula* (stinking chamomile, stinking mayweed), *Baileya multiradiata* (desert marigold), *Bigelowia* spp. (rayless goldenrod), *Brickellia grandiflora* (tasselflower brickellbush), *Centaurea solstitialis* (yellow star-thistle), *Flourensia cernua* (tarbush, blackbrush), *Gutierrezia microcephala* (snakeweed), *Helenium* spp. (sneezeweed), *Hymenoxys* spp. (rubberweed), *Oxytenia acerosa* (copperweed), *Psilostrophe* spp. (paperflower), *Rudbeckia laciniata* (cutleaf coneflower), *Sartwellia flaveriae* (glowwort), *Solidago* spp. (goldenrod), *Tanacetum vulgare* (common tansy), and *Tetradymia* spp. (horsebrush). Other toxic composites discussed elsewhere in this book include rough cocklebur (*Xanthium strumarium*) and ragworts (*Senecio* spp.). Interested readers should consult Fuller and McClintock (1986) and Frohne and Pfänder (2005) for detailed listings.

water hemlocks

Cicuta spp.
carrot family (Apiaceae)

Quick check. Erect herbaceous perennials of damp ground and shallow water; thick, fleshy underground stem base is divided internally by cross partitions, with a series of hollow chambers; leaves compound, with many toothed segments, and leaf veins in most species directed to the V between the teeth, rather than the tips; white flowers in umbrella-shaped clusters. Considered the most poisonous plant genus in North America. Entire plant, especially roots and rootstock, highly toxic, often fatal if ingested; poisoning occurs rapidly. Sometimes mistaken for edible look-alikes, with deadly results.

Description. The several species of water hemlock, also called cowbane, in North America all share similar diagnostic features, and all are very toxic. They are herbaceous perennials growing from a thickened, fleshy stem base or rootstock, which, when cut open lengthwise, is shown to be divided into chambers by a serious of cross partitions. These chambers are usually hollow, but in young plants they may be less obvious. A number of fleshy, tuber-like roots are clustered around the rootstock. The entire plant has a parsnip-like odor, which is pungent but not unpleasant. A yellow juice (the toxin itself) exudes from the white flesh of the rootstock when cut. The stems, 1–2 m (3–7 ft.) tall when mature, are often purple-striped or mottled, and are hollow except for cross partitions at the leaf nodes. The leaves are alternate, with stalks clasping the stem, and two to three times divided into many narrow, toothed leaflets, each usually 2.5–10 cm (1–4 in.) long. In most species (except *Cicuta bulbifera* and some varieties of *C. maculata*) the major leaf veins are directed toward the notches between the teeth, not at the tips as in other plants of the same family. The flowers are small and

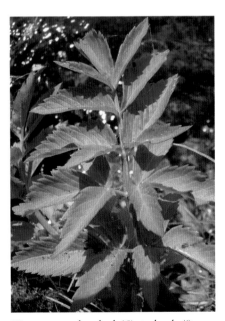

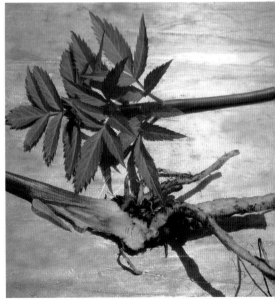

Western water hemlock (*Cicuta douglasii*).   Western water hemlock leaf and rootstock.

white, in umbrella-shaped clusters, as is typical for members of this family. There are often many flower clusters on a single plant, borne on branches at or near the top. The fruits are small, ribbed, and paired.

Occurrence. Various species are found throughout North America, in shallow ditches, wet meadows, lake and pond edges, marshes, and slow-running creeks. Common species include spotted water hemlock (*Cicuta maculata*) found from Alaska across Canada and the eastern United States; *C. bulbifera* (which bears clusters of bulblets in the axils of its upper leaves), found across Canada and the northern States; western water hemlock (*C. douglasii*) of western North America, from Alaska to southern California and Mexico; and Mackenzie's water hemlock (*C. virosa*), of northern Canada and Alaska.

Toxicity. Some authorities consider water hemlock to be the most violently poisonous plant genus of the north temperate zone; ingestion of one portion of root the width of a finger can be fatal to an adult. All parts of the plant are toxic, especially the fleshy rootstock and roots. The toxin, a yellowish, oily liquid, which exudes from the rootstock and roots when cut, is a mixture of polyynes, including cicutoxin, and cicutol, which are complex, highly unsaturated alcohols. They act directly and rapidly on the cen-

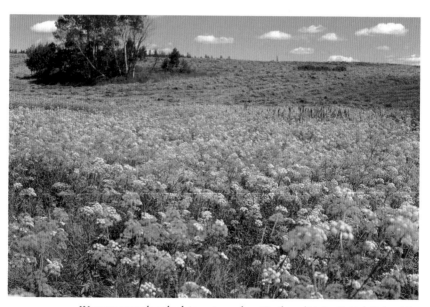

Western water hemlock in wet meadow, Cariboo district, British Columbia.

tral nervous system. Human poisoning is quite common, often occurring when water hemlock is confused with similar-looking edible species. Ironically, these plants can have a pleasant, celery or parsnip smell, which invites tasting. Many edible plants, including parsnip, carrot, celery, and wild edible roots such as waterparsnips (*Sium* spp.), and yampahs, or wild caraways (*Perideridia* spp.) are in the same family. Children have been poisoned from using the hollow stems for peashooters or whistles.

Symptoms of poisoning occur from 15 minutes to an hour from the time of ingestion, and include nausea, salivation and frothing at the mouth, vomiting, violent convulsions and spasms, fever, low heart rate, possible low blood pressure, tremors, severe abdominal pain, widely dilated pupils, delirium, coma, respiratory paralysis, and death, which often occurs before medical help can even be sought. If the first few hours are survived, the patient will usually recover.

Water hemlock is equally poisonous to all types of livestock and has caused severe losses of grazing animals, which may eat exposed rootstocks from cleared-out ditches or the dried edges of lakes and ponds. The leaves and stems are also sometimes browsed but are not as toxic.

Notes. Indigenous peoples of North America have long been aware of the poisonous qualities of water hemlock. A well-known indigenous antidote—said to be the only effective one for this and other highly poisonous plants—is feeding the victim salmon oil skimmed from salmonhead soup.

A toxin closely related to cicutoxin is found in another wetland plant, water parsley (*Oenanthe sarmentosa*), also of the carrot family. The European species *O. crocata* (hemlock waterdropwort), also known as dead men's fingers (for its thick whitish roots), has fatally poisoned humans and livestock in Britain and elsewhere; it is now introduced around Washington, D.C. Other *Oenanthe* species should be considered potentially toxic. Another toxic relative, often confused with water hemlock, is the introduced weed, poison hemlock (*Conium maculatum*), described earlier in this section.

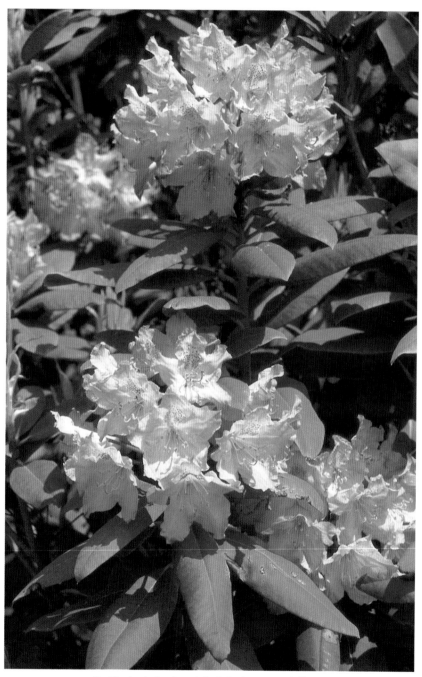

Pacific rhododendron (*Rhododendron macrophyllum*).

CHAPTER 4

Poisonous Garden and Crop Plants
Including common garden weeds

TREES AND TALL SHRUBS

apricot and other stonefruits
Prunus armeniaca and related spp. and genera
rose family (Rosaceae)

Quick check. Apricot trees produce pink blossoms early in spring. The yellowish to orange-colored fruit is sweet and edible, but seeds produce cyanide. Similarly poisonous are bark and leaves. Leaves are simple, oval-shaped. If swallowed in quantity, any of these plant parts can be fatal. Peaches, plums, and cherries also have potentially toxic seed kernels, bark, and leaves.

Description. Small deciduous tree with reddish bark and smooth twigs. The flowers, appearing before the leaves, are pinkish and up to 2.5 cm (1 in.) across. The leaves are oval, about 5 cm (2 in.) long, finely toothed at the edges, and with a pointed tip. The fruits, widely marketed, are fleshy and yellowish to orange, often flashed with red. Smaller than peaches, apricots are slightly flattened, with a characteristic groove along one side. Each fruit contains a large, single, brown stone, flattened and pointed at each end and grooved along the sides. The hard stone encloses one or two almond-like seed kernels.

Occurrence. Apricot, its larger relative, peach (*Prunus persica*), and hybrid nectarine are all common and important cultivated fruits in North America. There are many forms, some grown for their fruits, others for their blossoms. Apricot pits are sometimes sold in health food stores as herbal medicines but often without proper labeling as to their dangers.

Toxicity. Several of our common fruiting trees, including apricots, peaches, nectarines, cherries, and plums (*Prunus* spp.), apples (*Malus* spp.), and pears (*Pyrus* spp.), contain substantial amounts of the cyanide-producing

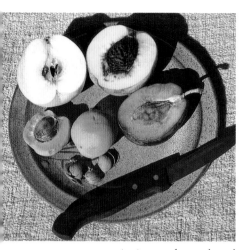

Apricot, apple, peach, and plum: all have seeds with cyanogenic glycosides.

glycoside, amygdalin, in their bark, leaves, and seeds or pits. Poisoning symptoms are difficulty in breathing, inability to speak, twitching, spasms, and in severe cases, coma and sudden death. Children have been poisoned from swallowing the seeds or seed kernels of these species, chewing on the twigs, or making tea from the leaves.

Notes. Several serious cases of poisoning have been reported from misuse of apricot seed kernels or pits as a source of the drug laetrile, widely promoted in the 1970s as a cure for cancer and for its reputed health benefits and since proven to be ineffective and dangerous.

Berries of another shrub in the same family, jetbead (*Rhodotypos scandens*; syn. *R. tetrapetalus*), also contain amygdalin and are highly toxic and potentially fatal if eaten. Other plants in the rose family have seeds and foliage that should be considered suspect: Saskatoon serviceberry (*Amelanchier alnifolia* and related spp.), mountain ashes, or rowans (*Sorbus* spp.), hawthorns (*Crataegus* spp.), firethorns (*Pyracantha* spp.), and cotoneasters (*Cotoneaster* spp.). These seldom cause poisoning but should be treated with caution. Saskatoon serviceberries are widely used edible fruit in many parts of North America, and mountain ash and hawthorn berries, though not very palatable, are sometimes used to make jelly.

black locust

Robinia pseudoacacia
pea family (Fabaceae)

Quick check. Deciduous tree with furrowed bark, compound leaves, whitish (or pink), fragrant flowers in hanging clusters, and bean-like seedpods. Entire plant potentially highly toxic from lectins, but human fatalities unknown.

Description. Black locust, or false acacia, is a deciduous tree up to 25 m (80 ft.) tall, with deeply furrowed, dark brown bark and thorny branches. The leaves are alternate and pinnately compound, with seven to 19 leaflets, arranged on either side of a central vein, or axis. The leaflets are oval or elliptical and up to 5 cm (2 in.) long. The flowers are whitish (pink in some varieties), up to 2 cm (0.8 in.) long, and very fragrant, growing in dense, hanging clusters. The fruits are flattened, hanging, bean-like pods, each containing several seeds. When mature they are dark brown to blackish and often remain on the branches over winter.

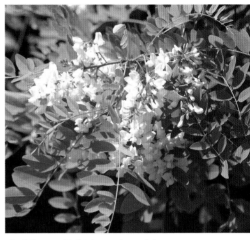

Black locust (*Robinia pseudoacacia*).

Occurrence. This tree is native to the woods of the eastern United States from Pennsylvania to Georgia and west to Iowa, Missouri, and Oklahoma. It is widely planted in gardens and along boulevards as a shade and ornamental tree. There are many cultivars, some with golden or purplish foliage, others with pink flowers.

Toxicity. The entire tree, particularly the bark and seeds, contains lectins, poisonous proteins similar to ricin in castorbean. These agglutinate red blood cells, interfere with protein synthesis in the small intestine, and cause disturbances in the glycogen level of liver and muscle cells. The toxic principles of this plant (formerly known as robin and phasin) are actually mixtures of different lectins, agglutinins, or isolectins. The flowers are the least toxic. Human poisoning from black locust seeds and pods is potentially serious, but fortunately rare, and fatalities are unknown. Symptoms appear after several hours and include lassitude, nausea, vomiting, abdominal pain, diarrhea, loss of appetite, dilation of pupils, delirium, confusion, stupor, seizures, diabetes, and in severe cases, respiratory depression, coma, and circulatory collapse, which can occur from two to several days after ingestion.

There have been many instances of serious, even fatal poisoning in animals from black locust.

Notes. A notorious case of human poisoning occurred in 1887, when 32 boys at a Brooklyn orphanage, for reasons unknown, ate the inner bark of black locust fence posts from the yard of the institution. Two boys were severely poisoned but eventually recovered.

Do not confuse black locust, which is sometimes called honeylocust, with the true honeylocust (*Gleditsia triacanthos*), a tall tree of the same family, but with branched thorns and narrower leaflets. The seed pulp of this latter tree is considered edible, pleasant and sweet.

burningbush and spindletrees

Euonymus spp.
bittersweet family (Celastraceae)

Quick check. Small trees or shrubs with perfect three- to five-parted flowers, and lobed fruits surrounded by a bright orange or red covering; leaves bright red or orange in fall; entire plants, especially attractive fruits, potentially dangerous but not known to be fatal.

Description. Leafy trees, shrubs, or rarely, vine-like climbers. The branches are usually four-angled, with conspicuous winter buds. The leaves are simple, opposite, and short-stalked, with smooth or toothed edges. *Euonymus* species are mostly deciduous, turning to brilliant red or orange in the fall. Male (pollen-producing) and female (seed-producing) flowers are borne separately. The flowers are small, greenish yellow or purplish, produced in small clusters at the leaf axils. The fruits are attractive three- to five-celled capsules, divided to the base into rounded lobes. The seeds, which are white, red, or black, are enclosed in a bright orange or red covering.

Occurrence. Several species of *Euonymus* are native to parts of North America, including bursting-heart, or strawberry bush (*E. americanus*), a common shrub of the eastern

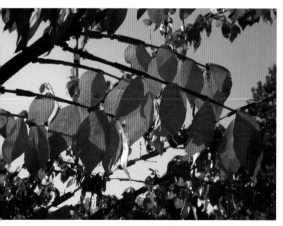

Burningbush (*Euonymus alatus*).

United States. The one most often encountered as an ornamental, however, is burningbush (*E. alatus*), a deciduous, spreading tall shrub, to 2.4 m (8 ft.) high, native to China and Japan; it has branches with characteristic corky wings and leaves that turn bright crimson in the fall.

Toxicity. All parts, including leaves, bark, and fruits, are poisonous and violently purgative, but human poisoning has been reported only from the fruit of European spindletree (*Euonymus europaeus*). It and probably all species contain several digitalis-like cardioactive glycosides (digitaloids), with digitoxigenin as the aglycone, and several peptide and sesquiterpene alkaloids, any of which may be responsible for their toxicity. A lectin that inhibits protein synthesis in cells has also been isolated. Symptoms of poisoning appear ten to 12 hours after ingestion of the fruit (or probably any part of the plant) and include watery diarrhea, persistent vomiting, fever, chills, weakness, hallucinations, convulsions, and coma.

Notes. Ingestion of *Euonymus* fruits by children is regularly reported from poison control centers, but fortunately, poisoning is rarely serious. American bittersweet (*Celastrus scandens*) is related to *Euonymus*; the attractive fruits of this climbing vine are considered toxic by the Iroquois and other indigenous peoples (Moerman 2003). They should not be eaten.

cherry laurel

Prunus laurocerasus and related spp.
rose family (Rosaceae)

Quick check. Small tree, tall shrub, or hedge plant, with large evergreen leaves, whitish flowers in elongated clusters, and blackish, cherry-like fruits. The leaves, bark, fruit, and seeds can cause cyanide poisoning; seldom fatal.

Description. Evergreen tree or shrub with thick, glossy, leathery leaves; often grown as a hedge plant. The leaves are lance-shaped to elliptical, short-stalked, pointed, finely toothed at the edges, and up to 15 cm (6 in.) long. The flowers are small and white or cream-colored, in dense elongated clusters borne in the leaf axils. The fleshy fruits are shiny, dark purple or blackish, each with a single, cherry-like stone in the center. There are many cultivars, with different growth habits and leaf sizes and colors.

Occurrence. A native of southeastern Europe and the Middle East, this bushy tree or shrub is widely planted in North American gardens and parks as an ornamental shade and hedge plant.

Toxicity. The bark, flowers, fruits, and especially the leaves and seed kernels of cherry laurel, like those of other *Prunus* species, contain considerable quantities of cyanide-producing glycosides, including amygdalin and prunasin. The fully ripe fleshy part of the cherries is generally the least toxic. The symptoms are the same as those of poisoning by apricot kernels, apple seeds, and other types of cherries, all due to cyanide poisoning. The symptoms may arise very quickly, and death can occur rapidly when large quantities are consumed, but fortunately, this is rare; the human body can handle small quantities without problem. Cherry laurel poisoning is not common, but children sometimes eat the small, black "cherries," or people sometimes mistake the leaves for those of sweet bay laurel (*Laurus nobilis*), and try to use them for flavoring food. The bitter, unpleasant taste is usually sufficient deterrent to eating large amounts of the leaves. Browsing animals are occasionally poisoned by eating the foliage or hedge trimmings of cherry laurel.

Notes. A related species, Carolina laurelcherry (*Prunus caroliniana*), native to moist valleys of the eastern United States from South Carolina to Texas, is planted as an ornamental in the southeastern states and southern California. It is an evergreen tree growing up to 12 m (40 ft.) high, with glossy

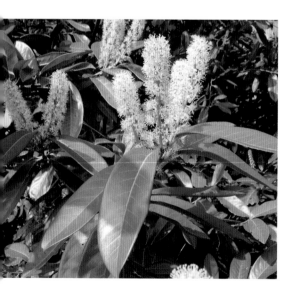

Cherry laurel (*Prunus laurocerasus*).

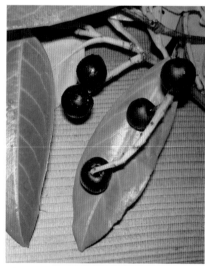

Cherry laurel fruits.

leaves, very small, white flowers in dense clusters, and black, shiny fruit. Its poisonous qualities are similar to those of cherry laurel.

Many other plants are called laurels, including the aforementioned sweet bay laurel (*Laurus nobilis*), whose leaves are used in flavoring soups and stews. Japanese laurel (*Aucuba japonica*), in the dogwood family (Cornaceae), is an evergreen landscaping shrub with large, coarsely toothed, often mottled leaves, and scarlet berry-like fruits, which are mildly poisonous due to triterpenoid saponins. Sheep laurel, mountain laurel, and alpine laurel (*Kalmia* spp.) and spurgelaurel (*Daphne laureola*) are unrelated laurels that, like cherry laurel, have leathery, evergreen leaves. Both *Kalmia* and *Daphne* are toxic.

chinaberrytree
Melia azedarach
mahogany family (Meliaceae)

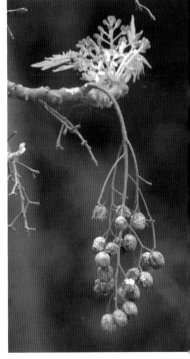

Quick check. Small to medium deciduous tree with large, divided leaves, small, purplish flowers, and yellowish, cherry-sized fruits; toxins variable in concentration; symptoms may be delayed; sometimes fatal.

Description. A deciduous tree up to 15 m (50 ft.) tall, with a thick trunk, furrowed bark, and spreading branches. The leaves are large, long-stalked, and compound, each divided into numerous, oval-shaped, toothed leaflets about 2.5–5 cm (1–2 in.) long. The overall leaf shape is roughly triangular. The flowers are lilac-colored, delicate, and fragrant, borne in open, long-stalked clusters. The fruits are fleshy, globular, cream-colored to yellow, and cherry-sized, each containing a single seed. Smooth at first, they persist after the leaves have fallen, becoming wrinkled.

Occurrence. A native of Southwest Asia, this tree is a common garden ornamental and shade plant of the southern United States, particularly from Virginia south to Florida, west to Texas, and in California. It

Chinaberrytree
(*Melia azedarach*).

also occurs at lower elevations in Hawaii. It is a frequent garden escape in woods, old fields, fencerows, and scrubby areas.

Toxicity. The leaves, bark, and fruit are toxic, although the concentration of toxins varies from one population to the next. Eating only six to eight berries can be lethal to a child. The toxins, tetranortriterpene neurotoxins (or meliatoxins) and as yet unidentified resins, irritate the digestive tract and cause degeneration of the liver and kidneys. Symptoms are often delayed. They include faintness, lack of coordination, confusion, and stupor, and in some cases severe stomach pain, diarrhea, vomiting, difficulty in breathing, convulsions, partial to complete paralysis, and death, which may occur within a day.

Notes. This tree has a variety of local names, including Indian lilac, bead tree, paradise tree, and pride of India. In some places the fruit is eaten without harm, but its use is definitely not recommended. Children may be poisoned from drinking tea made from the leaves. The seeds are sometimes used for rosaries.

golden chain tree

Laburnum anagyroides
pea family (Fabaceae)

Quick check. Ornamental tree or tall shrub with drooping clusters of bright yellow, pea-like flowers, and hanging pea-like pods. Green pods and seeds are a frequent, not usually fatal, cause of poisoning in children.

Description. Large shrub or small deciduous tree up to 10 m (30 ft.) tall, with spreading branches. The leaves, borne on long stalks, are alternate and compound, each with three elliptical to oblong leaflets. The flowers are bright yellow and pea-like, borne in dense, drooping clusters. The fruits are elongated several-seeded pods up to 8 cm (3 in.) long. The unripe pods resemble clusters of hanging beans. When ripe, they turn black, and often hang on the branches over the winter.

Occurrence. Golden chain tree is native to central and southern Europe. It is a popular winter-hardy ornamental throughout temperate North America, grown for its attractive hanging flowers. Occasionally it occurs as a garden escape in woods and fields.

Toxicity. All parts of the plant, especially the bark and seeds, contain quino-

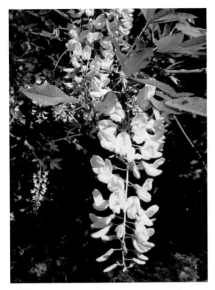

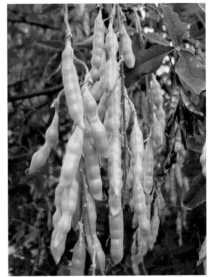

Golden chain tree (*Laburnum anagyroides*).   Golden chain tree pods.

lizidine alkaloids, mainly cytisine in the seeds, which is similar in its effects to nicotine. The concentration of this potent toxin varies considerably with season and genetic strain. All laburnum plants should be regarded as highly poisonous: 20 seeds are lethal for a small child. Usually, however, the rapid onset of vomiting after ingestion prevents absorption of large quantities of cytisine, so that fatalities are relatively rare.

Notes. Despite the bad reputation of this plant, documented fatalities are few (one being a man who died after consuming 23 laburnum pods, or 35–50 mg of cytisine). *Laburnum* is closely related to Scotch broom, also considered poisonous.

holly, English
Ilex aquifolium and related spp.
holly family (Aquifoliaceae)

Quick check. Dense, evergreen tree or tall shrub, with dark green, shiny, spiny leaves, small whitish flowers, and attractive, scarlet berries. Berries and leaves may cause digestive upset; berries an occasional cause of poisoning in children but not known to be fatal.

Description. *Ilex aquifolium* (English holly) is an evergreen shrub or tree, up to 15 m (50 ft.) tall, with smooth, gray bark and many spreading branches forming a dense, conical crown. The thick, leathery, dark green leaves are alternate and short-stalked, usually sharply spined at the tip and around the edges. Male and female flowers, borne on separate plants, are small, dull white, and clustered in the leaf axils. The fruits are scarlet, globular, and shiny, each containing two to four seeds. The many available cultivars are of different sizes, forms, and spine types; some have variegated leaves, with white or yellowish margins.

Occurrence. English holly is widely grown in temperate North America as an ornamental plant, especially for its decorative berries and foliage at Christmas. It is also used as a hedge species. Many other *Ilex* species, both evergreen and deciduous, occur in North America as native species or ornamentals.

Toxicity. Both the showy, scarlet berries and leathery leaves contain saponin and theobromine, a caffeine-like alkaloid. Eating the berries is the usual cause of poisoning. For young children, eating only a few berries can produce symptoms including abdominal pain, nausea, vomiting, diarrhea, and drowsiness. However, fatalities from holly are unknown, and its poisonous properties are possibly overstated. Mild doses of the leaves or berries stimulate the central nervous system; higher doses depress it.

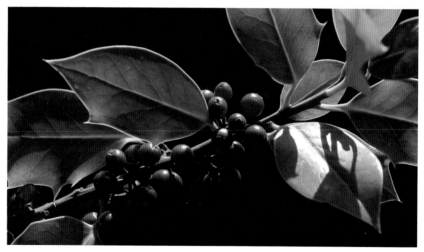

English holly (*Ilex aquifolium*).

Notes. Holly is well known as a decorative Christmas plant, with its bright red berries and dark green, shiny leaves. Several native holly species, with red, orange, or black fruits, occur in eastern and southern North America. All should be regarded with caution. One species, *Ilex vomitoria* (yaupon), is found along the coast of southeastern United States. The leaves can be made into a mild tea, but if drunk in a concentrated brew, it can cause hallucinations and vomiting. Southerners used it as a substitute for coffee and tea during the American Civil War. A related beverage plant is the South American yerba maté, or Paraguay tea (*I. paraguayensis*); rich in caffeine, it is still widely used as a stimulating tea.

horse chestnut

Aesculus hippocastanum
horse chestnut family (Hippocastanaceae)

Quick check. Large deciduous tree with palmately compound leaves, whitish or pinkish flowers in upright clusters, and chestnut-like seeds, enclosed in a prickly, greenish husk. The leaves and seeds are toxic but rarely fatal in humans.

Description. A large, much-branching, deciduous tree, up to 30 m (100 ft.) high, with smooth, gray bark and prominent sticky buds in winter and spring. The leaves are opposite and palmately compound, each with five to seven oblong leaflets radiating from the end of a long stalk. The flowers are borne in dense, often upright, elongated clusters, and are usually white blotched with red and yellow, but there are red- and pink-flowered varieties, as well as double-flowered types. The fruits are spherical capsules, each consisting of a leathery, yellowish green, spiny or warty covering enclosing one to three large, conspicuous nut-like seeds. The seeds bear large scars and are brown and glossy when first exposed, becoming duller with age.

Occurrence. Horse chestnut was introduced from Europe and is widely planted as an ornamental shade tree in North America.

Toxicity. Horse chestnut—especially the young leaves, sprouts, flowers, and seeds—contains more than 30 monodesmosidic saponins known collectively as aescin. Some of these (beta-aescin) can break down blood proteins. Unidentified alkaloids are also present. Poisoning is most com-

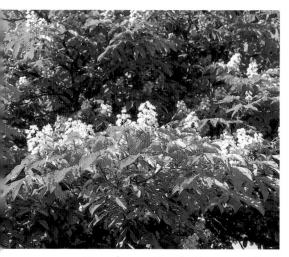

Horse chestnut (*Aesculus hippocastanum*).

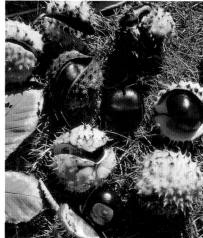

Horse chestnut fruits.

mon from children eating the seeds or "conkers," or from people mistaking horse chestnuts for edible sweet chestnuts (*Castanea* spp.), which look very similar. Animals are sometimes poisoned from eating the leaves and seeds. Symptoms of poisoning include inflammation of the mucous membranes, vomiting, thirst, weakness, lack of coordination, muscular twitching, dilated pupils, stupor, and paralysis. Coma and death from respiratory paralysis may occur in severe cases, but human fatalities are rare, usually resulting from repeated doses.

Notes. Horse chestnut is a relative of the native buckeyes (see Chapter 3) and is similarly toxic. Nevertheless, it is an important herbal medication to treat venous insufficiency (e.g., varicose veins and edema or fluid buildup in legs and feet due to poor vein function) and is considered safe and effective when used as prescribed (Blumenthal 2000; Suter et al. 2006).

tungoil tree

Vernicia fordii (syn. *Aleurites fordii*) and related spp.
spurge family (Euphorbiaceae)

Quick check. Deciduous tree with large, heart-shaped or lobed leaves, whitish, clustered flowers, with red or orange veins, nut-like seeds, and milky latex. Entire plant toxic and occasionally fatal; the seeds and oil are the most common cause of poisoning.

Description. Tungoil tree, or tung nut, is a deciduous tree to 20 m (60 ft.) high, with large, alternate, smooth-edged leaves that are long-stalked with heart-shaped blades. The flowers grow in large clusters and are usually white, sometimes with red or orange veins. The fruits, green when unripe and brown at maturity, are large and globular or somewhat pointed,

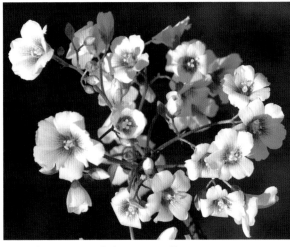

Tungoil tree (*Vernicia fordii*). James Miller

borne on drooping stalks. Tungoil fruits each contain three to seven rough-coated, chestnut-like seeds within the tough hull.

Occurrence. Native to central Asia, tungoil tree is now widely distributed in the tropics, and has been planted in large commercial orchards as an oil crop in the Gulf Coast region from northern Florida to Texas (as well as in Hawaii). It is also planted as an ornamental and shade tree in the southern United States.

Several species in the related genus *Aleurites* occur as ornamentals in parts of the continental United States and Hawaii. Of these, candlenut, or kukui (*A. moluccana*) is best known and is also considered toxic. It resembles tungoil tree, but its leaves are shallowly three- to five-lobed and often have a light, silvery cast.

Toxicity. All parts of tungoil tree are poisonous; the main toxic principles of tung seeds are esters of 16-hydroxyphorbol. The large, attractive, nut-like seeds are the most common cause of human poisoning; a single seed can cause serious illness, and many cases of poisoning have been reported over the years. Symptoms include discomfort and nausea, followed by very severe stomach pain, with vomiting, diarrhea, weakness, depressed reflexes and breathing, and sometimes death. Poisoning of cattle and other animals browsing the cut foliage is not uncommon.

Notes. Frohne and Pfänder (2005) cite an unusual case of tungoil poisoning, in which a baker in Hamburg, Germany, was inadvertently sold a barrel of the oil and used it to make pancakes, causing diarrhea and vomiting in 190 of his customers.

As well as tungoil tree, the spurge family contains a number of toxic and irritant plants, including spurges (*Euphorbia* spp.), castorbean, crotons, and at least three other trees occurring occasionally in the southern United States: Barbados nut, manchineel tree, and sandbox tree.

Barbados nut (*Jatropha curcas*), also aptly called purge nut or physic nut, is a small tree or coarse shrub with large, alternate, long-stalked, palmately veined leaves that are usually three- to five-lobed, small, yellow flowers, and brownish black fruiting capsules containing two to three black seeds. It and others in the genus are widely grown as tropical ornamentals and occur in Florida and Hawaii. They contain curcin, a toxic protein. The fruits and seeds, which are attractive to children, can cause severe gastrointestinal irritation and sometimes coma when ingested.

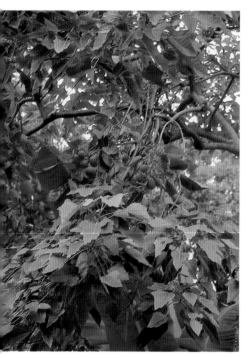

Kukui, or candlenut
(*Aleurites moluccana*).

Manchineel tree (*Hippomane mancinella*), native to the southern tip of Florida and the Keys but now restricted to remote areas like the Everglades, is a small to medium-sized tree with milky juice, large, oval dark green leaves with finely toothed margins, small greenish flowers in spikes, and round, green or yellowish green fruits about 4 cm (1.5 in.) across. The milky sap is extremely caustic to the skin and can cause temporary blindness, and the seeds cause severe gastroenteritis if ingested.

Sandbox tree (*Hura crepitans*) is a large, spiny tree occasionally grown for its curious, violently explosive fruits. Its seeds and milky juice contain huratoxin, a carcinogenic diterpene, and hurin, which is highly irritant, causing severe vomiting and diarrhea.

yews

Taxus spp.
yew family (Taxaceae)

Quick check. Evergreen, needled trees or shrubs with pollen cones and reddish berry-like "fruits" borne on separate individual plants; entire plant, except berry-like flesh around the seed, is highly toxic, but human fatalities are rare.

Description. Evergreen trees or shrubs with scaly, reddish brown bark. The branches have a flattened appearance, with the flat, needle-like leaves spreading out along the twigs. The needles are pointed, dark green above, pale green beneath. The plants are dioecious, with the male (pollen-producing) cones and the female (seed-producing) structures borne on separate plants. Each ripened seed is surrounded by a pinkish to scarlet, fleshy cup, or aril, giving it the appearance of a "berry" with the brown seed exposed at the top.

Occurrence. English yew (*Taxus baccata*), Japanese yew (*T. cuspidata*), and hybrid yew (*T. ×media*), the most commonly grown ornamental yews in North America, are found in gardens and hedges, lending themselves well to ornamental shaping. Three species are native to North America, growing in forests and woodlands: Pacific yew (*T. brevifolia*), in the west from British Columbia to California; Canada yew, or ground hemlock (*T. canadensis*) in the east from Newfoundland to Virginia and the midwestern states, and Florida yew (*T. floridana*), restricted to the Apalachicola River area in Florida.

Toxicity. All parts of yews, except the fleshy red aril around the seed, are toxic. The poisonous principles are derivatives of taxane, including Taxol, a compound isolated from the bark of Pacific yew that is used as an anticancer drug. Taxine B is a diterpene compound, a terpenoid alkaloid, which is most likely to be responsible for the high toxicity of yews. Yews also contain an irritating volatile oil and a cyanogenic glycoside, taxiphyllin.

Symptoms of yew poisoning include nausea, dry throat, severe vomiting, diarrhea, rash, pallor, drowsiness, abdominal pain, dizziness, trembling, stiffness, fever, and sometimes allergy symptoms. Acute abdominal pain, irregular heartbeat, dilated pupils, collapse, coma, and convulsions,

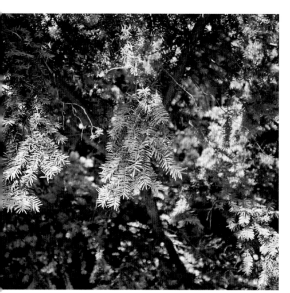

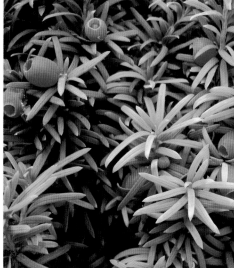

English yew (*Taxus baccata*).   Hybrid yew (*Taxus ×media*).

followed by slow pulse and weak breathing, are symptoms of severe poisoning. Death is from respiratory and heart failure. Occasional fatalities occur when large quantities are consumed, or when children eat the "berries," chewing up the seeds. In the last case, even one or two seeds could be lethal for a small child. Parents of small children should remove the decorative "berries" from any nearby ornamental yews. Browsing animals are frequently fatally poisoned by yew.

Notes. Yews have been used since prehistoric times in folk medicine, both in Europe and North America. English yew has long been known as a tree of death and has been used since antiquity as a poison and for committing suicide. Occasional deaths have occurred from misuse of herbal preparations from yew leaves. The fleshy red aril, or "berry," is pleasant-tasting and edible, at least in small quantities and as long as the seed is not eaten with it. Even then, there have been cases of as many as 40 berries being eaten, with the seeds, without any symptoms of poisoning being evident, apparently because the seeds were swallowed without being chewed and passed through the digestive tract without releasing their toxins.

MEDIUM TO LOW SHRUBS

box, common
Buxus sempervirens
boxwood family (Buxaceae)

Quick check. Evergreen shrub with simple, leathery leaves, commonly grown as a hedge plant; potentially fatal in large quantities.

Description. Evergreen shrub or small tree (rarely) up to 8 m (25 ft.) high, with four-angled or slightly winged branches. The leaves are short-stalked, opposite, and leathery, up to 4 cm (1.5 in.) long. The flowers, formed in early spring, are small, pale green, and inconspicuous. The fruit is a small, ovoid capsule. Its numerous cultivars differ in growth form and leaf size and color; some have variegated foliage or leaves that are edged with yellow or silvery white. A few other *Buxus* species are grown in North America; all should be considered suspect.

Occurrence. A native of western Europe and the Mediterranean, box is extensively used in North America for hedges and borders because it stands pruning and shaping well. It is also sometimes grown as a single specimen shrub or small tree.

Toxicity. All parts of the plant contain buxines, steroidal alkaloids. Eating the leaves and branches can cause abdominal pains, vomiting, diarrhea, and, in large doses, lack of coordination, convulsions, coma, and death from respiratory failure. Fortunately, the plant is not particularly conspicuous and seldom causes poisoning in humans. Browsing animals such as pigs, however, have been fatally poisoned from box hedge clippings, and in one instance, aquarium fish were killed when branches were placed in the tank as decoration.

Notes. Although quite toxic, box is usually avoided by animals because of its disagreeable odor and acrid taste. It is sometimes confused with *Paxistima myrsinites* (Oregon boxleaf, or false box), a low, evergreen shrub native to western North America. This latter shrub, often used in floral decorations, is related to the poisonous burningbushes and spindletrees (*Euonymus* spp.) but has not itself been implicated as poisonous.

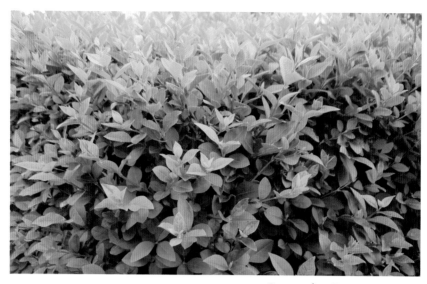

Common box (*Buxus sempervirens*).

Two other ornamentals from the boxwood family, Japanese spurge (*Pachysandra terminalis*) and sweet box (*Sarcococca hookeriana*), also contain steroidal alkaloids and should be considered suspect.

daphnes

Daphne mezereum and related spp.
mezereum family (Thymelaeaceae)

Quick check. Deciduous shrub with simple, alternate leaves; purple or white, fragrant flowers appear in spring before the leaves; scarlet, or occasionally yellow, single-seeded, berry-like fruits. Entire plant, especially the attractive fruits, is highly toxic; fruits may be fatal even if only a few are eaten.

Description. *Daphne mezereum* (paradise plant, mezereon, spurge olive) is a deciduous shrub up to 1.2 m (4 ft.) high, with simple, alternate, bright green leaves 5–8 cm (2–3 in.) long. The small flowers are fragrant, lilac-purple or sometimes white, growing in clusters and appearing in spring before the leaves. They are funnel-shaped and four-lobed, flaring at the mouth. The fruits are attractive, scarlet or yellow berry-like drupes. A related shrub, spurgelaurel or daphne laurel (*D. laureola*), has dark green, leathery, evergreen leaves, yellowish green, scented flowers, and bluish black fruits.

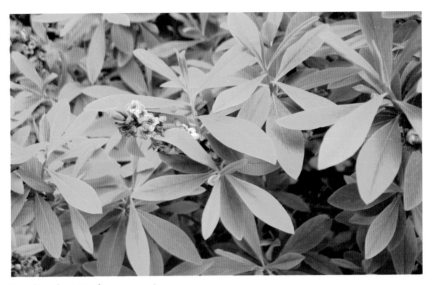

Paradise plant (*Daphne mezereum*).

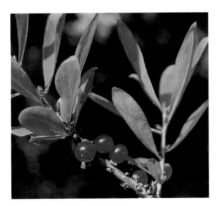

Paradise plant fruits.

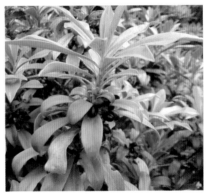

Spurgelaurel (*Daphne laureola*).

Occurrence. A native of Eurasia, paradise plant is cultivated as an ornamental throughout much of North America and occurs as a garden escape in the northeastern states and eastern Canada. Spurgelaurel and other *Daphne* species are also widely grown as ornamentals and are sometimes found as escapes.

Toxicity. All parts of daphnes, particularly the bark and the berry-like fruits, are toxic, due to an acrid, irritant sap. Most of the daphnetoxins, the toxic compounds found in the bark, are esters with a diterpenoid (daphnane) skeleton. Several other poisonous compounds are present, including daph-nin, a lactone glycoside, and its related product, daphnetin. Toxins restricted to the fruits include mezerein, a compound related to phorbols.

Chewing the bark, flowers, or fruits causes painful blistering of the lips, mouth, and throat, with salivation, thirst, and inability to eat or drink, fol-lowed by swelling of the eyelids and nostrils, intense burning and ulcer-ation of the digestive tract, vomiting, bloody diarrhea, weakness, head-aches, and in severe cases, delirium, convulsions, coma, and death. Eating only a few fruits can be fatal to a child. The sap of daphne may cause severe skin irritation and ulceration, and the poison may enter the body through skin contact.

Notes. Reference to daphne as a poisonous plant is found in the writings of the early Greek herbalist Dioscorides. Cases of daphne poisoning in North America are rare, but the brightly colored fruits and sweet-smelling flow-ers may attract young children. Since only a few berries are enough to kill a child, people growing *Daphne* in conspicuous places should take care to remove the berries or restrict access to young children.

pieris, Japanese

Pieris japonica
heather family (Ericaceae)

Quick check. Low to tall shrub with simple leathery leaves, often reddish when young, and dense sprays of white (or pinkish), urn-shaped flowers; occasionally fatal to children.

Description. Evergreen shrub, rarely as high as 10 m (30 ft.). The leaves are simple, leathery, smooth, toothed, and up to 8 cm (3 in.) long. The young leaves are often scarlet or pinkish, clustered in dense, showy sprays. The flowers are white or pinkish and urn-shaped, borne in dense clusters. The fruits are small five-parted capsules.

Occurrence. This shrub is native to Japan. Many are planted as ornamentals in North American gardens, including a dwarf bonsai cultivar and one with variegated leaves. There are several other species, including two native to North America. All should be considered dangerous.

Toxicity. Like many other plants in the heather family, Japanese pieris con-tains grayanotoxins, toxic diterpenoids that are derivatives of acetyl-

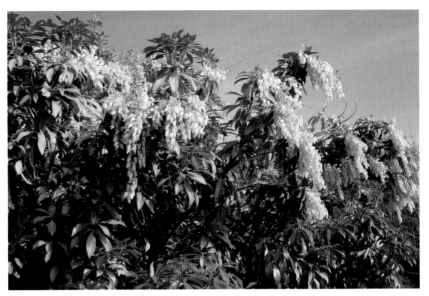

Japanese pieris (*Pieris japonica*).

andromedol. The leaves, and even honey made from the flower nectar, are toxic. Symptoms begin with a burning sensation in the mouth, followed by salivation, copious tears, runny nose, vomiting, stomach cramps, diarrhea, and "prickly" skin after several hours. Headache, dim vision, weakness, and slow heartbeat, followed by severe hypotension, coma, and convulsions may also occur. Fatalities in children eating the leaves have been reported.

Notes. Japanese pieris is related to several other poisonous shrubs with similar toxins and symptoms, including rhododendrons and azaleas, and sheep laurel, mountain laurel, and relatives.

privet, European
Ligustrum vulgare
olive family (Oleaceae)

Quick check. Deciduous (sometimes evergreen) shrub and hedge plant with medium-sized leaves, small, white, clustered flowers, and small, shiny black berries. Leaves and berries potentially, but rarely, fatal.

Description. Densely growing hedge plant or open shrub up to 5 m (16 ft.) tall, with smooth bark, slender branches, and young shoots having a light covering of hairs. The more trimming the shrubs receive, the denser their branches. The leaves, usually 3–6 cm (1–2.5 in.) long, dark green above, lighter beneath, are borne in pairs. They are simple and elliptical, with short stalks and smooth edges. Although classed as deciduous, the plant is partially evergreen in some varieties. The flowers, which appear in summer, are small, creamy white, tubular, and fragrant, in dense pyramidal clusters. The tightly clustered berries are dark blue or black, and shiny, the size of small peas. They may remain on the shrubs over the winter, making them conspicuous to children after the leaves have fallen.

Occurrence. Native to southern England, European privet is one of the most widely cultivated hedge plants in North America and is also grown singly as an ornamental shrub. It is sometimes found as a garden escape in woodlands near settled areas. Its many cultivars offer dwarf habit, variegated leaves, and small leaves.

Toxicity. It is not clear whether the bitter iridoid substances or alkaloids known to be present in this species are in quantities sufficient to cause poisoning. Occasional fatalities, preceded by severe gastrointestinal irritation, with vomiting and diarrhea, and convulsions, were reported in the past, but there have been few if any substantiated cases of privet-caused deaths within the last century. In fact, human poisoning is so rare, it is uncertain whether it occurs from children eating the berries or adults chewing on the

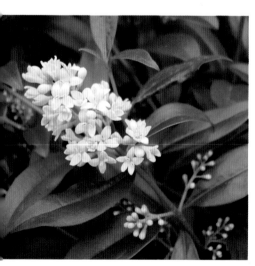

European privet (*Ligustrum vulgare*).

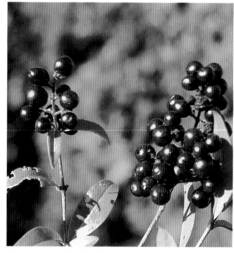

European privet berries.

leaves. Animal poisoning, usually from eating the hedge trimmings, is also unusual; however, when it does occur, it is often severe or even fatal. Privet may also cause severe dermatitis in people trimming hedges or shrubs.

Notes. Other species, including California privet (*Ligustrum ovalifolium*) and Japanese privet (*L. japonicum*), are commonly grown as ornamentals and should also be considered potentially toxic.

rhododendrons and azaleas

Rhododendron spp.
heather family (Ericaceae)

Quick check. Evergreen shrubs or small trees (mostly rhododendrons), or deciduous shrubs (mostly azaleas), with simple leaves and large, showy, bell-shaped or funnel-formed flowers of various colors; leaves, flowers, and flower nectar toxic, but rarely fatal for humans.

Description. This large genus of evergreen or deciduous shrubs, or rarely small trees, with prominent, tightly scaled buds, is generally divided into two groups: rhododendrons, most with leathery, evergreen leaves, and azaleas, most with thinner, deciduous leaves. The leaves of both are short-stalked, simple, and alternate, and the showy flowers are large, bell-shaped or funnel-formed, and borne in dense clusters. They come in many colors: white, cream, pink, mauve, red, orange, yellow, and purple. The fruits are dry capsules containing numerous tiny seeds.

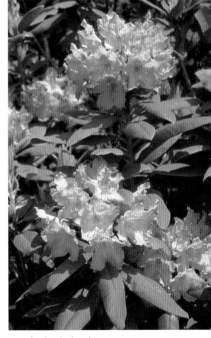

Occurrence. The approximately 800 species of *Rhododendron* occur naturally in temperate regions of the northern hemisphere and in the mountains of Southeast Asia and Australia. More than 25 species are native to North America. Rhododendrons and azaleas are extremely popular as ornamentals in North American gardens, and the hybridization of various species is a major horticultural industry, yielding innumerable cultivars.

Pacific rhododendron
(*Rhododendron macrophyllum*).

Toxicity. The leaves, flowers, pollen, and nectar of many *Rhododendron* species contain several grayanotoxins, all of which are derived from aceylandromedol. One of these toxic diterpenoids, grayanotoxin 1, or rhodotoxin, is prevalent in rhododendron flower nectar, and has caused poisoning of bees and the honey they produce from it. Human poisoning from eating the plant itself is unusual but has been reported in children who chewed the leaves. Symptoms of poisoning include initial burning of the mouth, salivation, watering eyes, and runny nose, followed up to several hours later by vomiting, convulsions, headache, "prickly" skin, muscular weakness, drowsiness, slow and irregular heartbeat, very low blood pressure, and paralysis. Chronic poisoning, from drinking tea of rhododendrons or their relatives, or using rhododendron honey, may occur, with persistent low blood pressure and episodes of high blood pressure.

Notes. As early as 400 B.C. a report was made of Greek soldiers being poisoned by wild rhododendron honey. The Turkish species *Rhododendron luteum* and *R. ponticum* have been implicated in cases of honey poisoning (Sütlüpmar et al. 1993). Sir Edmund Hillary complained of being mildly poisoned by tea sweetened with rhododendron honey in the early stages of the first successful ascent of Mt. Everest. Bees may also be affected; in parts of Scotland, ornamental rhododendron plantings have made beekeeping uneconomic because of serious loss of bees in the spring from rhododendron nectar. Notably, however, the level of toxicity in rhododendrons is variable, and some species evidently do not contain grayanotoxins. Labrador tea (*Ledum palustre*) is closely related to *Rhododendron* but is apparently safe in moderation (see Appendix 2).

VINES

clematis

Clematis spp.
buttercup family (Ranunculaceae)

Quick check. Trailing or climbing woody vines (occasionally erect) with usually compound leaves and showy flowers of various colors; the plants contain a severe irritant; seldom fatal.

Description. Most clematis, also known as virgin's bower or leather flower, are woody vines, climbing by clasping leafstalks; some few are erect, herbaceous perennials. The leaves are opposite, and usually divided into three or more segments. The flowers range from small to large and very showy, with colors from white to pink to reddish to purple. Some are urn-shaped or bell-shaped; most open flat at maturity, revealing numerous stamens. The colored portions are actually sepals; petals are lacking. In some species, the flowers are clustered, but most ornamental types have large, singly borne flowers. The densely clustered fruits are small and single-seeded, each with a long, feathery style.

Occurrence. Over 50 *Clematis* species occur in North America. Species grow wild in many regions of the continent, but the plants are usually encountered as cultivated ornamental vines on walls, fences, and trellises. Many horticultural varieties are available, with large attractive flowers in a wide range of colors.

Toxicity. Clematis and many other plants in the buttercup family contain an irritant compound, protoanemonin, in the fresh leaves and sap. Produced from a glycoside, ranunculin, protoanemonin is a highly reactive lactone that binds with sulfydryl groups. It can cause irritation and blistering of the skin with handling of the plant, and, if the fresh leaves are eaten, it causes intense burning and inflammation of the mouth and digestive tract, with profuse salivation, inflamed eyes, blistering, and ulceration, followed by abdominal cramps, weakness, vomiting of blood, and bloody diarrhea. The kidneys may also be affected; initially, there may be excessive, painful urination with the presence of blood in the urine, followed by a depletion in urine output. The victim may also feel dizzy and confused and, in severe cases, suffer fainting and convulsions. Fortunately, the initial burning of the mouth usually precludes eating large, or fatal doses. Animals are occasionally poisoned from eating clematis, but because of the acrid taste and irritation of the mouth caused by the plant, fatalities are not common.

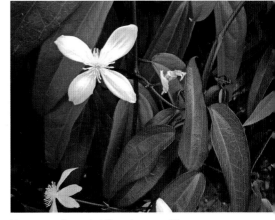

Notes. Protoanemonin is present only in fresh plant material; drying or cooking apparently deactivates it.

Evergreen clematis (*Clematis armandii*).

ivy, English
Hedera helix
ginseng family (Araliaceae)

Quick check. Evergreen vine of gardens and woods, with dark green or mottled, leathery leaves, usually three- to five-lobed; flowers are small, greenish, clustered; fruits pea-sized and black. Leaves and berries moderately poisonous, seldom fatal. Keep small children away from berries.

Description. English ivy is a creeping or climbing evergreen vine with many short, clinging aerial roots along the stems. Leaves leathery, pungent-smelling when crushed, usually dark green and three- to five-lobed, but there are cultivars with leaf form varying from simple shield-shaped to long, pointed star-shaped, and leaf color from dark green to variegated white, cream, or yellow. The leaves are 4–10 cm (1.5–4 in.) across. The flowers are whitish to greenish and small, in rounded clusters, with male and female flowers on separate plants. The fruits are round, black, bitter-tasting, pea-sized berries, each containing three to five seeds.

Occurrence. Native to Europe and the United Kingdom, this ivy is widely planted as a ground and wall cover throughout North America. A common garden escape and often invasive, growing in patches on the ground and climbing trees in woods near settled areas. Many cultivars are grown as houseplants.

Toxicity. The entire plant contains triterpene saponins—hederasaponins A, B, and C—which undergo partial hydrolysis with loss of sugars, form-

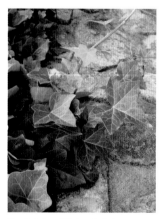

English ivy (*Hedera helix*).

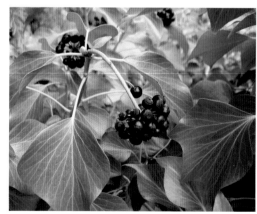

English ivy fruits.

ing hederins, toxic saponin glycosides. The berries occasionally poison children who eat them in quantity. Symptoms include vomiting, diarrhea, labored breathing, excitability, convulsions, and coma, but there have been few recent cases with such drastic results. The leaves are harmful to browsing livestock if large amounts are eaten, with symptoms of vomiting, diarrhea, spasms, staggering, and paralysis; animals usually recover after a few days. The sap can cause dermatitis, sometimes with severe blistering and inflammation.

Notes. A related plant of the eastern United States, Hercules' club, or devil's walkingstick (*Aralia spinosa*), has black berries that may also be poisonous. The prickly red-colored berries of another relative, devilsclub (*Oplopanax horridus*), are also reputedly poisonous or at least strongly laxative. This latter plant is widely used in the traditional medicine of western indigenous peoples. These species and English ivy are all related to ginseng (*Panax* spp.), a well-known Chinese herbal medicine and tonic. English ivy extracts have been shown in clinical trials to be beneficial in treating childhood bronchial asthma (Milot 2004).

morning-glory, beach moonflower, and grannyvine

Ipomoea tricolor and *I. violacea*
morning-glory family (Convolvulaceae)

Quick check. Annual or perennial vines with large, showy, flaring flowers. Seeds hallucinogenic, potentially dangerous to children, but not fatal.

Description. Vigorous annual or perennial vines without hairs on the stem or leaves. The twining stems grow up to 3 m (10 ft.) high. The leaves are heart-shaped, usually 10–25 cm (4–10 in.) long. The funnel-shaped flowers are large and showy, up to 10 cm (4 in.) across, varying in color from pale to sky blue, blue-and-white striped, pink, and rose (all with paler centers), or white, depending on the variety. Each flower lasts only one day. The fruiting

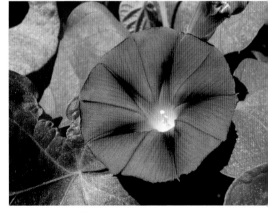

Morning-glory (*Ipomoea* sp.).

capsules contain numerous seeds. *Ipomoea tricolor* and *I. violacea* are very similar and sometimes considered synonymous.

Occurrence. Morning-glory cultivars are often grown in North America as ornamental vines. Several, including 'Heavenly Blue', 'Pearly Gates', 'Flying Saucers', 'Wedding Bells', 'Summer Skies', and 'Blue Star', have attained popularity because of their hallucinogenic effects.

Toxicity. The seeds of various cultivars of *Ipomoea tricolor* and *I. violacea* (but not necessarily of other species of the genus *Ipomoea*) contain amides of lysergic acid, which are similar to but not nearly as potent as LSD in their hallucinogenic effects. They are sometimes eaten or drunk as an infusion by those seeking a high. Ingestion of the seeds can cause nausea and hallucinations. Their main danger is when small children ingest relatively large quantities, which is, fortunately, not a common occurrence. Additionally, those wishing to experiment with these seeds should be warned that some suppliers dust them with a noxious chemical fungicide.

Notes. The seeds of morning-glory vines and some relatives have been used for centuries in Central America and elsewhere for their hallucinogenic effects. Characteristic visions of the "little people," common to those who use morning-glory seeds or any of a number of other hallucinogens, may well account for the worldwide traditions of elves, leprechauns, gnomes, and other tiny people of folk tales.

sweetpea

Lathyrus odoratus and related spp.
pea family (Fabaceae)

Quick check. Herbaceous climbing vine with showy, clustered, fragrant flowers in a variety of colors, and narrow seedpods resembling peapods; seedlings, pods, and seeds cause paralysis and may be fatal if eaten in large quantities.

Description. Herbaceous annual vine, with hairy, winged or strongly angled stems up to 2 m (6 ft.) or more high. The leaves consist of a single pair of elliptic to lance-shaped or oval leaves, with well-developed, branching tendrils at the tip. The flowers are large, showy, and fragrant, borne in clusters of two to five on long stalks growing from the leaf axils. Occurring in a wide variety of colors, from red to white to dark purple or bluish, the flowers are typical of the pea family, with a large upper petal, or banner, two outer petals at the sides (wings), and a keel of two inner petals, joined together. The pea-like seedpods are narrow, elongated, and hairy, containing four to ten pea-like (this time dangerously so) seeds. There are many other *Lathyrus* species, most with pinkish or purple flowers, some white- or yellow-flowered. All and all their parts should be considered inedible in large quantities.

Occurrence. This attractive herbaceous Mediterranean plant, originating from Sicily east to Crete, is widely grown in North American flower gardens, and its fragrant blooms are popular as cut flowers. It occasionally also occurs as a garden escape. There are many wild relatives of the sweetpea, some native and some naturalized from other regions.

Toxicity. Sweetpea and its relatives contain numerous lathyrogens, toxic amino acids, and their derivatives, notably beta-aminopropionitrile. The highest concentrations are in the seedlings and pods, and, especially, the seeds. Sweetpea seedlings also contain isoxazolin-5-one derivatives, which makes them even more poisonous than dry seeds. Lathyrogens have been responsible for lathyrism, a disease characterized by paralysis, weak heartbeat, shallow breathing, muscular tremors, and convulsions in both humans and animals who have eaten the seeds or plants of sweetpea or other *Lathyrus* species. Animals fed the seeds have also developed severe skeletal abnormalities, dilation and rupture of arteries, and damage to connective tissue. Fortunately, poisoning occurs only after large quantities of seeds or plants are eaten; when small quantities are eaten, the effects are said to be negligible.

Notes. The pea-like seeds of sweetpea are commonly eaten by children, and poison control centers are frequently contacted about them. They are apparently not dangerous unless large quantities are eaten, but nevertheless, children should be warned against them.

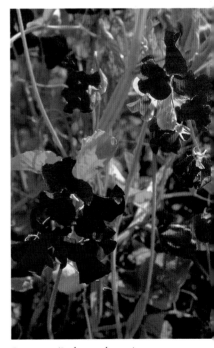

Sweetpea (*Lathyrus odoratus*).

Virginia creeper

Parthenocissus quinquefolia
grape family (Vitaceae)

Quick check. Woody vine with palmately divided, compound leaves and small, blue or blackish, clustered fruits; berries toxic, suspected of causing fatalities in children.

Description. Virginia creeper, or American ivy, is a woody vine, climbing by many-branched tendrils, with long-stalked, alternate, compound leaves divided into three to six radiating leaflets, each pointed and toothed along the margins. The flowers are small, greenish, and clustered, and the fruits are small, blue or blackish, grape-like berries. Woodbine (*Parthenocissus vitacea*) can be distinguished by having few-branched tendrils.

Occurrence. Native to woods of eastern and central North America. Virginia creeper grows on walls, fences, and trees throughout much of the United States and southern Canada. It and its several cultivars are commonly grown for their decorative foliage, which turns scarlet in the fall.

Toxicity. This plant has been implicated in several cases of poisoning, and at least one fatality of a child who ate the berries. The actual toxins are unknown (Frohne and Pfänder 2005). In one study, however, a guinea pig fed 12 berries died within 36 hours, and parakeets have also been poisoned from the berries. The plants also contain raphides, irritant needle-like crystals similar to those of members of the arum family, which can cause irritation and swelling of tissues of the skin, mouth, tongue, or eyes. Symptoms of poisoning include nausea, vomiting, diarrhea, and feeling a need for urination or a bowel movement.

Notes. Virginia creeper is sometimes confused with poison ivy, but the latter has three leaflets per leaf. Another potentially toxic species, common in gardens as an ornamental vine, is Boston ivy (*Parthenocissus tricuspidata*); it too contains irritant raphides and has simple, glossy, three-lobed

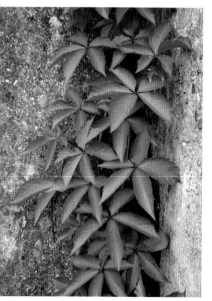

Virginia creeper
(*Parthenocissus quinquefolia*).

(sometimes three-parted) leaves. *Parthenocissus* is in the same family as grape (*Vitis vinifera*), whose fruits and leaves are edible.

wisterias

Wisteria spp.
pea family (Fabaceae)

Quick check. Woody vines with pinnate leaves and purplish to white pea-like flowers in hanging clusters; entire plant, especially seeds and seedpods, toxic but seldom fatal.

Description. Woody, deciduous climbing vines, occasionally grown as shrubs or trees. The leaves are pinnately compound, and the fragrant, pea-like flowers are produced in large, showy, hanging clusters. They are usually mauve to blue-violet, but white- and pink-flowered varieties also exist. The hanging, flattened fruiting pods are bean-like and smooth or velvety, depending on the species. The seeds are dark brown, oval, and flattened.

Occurrence. Several *Wisteria* species occur in North America, including the native *W. frutescens*, growing in rich woods and around wooded swamps of the eastern United States. The major cultivated types, Chinese wisteria (*W. sinensis*) and Japanese wisteria (*W. floribunda*), are introduced from Asia and are often planted as twining ornamentals around patios, trellises, and walls,

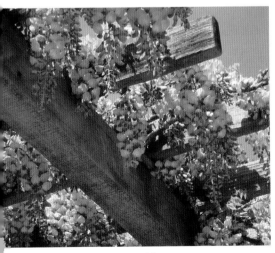

Wisteria (*Wisteria sinensis*).

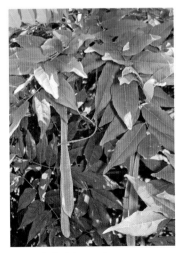

Wisteria fruiting pods.

or sometimes grown as bushy specimens on lawns. The cultivated species are common garden escapes, especially in the southeastern United States.

Toxicity. All parts of the plant, especially the seeds and seedpods, are poisonous. Wisterias contain toxic lectins; these agglutinate red blood cells and interfere with protein synthesis. The same toxins occur in black locust (*Robinia pseudoacacia*) and several other genera in the pea family. Other toxins include a glycoside, wistarin. The seeds are the most notorious in toxicity. Eating one or two seeds, which resemble dark brown lima beans, can cause serious illness in a child. There are dozens of records of poisoning of children from these seeds, with symptoms of serious gastrointestinal problems: nausea, abdominal pains, and repeated vomiting, sometimes with mild diarrhea. Ingesting large amounts of the bark has caused hypovolemic shock from fluid loss. Even in severe cases, however, recovery is usually complete in 24 hours, but headache and giddiness can continue for days.

Notes. Wisteria flowers were eaten in China (Hedrick 1972); however, they should be considered as toxic as the rest of the plant until proven otherwise.

HERBACEOUS PLANTS

autumn crocus
Colchicum autumnale
lily family (Liliaceae)

Quick check. Showy autumn-flowering corm plants with long, tubular, mauve to purplish flowers; entire plant highly toxic.

Description. A perennial growing from a corm up to 5 cm (2 in.) across. The leaves are glossy and bright green, up to 30 cm (12 in.) long, and 2.5 cm (1 in.) or more wide. They are produced in the spring then die back before the flowers emerge, in the late summer and fall. The flowers, usually produced in quantity from many clustered corms, are showy, long, tubular at the base, and pale purple (or sometimes almost white). The flowers die down soon after opening, and an oval fruit is formed at the base of the flower tube, close to the ground, where it remains until the following spring. The fruiting stalk then elongates, and the ripened capsules appear above the leaves, splitting open to reveal many small seeds.

Occurrence. Commonly grown in gardens and as a potted bulb indoors.

Toxicity. All parts of the plant, particularly the corm and seeds, are toxic, containing the pseudo-alkaloid drugs colchicine and colchiceine. Colchicine affects the nervous system and prevents normal cell division. Symptoms of poisoning include burning pain in the mouth and throat, intense thirst, nausea, and violent vomiting. Severe abdominal pain and profuse, persistent diarrhea, followed by lethargy, low blood pressure, shock due to fluid loss, and collapse, have been reported. Kidney damage (with scanty and blood-stained urine), convulsions, coma, and death from respiratory failure may occur. Colchicine is slow to be absorbed, and signs of poisoning may be delayed for two to six hours, or even as long as 48 hours. Temporary hair loss may occur after about two weeks. All classes of animals are susceptible to colchicine poisoning. Children and young animals may be poisoned from colchicine-contaminated milk.

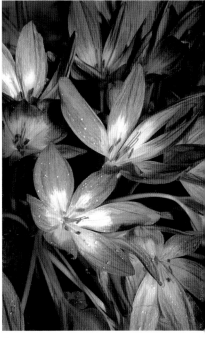

Autumn crocus
(*Colchicum autumnale*).

Notes. Frohne and Pfänder (2005) describe numerous cases of colchicine poisoning, including several that were fatal. In Europe, people often confuse autumn crocus leaves with those of ramsons, or bear garlic (*Allium ursinum*), with occasional deadly results. Autumn crocus has also been implicated in many suicides, and in one notorious murder: a former lecturer in pharmacy added colchicine to his wife's favorite currant liqueur, and she became ill and died four days later.

Autumn crocus is the commercial source of the drug colchicine, which is used as a suppressant for gout and rheumatism. *Colchicum* is grown commercially in central and southern Europe and northern Africa. The genus name comes from Colchis on the Black Sea, where the plant is abundant. Autumn crocus should not be confused with the spring-blooming crocuses of the genus *Crocus*; these belong to the iris family (Iridaceae).

belladonna

Atropa bella-donna
nightshade family (Solanaceae)

Quick check. A branching, herbaceous perennial with oval, pointed leaves, tubular purplish flowers, and black, shining berries. Entire plant, particularly berries, contains toxic alkaloids; potentially fatal, especially in children.

Description. Belladonna, or deadly nightshade, is a smooth, or slightly hairy, herbaceous perennial with upright, branching stems up to 1.5 m (5 ft.) high. The leaves are short-stalked and usually arranged alternately or in pairs, with one leaf much smaller than the other. Generally oval, and pointed, they grow up to 20 cm (8 in.) long. The flowers, borne singly from the leaf axils or forks of branches, are tubular, up to 2.5 cm (1 in.) or more long, widening into five lobes at the mouth. They are commonly dull brownish purple to pale bluish purple, violet, or greenish. The fruit, at first green and then red, ripens to a shiny, black or dark purple berry partially enclosed by the five-lobed calyx.

Occurrence. A native of Europe and Asia Minor, belladonna is sometimes grown as a garden ornamental and herbal plant in North America.

Toxicity. The entire plant contains several toxic components, including varying quantities of tropane alkaloids: atropine, scopolamine, and hyoscyamine. Atropine is found throughout the plant, scopolamine in the roots,

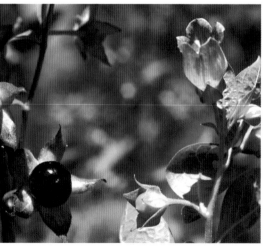

Belladonna (*Atropa bella-donna*).

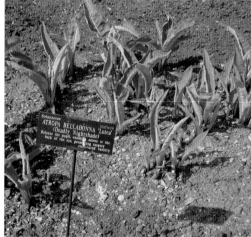

Young plants of yellow-flowered belladonna (*Atropa bella-donna* var. *lutea*).

and hycoscyamine in the flowers, fruits, and seeds. Most cases of human poisoning involve children eating the berries, but adults also occasionally consume concoctions of the leaves or the berries, sometimes mistaking them for edible types such as bilberries. Symptoms of poisoning include abdominal pain, vomiting, dilated pupils, and rapid pulse. Hallucinations sometimes occur, especially in children. In severe cases, convulsions, coma, and death from respiratory failure may result. Fatalities are rare, but as few as three berries have been reported to be lethal to a child. Animals seldom eat the plant, but deaths in livestock are known.

Notes. The common and species name come from the Italian *bella* ("beautiful") and *donna* ("lady"): women of fashion used to drop juice from belladonna into their eyes to dilate their pupils and make them more attractive. The leaves and fleshy root of belladonna, and the alkaloids they contain, have been valued for centuries as painkillers and sedatives. When used in correct doses, belladonna tropane alkaloids have many applications—for example, controlling spasms of the urinary tract and excess motor activity of the digestive tract, correction of hypotension associated with slow heart rate, and dilation of the pupil of the eye for ophthalmic diagnosis and treatment. The same class of alkaloids is found in other members of the nightshade family, including black henbane, black nightshade, and jimsonweed. All should be considered highly toxic. There are instances of botanical gardens having to remove belladonna plants from their exhibits to prevent access to them by those wishing to commit suicide.

cardinalflower
Lobelia cardinalis and related spp.
lobelia family (Lobeliaceae)

Quick check. Tall herbaceous perennial with showy, bright red flowers; entire plant toxic, potentially fatal.

Description. Cardinalflower is a green or reddish-colored, sometimes branching, herbaceous perennial growing up to 1 m (3 ft.) or more tall. If cut or bruised, the plants exude a white sap and give off an unpleasant acrid odor. The leaves are alternate and lance-shaped, with undulating, slightly toothed margins, and bases running down the stem. The flowers are borne in dense, terminal clusters; they are bright red (occasionally pure white), and irregu-

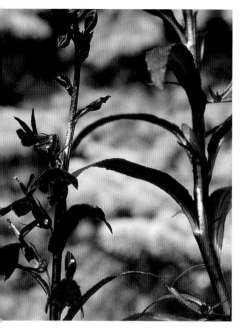

Cardinalflower hybrid.

lar, with a tubular portion, a two-cleft upper lip, and a three-cleft lower lip. The fruits are two-celled capsules containing numerous seeds. Several cultivars of cardinalflower are grown, some with deep red foliage.

Occurrence. Native to moist areas of central, eastern, and southern North America, cardinalflowers are often grown as garden ornamentals for their brilliant red flowers.

Toxicity. The entire plant is poisonous, containing a mixture of pyridine alkaloids, particularly alpha lobeline, which are chemically and functionally similar to nicotine in tobacco. Symptoms of poisoning include nausea, vomiting, salivation, abdominal pain, diarrhea, headache, sweating, dilation of the pupils, lack of coordination, confusion, paralysis, lowered temperature, initial high blood pressure followed by low blood pressure, rapid or irregular heartbeat, and in severe cases, convulsions, collapse, coma, and death. The sap can irritate the skin. Livestock are also susceptible to poisoning by this plant.

Notes. Cardinalflower, like Indian-tobacco (*Lobelia inflata*), was used in American folk medicine for a variety of ailments, including syphilis and worms; however, since overdoses resulted in severe illness and sometimes death, its use was discontinued. There are several other species of *Lobelia*, including great blue lobelia (*L. siphilitica*), and many short or trailing, blue-flowered cultivars commonly grown in borders and in hanging baskets. All should be considered toxic.

celandine

Chelidonium majus
poppy family (Papaveraceae)

Quick check. Yellow-flowered herb, with reddish, acrid juice; entire plant poisonous, occasionally fatal; juice may irritate the skin.

Description. An erect, branched biennial or perennial herb, with smooth or slightly hairy stems up to 1.2 m (4 ft.) high and leaves deeply divided into oval segments with irregularly scalloped edges. The flowers, borne throughout the summer in loose, terminal clusters, are bright yellow, four-petalled, with greenish yellow stamens, and up to 2.5 cm (1 in.) across. Some varieties are double-flowered. The elongated fruiting capsules contain white-tipped black seeds. When cut, the stems exude a yellow-orange latex, or sap, which turns red upon exposure to the air.

Occurrence. A native of Eurasia, celandine is found as a garden plant in various parts of North America and also occurs as an escape in some localities, particularly around old gardens.

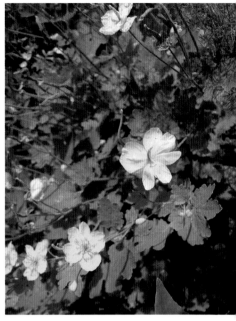

Celandine (*Chelidonium majus*).

Toxicity. This plant contains many toxic isoquinoline alkaloids, most notably coptisine, chelidonine, and berberine, all of which are chemically related to papaverine, found in poppy species. Fortunately, the plant is rarely eaten because of its pungent, unpleasant smell and acrid taste. However, children have been poisoned from it, and deaths in both humans and livestock have been reported. Symptoms may not develop for 12 or more hours. They include drowsiness, headache, salivation, and thirst, followed in about six hours by fever, vomiting, diarrhea, and in severe cases, coma and heart failure. The seed capsules are especially potent. An entire herd of cattle in Britain was severely poisoned, some individuals fatally, from eating the plants at the fruiting stage. The latex can cause irritation and blistering of the skin.

Notes. In the United Kingdom, this plant is referred to as greater celandine, and the unrelated *Ranunculus ficaria* (fig buttercup) is called lesser celandine. Greater celandine is also known as rock poppy, or wart wort (alluding to the former use of the latex to eliminate warts and corns).

corncockle

Agrostemma githago
pink family (Caryophyllaceae)

Quick check. Erect, grayish colored annual with thin, pointed leaves and showy purplish pink flowers; entire plant contains saponins; seeds can contaminate grain; potentially fatal in large quantities.

Description. An erect annual, 30 cm (1 ft.) to 1 m (3 ft.) tall, with a simple or sparsely branched stem and narrow, pointed leaves. The stem and leaves are covered with white hairs, giving the plant a grayish green coloring. The leaves, up to 12 cm (5 in.) long, arise in pairs, clasping the stem at their base. The purplish pink, five-petalled flowers are borne singly at the ends of the stems, and are about 2.5 cm (1 in.) across, with a bulbous base and narrow, pointed sepals that extend beyond the petals. The fruiting capsules dry to a light brown and open by five teeth to reveal many black seeds, each about 3 mm (0.1 in.) long, with a pitted surface.

Occurrence. Native to Europe, corncockle is widely established in North America as a weed of cultivated grain fields and wastelands. It is sometimes grown in gardens as an ornamental.

Toxicity. The entire plant contains soap-like saponins. These do not dissolve in water but remain suspended, giving the water a frothing or lathering action. The active compounds are githagoside and other triterpenoid saponins. When the seeds contaminate grain, they can cause a chronic form of poisoning, githagism, with symptoms of drowsiness, yawning, weight loss,

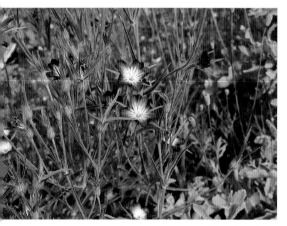

Agrostemma githago. Allan Armitage

digestive disturbances, weakness, and even death if the contaminated diet is continued. Acute poisoning is rare, because the plant and its seeds are bitter-tasting, and highly contaminated flour has a grayish color and unpleasant odor as well as a bad taste. Acute symptoms of poisoning include severe stomach pain, vomiting, diarrhea, dizziness, weakness, and slow breathing. If the aglycone gypsogenin enters the bloodstream, it causes the breakdown of red blood cells. Animals of all types, particularly poultry, are susceptible to corncockle poisoning, especially when the seeds contaminate their food.

Notes. All members of the pink family contain saponins, but few except corncockle have been associated with human poisoning. Bouncingbet (*Saponaria officinalis*) and cow soapwort (*Vaccaria hispanica*) are two relatives notable for their high saponin content. They should be treated as poisonous, although few documented cases of poisoning implicate them. The main danger from corncockle is in the seeds contaminating grain, especially wheat: since highly contaminated grain cannot be sold, this weed has caused severe economic losses to North American grain growers. However, with modern agricultural methods and herbicides, corncockle is not as common as it once was.

daffodils

Narcissus spp.
lily family (Liliaceae)

Quick check. Showy, yellow- or whitish-flowered spring bulbs; entire plants toxic, but seldom fatal.

Description. There are many varieties of daffodils, or jonquils. They grow from onion-like bulbs and have long, narrow, often somewhat fleshy basal leaves; the showy flowers are borne singly or in small clusters at the end of tall, erect, fleshy stalks. The flowers are usually yellow, or whitish, with a characteristic flaring tube emerging from the center of six spreading petals. The tube in some cultivars is bright orange. Some are very fragrant.

Occurrence. The wild precursors of the many cultivated forms of *Narcissus* are native to Europe and North Africa. These spring-flowering plants are grown in gardens throughout temperate North America and are also found indoors as cut flowers and forced winter bulbs.

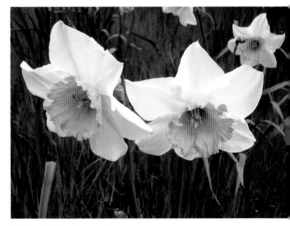

Daffodil (*Narcissus* sp.).

Toxicity. The entire plant, particularly the outer scale leaves of the bulbs, contains a rich diversity of toxic alkaloids, including narcissine, lycorine, and galanthamine. The bulbs are sometimes mistaken for onions and eaten raw or cooked. They cause dizziness, abdominal pain, nausea, vomiting, and sometimes diarrhea. Trembling, convulsions, and death may occur if large quantities are consumed, but usually recovery occurs within a few hours.

Notes. In the Netherlands, cattle were fatally poisoned after being fed *Narcissus* bulbs during World War II food shortages. *Hippeastrum* spp. (amaryllis) and *Crinum* spp. (cape lily), flowering bulbs of the same family, are widely grown in gardens in warm areas and potted indoors throughout North America; they are reported to contain narcissine and related alkaloids, and should also be considered dangerous. *Tulipa gesneriana* is another popular species of the lily family that is poisonous; it and other tulip species are known to cause allergic skin irritation, especially to those who handle the bulbs, and can also cause gastrointestinal upset if the bulbs are eaten; but such poisoning is rare and no fatalities are reported.

foxglove, purple

Digitalis purpurea
figwort family (Scrophulariaceae)

Quick check. Biennial with large, oval basal leaves and tall flowering stalks with many purplish (or white) tubular flowers, maturing from bottom to top of the stalk; entire plant contains potent glycosides affecting the heart; potentially fatal.

Description. An erect biennial (or occasionally perennial) herb, with flowering stem 1.5 m (5 ft.) or more high. In the first year the leaves form a rosette at ground level. The basal leaves are large, oval, pointed at the tip, prominently veined, and finely toothed around the margins. Especially on the undersides, they are covered with short, soft hairs, giving the plant a grayish green cast. The flowering stems bear leafy bracts similar to, but smaller than, the basal leaves. The flowers are borne in a terminal, many-flowered spike, itself up to 60 cm (2 ft.) long. The flowers are drooping and mature in sequence from bottom to top. They are purplish pink, or sometimes white or yellowish, with a lower, paler colored, projecting lip, which is usually spotted with purple or brown. The fruits are oval capsules, which dry to a light brown and split open to reveal numerous tiny, dark brown seeds.

Occurrence. Purple foxglove is a hardy plant, originating in southern Europe and Central Asia and now widely distributed in North America. It is grown in gardens and is found as an escape along roadsides, in fields, and in burned or logged over areas. It is also cultivated in quantity as a medicinal drug plant.

Toxicity. Purple foxglove contains potent digitaloids, or steroid glycosides, including digitoxin and digitalin. These cardioactive compounds break down in the body to a sugar and a non-sugar component (aglycone). Acting together, they have a direct influence on the muscles of the heart. Even when dried or boiled, foxglove retains its active compounds. Children have been poisoned from eating the flowers, sucking the nectar, or even drinking water from vases containing the flowers. Occasional poisonings in adults occur from misuse of herbal

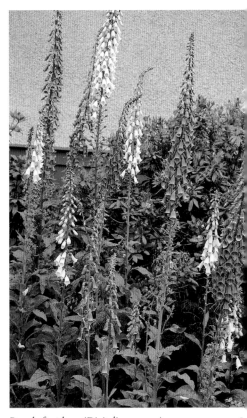

Purple foxglove (*Digitalis purpurea*).

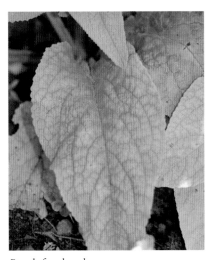

Purple foxglove leaves.

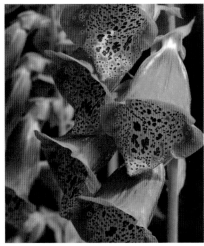

Purple foxglove flowers.

preparations of the plant, misidentification of the plant, or overdoses of digitalis in the form of heart medications.

Symptoms of poisoning include pain in the mouth and throat, nausea, vomiting, abdominal cramps, diarrhea, severe headache, irregular heartbeat and pulse, tremors, and in severe cases, convulsions and death due to cardiac arrest. Animals seldom eat foxglove, but it may be eaten in times of food scarcity or as a hay contaminant, sometimes with fatal results.

Notes. In the United Kingdom and especially Scotland, where foxglove tea was used to treat coughs, colds, and fevers, there were numerous records of fatalities among children through drinking this tea. Purple foxglove leaves closely resemble those of both common borage (*Borago officinalis*) and common comfrey (*Symphytum officinale*), especially when the plants are young. Confusion between foxglove and these plants has resulted in serious poisoning, since some people make herbal teas from borage and comfrey. (Comfrey tea is not recommended, due to the potential presence of liver-damaging pyrrolizidine alkaloids in some forms of comfrey, but those who do drink comfrey tea should learn to distinguish comfrey from foxglove.) Foxglove leaves are finely toothed along the edges, whereas comfrey leaves, though hairy, are smooth-edged. Borage leaves, on the other hand, are toothed like those of foxglove and extremely difficult to distinguish from them in the young stages of these plants.

Digoxin, digitoxin, and other substances isolated from digitalis, are highly important drugs in modern heart treatment, but the doses must be carefully monitored. Of course, people taking these medications should take care to keep them out of reach of children.

hellebore, black

Helleborus niger and related spp.
buttercup family (Ranunculaceae)

Quick check. Winter-blooming herbaceous perennial with deeply divided leaves and large whitish or purplish flowers. Entire plant contains foxglove-like cardiac glycosides; poisoning rare but may be fatal.

Description. Herbaceous perennial with thick, fibrous roots and long-stalked, compound leaves, the segments coarsely toothed. The flowering stems, up to 45 cm (18 in.) high, are simple or forked, bearing small leaves or bracts. The flowers bloom in winter and early spring. They are large and nodding, with five white, pinkish, or dark reddish purple, petal-like sepals. The fruit is a small capsule containing many glossy, black seeds.

Occurrence. Black hellebore, or Christmas rose, is native to Europe, and is widely cultivated. It and related species and their hybrids are grown in gardens throughout temperate North America, valued for their winter interest. In some places plants have naturalized.

Toxicity. Plants in the genus *Helleborus* contain a mixture of toxic compounds, including bufadienolides, saponins, and protoanemonin. In the past, human and animal poisoning frequently occurred from misuse of herbal preparations of hellebores as purgatives, local anaesthetics, or abortives, or to rid the skin of parasites. Because of the health risks, such medicinal use has been largely abandoned, and instances of poisoning by hellebores are rare. Symptoms, which may be delayed depending on the quantity ingested, include pain of the mouth and abdomen, nausea, vomiting, cramps, diarrhea, visual disturbances, loss of appetite, slow heartbeat, and possible abortion in pregnant women. Drinking milk from poisoned cows can cause vomiting and diarrhea.

Notes. Hellebore and its relatives are sometimes confused with another, unrelated plant in the lily family, green false hellebore (*Veratrum viride*), which is also very poisonous. There is also a *Helleborus* species, *H. viridis*, whose common name is green hellebore.

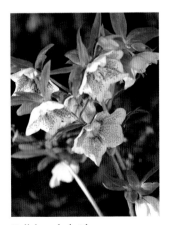

Hellebore hybrid.

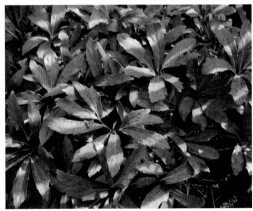

Black hellebore (*Helleborus niger*).

henbane, black

Hyoscyamus niger
nightshade family (Solanaceae)

Quick check. Hairy, herbaceous weed with disagreeable odor, large basal leaves, and funnel-shaped yellowish or mauve flowers borne along upper stems; entire plant toxic, but seldom fatal in humans; dangerous as a medicinal herb.

Description. Hairy, somewhat sticky annual or biennial weed about 60 cm (2 ft.) high, with a woody stem base. The entire plant has a strong, disagreeable smell. The basal leaves are stalked, up to 20 cm (8 in.) long, and with large irregular teeth on the margins. The stem leaves are stalkless, alternate, and unevenly lobed. The flowers, produced singly from the stems just above the leaves, are subtended by leafy bracts. The flowers are funnel-shaped, about 2.5 cm (1 in.) across, and greenish yellow to whitish, or occasionally mauve, conspicuously marked with a network of dark purplish veins. In fruiting, the calyx grows around the fruit and hardens into five pointed spines. The exposed cap of the ripened fruiting pod comes off, revealing numerous seeds.

Occurrence. A native of Europe, black henbane is a widespread weed of wastelands in the northeastern United States and is found sporadically across the continent, sometimes grown for herbal use.

Toxicity. All parts of the plant, particularly the roots and seeds, are poisonous. They contain tropane alkaloids of the same group as those in jimsonweeds and thorn-apples (*Datura* spp.) and belladonna (*Atropa belladonna*), namely hyoscyamine, scopolamine, and atropine. Symptoms of poisoning, which may persist for 12 hours or more, include dry mouth, dry skin, fever accompanied by rash, blurred vision, dilated pupils, rapid heartbeat, excitability, dizziness, delirium, confu-

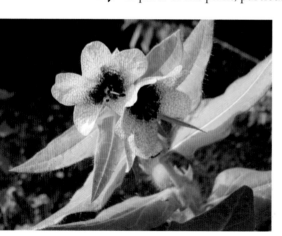

Black henbane (*Hyoscyamus niger*).

sion, headache, and, especially in children, hallucinations. Most incidents of accidental poisoning in humans are from earlier times in England and Europe, when henbane was commonly used medicinally. Occasional cases are still reported, either from misidentification of the plant or its roots as edible types, or from its misapplication as a medicine. The plant is unattractive to animals, but sometimes cattle and other livestock are poisoned by it, with symptoms similar to those of human poisoning.

Notes. Henbane has long been known in Europe as a medicinal plant, used for eye disorders, rheumatism, and as a sedative. In the Middle Ages it was also used in sorcery.

irises

Iris spp.
iris family (Iridaceae)

Quick check. Erect herbaceous perennials growing from rhizomes (or bulbs), with showy, colorful flowers in a distinctive formation: three outer spreading sepals and three erect inner petals. Entire plants, especially the rhizomes, are poisonous, but seldom fatal in humans.

Description. Irises, or flags (not to be confused with *Acorus americanus*, sweetflag, a plant with similar leaves but green flower spikes, not at all showy), are perennials that grow from thick rhizomes or bulbs, often occurring in dense clumps or patches. The stems are erect, either simple or branched, and the leaves are mostly basal. They are smooth-edged, long, narrow, and pointed, grass-like in some, broader in others. They often form two opposite ranks, in one plane in a fan-like formation. The showy, short-lived flowers are borne singly or in small clusters at the ends of the stems. The formation of the flowers is distinctive, with three outer sepals (falls), which are hanging or reflexed, and three inner petals (standards), usually erect and often arched. The flowers of *Iris pseudacorus* (yellow iris) are bright yellow; those of *I. germanica* (German iris) and its cultivars come in a wide variety of colors, including white, yellow, blue, purple, reddish, brownish, and variegated. Other species have yellow, blue, or purple flowers. The fruits are oblong, many-seeded capsules.

Occurrence. There are some 200 species of *Iris*, most native to the north temperate zone. Several species grow wild in parts of the continent, and many types and their cultivars are widely grown as garden ornamentals. *Iris pseudacorus* is a widespread garden escape, found commonly in ditches and marshes and along lake edges.

Toxicity. All parts of wild and cultivated irises, especially the rhizomes, are poisonous. *Iris pseudacorus* is probably the best known. It contains acrid poi-

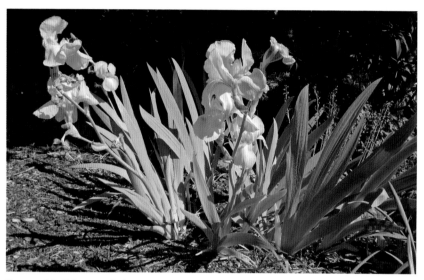

German iris (*Iris germanica*).

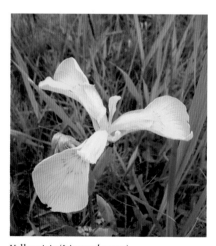

Yellow iris (*Iris pseudacorus*).

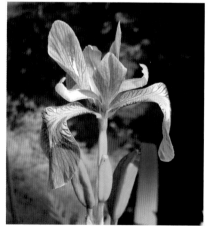

Virginia iris, or blue flag (*Iris virginica*).

sonous principles that cause gastrointestinal troubles for both animals and humans when the plants are consumed. They remain even when the plants are dried. Fresh rhizomes also contain triterpene-aldehyde. During storage, the scents alpha- and gamma-irone are formed. Eating iris rhizomes or leaves can cause severe digestive upset, with abdominal pain, nausea, vomiting, diarrhea, and fever. Humans are seldom poisoned, but there are numerous cases of fatalities in livestock from iris poisoning. Children should be warned against chewing on the leaves or fleshy portions of wild or cultivated iris plants, and gardeners should know that iris sap can irritate the skin, sometimes causing blistering.

Notes. A major danger from irises growing in marshes is the similarity of their leaves to those of cattails (*Typha* spp.), which are often found growing side by side with *Iris pseudacorus* or other wetland species. Cattails have edible rootstocks, shoots, and leaf bases, but those wishing to use them should be careful not to take iris instead.

larkspurs

Delphinium spp.
buttercup family (Ranunculaceae)

Quick check. Herbaceous annuals or perennials with deeply lobed, palmate leaves and purple (sometimes white or pink), spurred flowers in elongated clusters; entire plants highly toxic, potentially fatal.

Description. *Delphinium* offers considerable variation in the size and form of species. Some are tall and leafy-stemmed and grow in clumps; others are short and single-stemmed. Some are annuals, but most are perennials. The leaves of both types are usually deeply palmately lobed and long-stalked. The flowers are showy, borne in dense, elongated clusters, or racemes. The most common flower color is blue, ranging in shade from light sky blue to deep purplish blue; there are also white, mauve, and pink shades. The flowers have flaring petals, and each has a char-

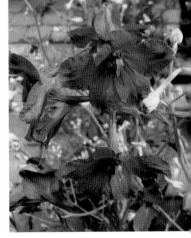

Larkspur (*Delphinium* sp.).

acteristic spur projecting backward from the upper part. The fruits are a cluster of dry, many-seeded follicles, with each capsule splitting along one side.

Occurrence. Hybrid perennial larkspurs feature in gardens throughout North America, and many native species grow in the wild in different parts of the continent.

Toxicity. Delphiniums contain toxic alkaloids similar to the aconitines found in monkshood, including 14-deactylnudicauline, methylaconitine, and nudicauline, which may be present with other alkaloids. The young plants can cause severe and often fatal poisoning of animals, especially range animals in the wild, but since humans seldom consume them, there are few reports of people being poisoned. In one instance, a man ingested delphinium leaves and seeds and five hours later developed symptoms of nausea, vomiting, abdominal pain, blurred vision, and dry skin and mouth. Restlessness, agitation, and dilation of the pupils lasted for 12 hours, after which recovery occurred.

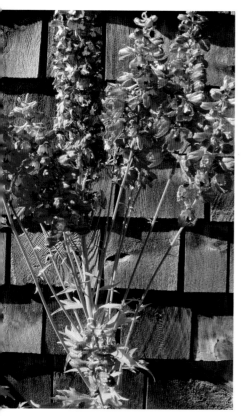

Larkspur hybrid.

Notes. Several other members of the buttercup family are toxic. As well as baneberry, buttercups, clematis, black hellebore, and monkshood (all described in this book), others are found both in the wild and in the garden: anemones (*Anemone* spp., *Pulsatilla* spp.), columbines (*Aquilegia* spp.), marsh marigolds (*Caltha* spp.), meadow-rues (*Thalictrum* spp.), and bugbanes (*Trautvetteria* spp.). Most contain irritant protoanemonins; columbines contain cyanogenic glycosides. Another poisonous garden plant in this family, with showy yellow or crimson flowers, is pheasant's eye (*Adonis* spp.); the whole plant contains digitalis-like glycosides and is still used in Europe as a medicinal herb.

lily of the valley, European

Convallaria majalis
lily family (Liliaceae)

Quick check. Herbaceous perennial with smooth-edged, elliptical leaves, prized in gardens for its fragrant, dainty, bell-like white flowers arranged along one side of the stalk. Entire plant toxic; sometimes fatal.

Description. Low, herbaceous perennial growing from creeping underground rootstocks, often forming extensive patches. The stems are upright, bearing two oval to elliptical, pointed, bright green leaves, smooth-edged, up to 20 cm (8 in.) long, and tapering to clasp the stalk. The white, delicate flowers are fragrant, bell-like, and globular. They are borne in a cluster of six to 12 along one side of a slender stalk, usually no more than 10 cm (4 in.) long. The fruits are fleshy, orange-red berries.

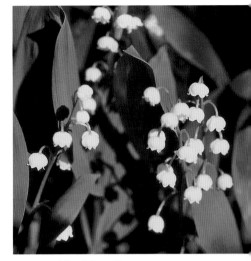

European lily of the valley
(*Convallaria majalis*).

Occurrence. A native of Eurasia, this species is frequently cultivated in gardens throughout temperate North America. It is also found as a garden escape in eastern North America. *Convallaria majuscula* (American lily of the valley), a related species, is native to the montane woods of North Carolina, Tennessee, Virginia, and West Virginia.

Toxicity. The entire plant is poisonous, containing more than 20 digitalis-like cardiac glycosides, including convallatoxin, convallarin, and convallamarin, as well as volatile oils, resins, and asparagine, a crystalline

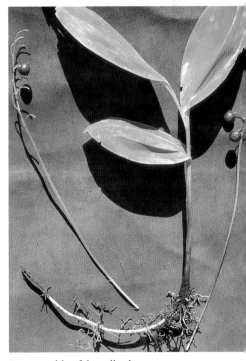

European lily of the valley leaves,
fruits, and rootstock.

amino acid. Convallatoxin is one of the most toxic of all naturally occurring substances that affect the heart. In addition to these glycosides, there are also saponins, which, together with volatile oils present in the plant, act as digestive tract irritants. Symptoms of poisoning are burning pain in the mouth and throat, heavy salivation, nausea, vomiting, abdominal pain, cramping, diarrhea, headache, dilated pupils, cold clammy skin, dazedness, and slow irregular heartbeat, sometimes leading to coma and death from heart failure. Depending on the quantity consumed, there may be a latent period before some of these symptoms are experienced. Children have been poisoned, some fatally, from eating the berries or chewing on the leaves. In one instance, the leaves were mistaken by adults for wild garlic leaves and were cooked in soup; those eating it became hot and flushed, and developed headache and hallucinations. Even water in which the cut flowers have been kept can be dangerous to drink.

Notes. Lily of the valley was formerly employed medicinally as a heart stimulant and diuretic but is now largely superseded by digoxin and digitoxin from foxglove, whose effects are more reliable.

lupines

Lupinus spp.
pea family (Fabaceae)

Quick check. Perennial or annual herbs or woody-based shrubs with palmately compound leaves, and smallish, pea-like flowers in elongated, terminal clusters, and flat, often hairy or silky, pea-like fruiting pods.

Description. Most lupines are herbaceous perennials, but some are annuals and some are shrubby, with a woody base. The leaves are alternate, and palmately compound, with five to 15 elongated, pointed leaflets radiating from the end of the leaf stalk. The flowers are like those of peas and similar legumes, crowded in showy, elongated terminal clusters, with the most mature flowers at the bottom and the last-opening at the top. Attractively colored, they range from blue to yellow, pink, white, or variegated. The pods, resembling peapods, are flattened, brownish or blackish when ripe, and often hairy or silky. They contain several flattened seeds.

Occurrence. There are about 200 species of lupine, most native to western North America and the Mediterranean region. Many varieties are grown as garden ornamentals, the most common being forms of bigleaf lupine (*Lupinus polyphyllus*). These often become naturalized around old gardens and homesteads, and some lupines are now being sown along highways for roadside stabilization.

Toxicity. Lupines contain a large number of potent alkaloids, including lupanine, anagyrine, and sparteine, which act on the nervous system. Some lupines also contain enzyme inhibitors and other toxins. The toxicity of the plants varies with species, time of year, and part of the plant. The seeds and pods, and the young leaves and stems in spring, are the most dangerous. Many species are toxic to grazing livestock, causing deaths and birth deformities, and some

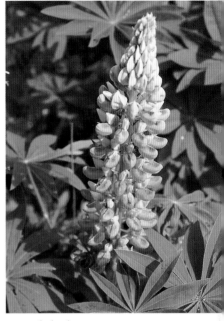

Lupine hybrid.

have been harmful to humans as well. The main danger of human poisoning is in eating the green, unripe seeds or pods, which may be mistaken for peas or beans, or the ripe seeds, whose pods may attract children because of their silky covering. The symptoms of poisoning are similar to those of golden chain tree (*Laburnum anagyroides*) but not as severe. They include vomiting, excessive salivation, nausea, dizziness, headache, and abdominal pain. Slowed breathing and heartbeat may also occur. In extreme cases, death through respiratory failure may result, but this is rare.

Notes. One species of lupine, *Lupinus latifolius*, which formed the main forage in an area heavily browsed by milk goats in Trinity County, California, was linked in 1981 to deformities in a human baby and in puppies when the mothers drank the goats' milk during their pregnancies, and to deformities and stillbirths in the goats during the same time period. The seeds and dried leaves of this species are known to have a high content of anagyrine, a quinolizidine alkaloid.

marijuana

Cannabis sativa
hemp family (Cannabaceae)

Quick check. Weedy, erect annual with palmately compound leaves with narrow, toothed leaflets. Entire plant contains toxic resins, which produce mind-altering symptoms ranging from mild to intense. Injection of hash oil can be fatal.

Description. Marijuana, or hemp, is an erect, herbaceous annual, with fluted or angled stems often 1.2–1.5 m (4–16 ft.) tall. The leaves on the lower part of the plant are borne from thickened nodes at intervals along the stem. They are palmately compound, with usually seven narrow, pointed, coarsely toothed leaflets, 5–15 cm (2–6 in.) long, arising like fingers on a hand from a single point at the end of the stalk. Male and female flowers are produced on different plants. They are inconspicuous, hidden among small leaves at the ends of branches. After flowering, the male plants turn yellow and die; the female plants remain dark green for about a month longer and produce small fruits (hemp seeds).

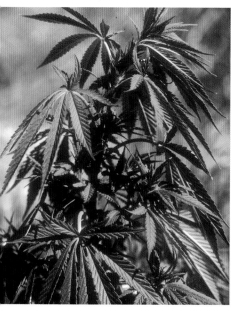

Marijuana (*Cannabis sativa*). Paul Kroeger

Occurrence. It is difficult to know where to place marijuana in this book, because it is grown (illegally) both indoors and outdoors for its narcotic effect and is also a persistent weed of roadsides and wastelands in parts of central and eastern North America. In some parts of Canada a tall strain of this plant is cultivated for fiber production. It is also grown for its oil-rich seeds, as well as for production of the narcotic cannabis.

Toxicity. Marijuana plants, both fresh and dried, contain toxic resins including tetrahydrocannabinol (THC). The concentration of these compounds varies considerably with the strain of the plant, part of the plant, its growth stage, how it is consumed, and the individual taking it. This variability comes mainly from the instability of some of the constituents. Smoking marijuana cigarettes, or joints, is about three times more powerful than ingestion. In small amounts, THC and its related compounds produce mild visual effects, brief mood elevation, and sedation; concentrated doses can cause confusion, depression, paranoia, panic, memory loss, rapid heartbeat, high blood pressure, psychosis, and coma. Smoking marijuana can cause throat irritation and coughing, as well as dry mouth, eye irritation, nausea, and vomiting. Injection of hash oil (a crude extract of hashish, or marijuana resins) can be fatal. The plant is bitter-tasting and is seldom touched by animals, but it has caused fatal poisoning of horses, mules, and cattle. Dogs fed marijuana products by their owners have shown serious symptoms—in some cases, muscular tremors, convulsions, prostration, and coma—but recovered within 24 hours in the cases reported. Children are at risk mainly from irresponsible behavior of adults feeding them marijuana biscuits or blowing marijuana smoke at them.

Notes. Cannabis is one of the earliest recorded narcotics. It is usually taken in the form of a tea, by chewing the plant parts, or by smoking the dried leaves or extracted resins. Until the late 1800s, it was used in human and veterinary medicine as a sedative and hypnotic. Now it is used mainly as an illicit recreational drug but also for its medicinal qualities; specifically, marijuana is recognized for its therapeutic value in pain relief, control of nausea and vomiting, and appetite stimulation. Mark Blumenthal (2006) reported on a product based on cannabis that was shown to be effective in reducing pain and sleep disturbance in people with multiple sclerosis (MS). Those wishing to smoke marijuana recreationally should be advised, however, that this is not only illegal but that the effects can be highly variable and unpredictable, and are not necessarily pleasant.

monkshood

Aconitum napellus and related spp.
buttercup family (Ranunculaceae)

Quick check. Herbaceous perennials similar to delphiniums, with deeply divided leaves and bluish, helmet-shaped flowers in elongated, terminal clusters; entire plant highly toxic and potentially fatal.

Description. All the approximately 100 species of monkshood, or aconite, are native to the north temperate zone. All are herbaceous perennials, growing from a dark, tuberous taproot, with usually unbranched stems up to 1 m (3 ft.) or more high. The leaves are more or less triangular in outline but deeply divided into narrow, pointed segments. The flowers, each with an enlarged, hood-like sepal forming a cap over the rest of the flower, are borne in an elongated cluster at the end of the stem. Flower colors range from blue and purple to yellow to white. The fruits usually form a tight group of three follicles, each splitting along the inside and containing many sharply angled seeds. These plants differ widely in chemical constituents, but all should be considered poisonous.

Occurrence. Several species of *Aconitum* are native to North America, most occurring in moist, montane areas. These are widely recognized as toxic by indigenous peoples (Moerman 2003). *Aconitum napellus* (Venus' chariot), native to Europe, is grown as an ornamental in gardens, as are several other species.

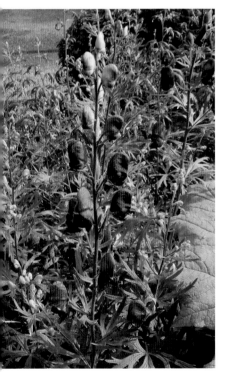

Venus' chariot
(*Aconitum napellus*).

Toxicity. *Aconitum napellus* contains several potent closely related diterpenoid alkaloids, especially aconitine, mesaconitine, napelline, and hypaconitine. It is often regarded as among the most poisonous plants in European flora. The similarity of monkshood to some species of larkspurs (*Delphinium* spp.), also toxic and more common than monkshood, has occasionally resulted in confusion in identification of poisoning causes. People are sometimes poisoned from misuse of herbal preparations containing monkshood, or from mistaking it for another plant. In one instance, a fatal human poisoning occurred when the roots of monkshood were mistaken for those of horseradish. The roots have also reportedly been mistaken for celery, and the leaves for parsley. Symptoms include tingling and burning of the lips, tongue, mouth, and throat, abdominal pain, excessive salivation together with intense thirst, severe vomiting, diarrhea, headache, cold feeling, slow heart rate, paralysis, confusion, restlessness, visual disturbances, convulsions, and delirium. Coma and death may occur rapidly from asphyxiation and circulatory failure, but in some cases the patient recovers fully within 24 hours. Animals seldom eat monkshood, but it does cause poisoning and occasional fatalities in livestock. A fatal dose for a dog has been estimated at 5 g (0.2 oz.), for a horse, 350 g (12 oz.).

Notes. The poisonous nature of monkshood has been known since ancient times, and plants have a long history of use in folk medicine. *Aconitum* species play a particularly important role in Indian and Chinese traditional medicine and have occasionally caused poisoning from improper dosage. Traditional doctors sometimes gauge the potency of aconitum by tasting it (Boesi and Cardi 2006). Wolfsbane (*Aconitum vulparia*) was formerly used as a poison for wolves.

poppy, opium
Papaver somniferum and related spp.
poppy family (Papaveraceae)

Quick check. Tall, large-flowered annual, with white to pale lilac to reddish or orange flowers and globular seed capsules; the numerous, small seeds are harmless in small amounts; eating other parts of the plant, especially the unripe seed capsules, may cause deep sleep and coma; seldom fatal.

Description. Erect, robust annual, up to 1.2 m (4 ft.) tall, with a uniformly bluish green cast. The leaves, up to 25 cm (10 in.) long, are alternate, lobed or toothed, with undulating margins. They are elongated or heart-shaped, with a clasping base. The flowers are borne singly, or two or three together, at the ends of the stems. The flower buds are nodding, the open flowers upright. They are large and showy, ranging in color from white to pale lilac to reddish or orange, often with dark blotches at the base of the petals. The fruit is a large, smooth, spherical or oval capsule, with a scalloped "lid." The small black or white seeds are numerous. The entire plant, especially the unripe capsules, exudes a milky sap when cut. Many cultivars are available, including popular double-flowered ones.

Occurrence. Although growing opium poppy is restricted by law because of its narcotic properties, it is nevertheless found in many North American gardens (especially cottage-style gardens) and as an escape in wastelands.

The species originated in Eurasia, and in some areas of the world it is cultivated as a medicinal plant and for its edible seeds. It is also grown for the illicit drug trade, mainly in the Middle East, Afghanistan, and Southeast Asia. Other poppies are also common garden flowers, and a few are native to North America; cultivated species include Iceland poppy (*P. nudicaule*), Oriental poppy (*P. orientale*), corn poppy (*P. rhoeas*), and California poppy (*Eschscholzia californica*).

Toxicity. The entire plant contains the drug opium—a crude resin that consists of a mixture of many potent isoquinoline alkaloids, including the well-known compounds morphine and codeine—as well as papaverine and various related substances. The unripe fruiting capsules are the main commercial source of opium, which exudes when the outside of the growing capsule is scored or cut. The ripe seeds contain only minute concentrations of opium; harmless in small amounts, they are used as a condiment and for decorating baked goods. Human poisoning occurs from eating the unripe capsules, from drinking tea made from these capsules, and from overdoses of opium or its manufactured derivatives, morphine, heroin, and codeine. These drugs are highly addictive, and illegal trafficking of them is a major problem in North America.

Symptoms of poppy poisoning include initial restlessness, excessive salivation, loss of appetite, stupor, shallow and slow breathing, deep sleep, and coma. Although poisoning is seldom fatal, recovery can be slow. Further-

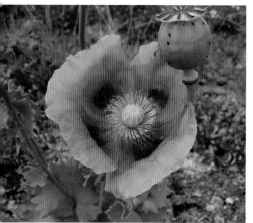

Opium poppy (*Papaver somniferum*).

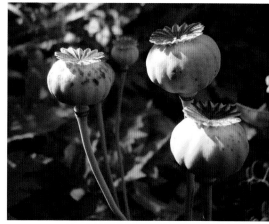

Opium poppy, mature seed capsules.

more, opiates are strongly addictive, and withdrawal is a ghastly experience. Large doses of opium or its derivatives can cause death through respiratory failure. Plants have caused poisoning in livestock, with severe economic losses through slow recovery and permanently depressed milk yield in lactating females. All poppies should be considered potentially toxic, although reports of poisoning from other species are very rare.

Notes. Opium is possibly the oldest narcotic known; records of its use go back as early as 4000 B.C. It was used as a painkiller and sleep-inducing drug by the ancient Greeks and Romans. By the 19th century innumerable patent medicines containing opium were popular in Europe and North America; opium-based teething syrups, cough medicines, sedatives, painkillers, and cures for diarrhea accounted for a major portion of prescription medicines, and many people became addicted to these medications. In China, opium smoking became a habit of millions, due to aggressive importation of the drug by British and American merchants. In 1838 a Chinese official attempted to enforce a ban on the opium trade and precipitated the Opium Wars, in which the British retained the right to import opium to China. Afghanistan currently produces 93% of the world's opium, with Myanmar next at 5%.

Several other members of the poppy family occurring in the southern United States and Mexico are toxic, including celandine (*Chelidonium majus*), bloodroot (*Sanguinaria canadensis*), and pricklypoppies (*Argemone* spp.). All

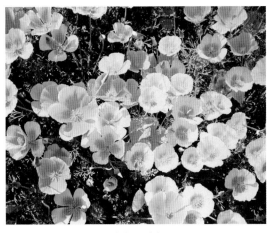

California poppy (*Eschscholzia californica*).

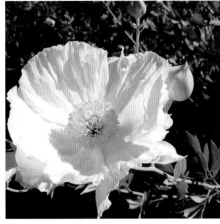

Bluestem pricklypoppy
(*Argemone albiflora*).

have prickly, yellowish or white flowers and exude a yellowish to reddish sap when cut. Pricklypoppy seeds are highly toxic and may cause severe poisoning when they contaminate home-ground grain.

potato
Solanum tuberosum
nightshade family (Solanaceae)

Quick check. Potato tubers are one of the world's most important foods, but the sprouts, green tubers, leaves, and berries can be dangerous; not usually fatal to humans.

Description. Tuber-bearing herbaceous perennials with dark green, compound leaves, and clustered whitish to purplish flowers with reflexed petals and protruding, yellow stamens. The tubers are of different shapes, colors, and textures, depending on their age and variety. Most commonly, they are brownish and ovoid. Red, yellow, and purplish tubers are also grown. The seldom-produced fruits are globular, yellow berries.

Occurrence. Potatoes are native to the montane regions of South America but are now a major crop plant in North America, Europe, and Asia and a major produce item in grocery stores everywhere.

Toxicity. Potato tubers are ubiquitous in the diets of North Americans. However, the plant is in the same genus as climbing nightshade (*Solanum dulcamara*) and black nightshade (*S. nigrum* and *S. americanum*) and, like them, contains steroidal alkaloids, such as solanine and related compounds, including some similar to atropine. Most cases of potato poisoning result from eating tubers that have turned green through exposure to light, or which have sprouted. In these tubers, the solanine content is many times higher than in normal, properly stored potatoes. The highest concentration of the toxins is in the skin, eyes, and sprouts of the tubers. Infection with potato blight fungus increases the concentration

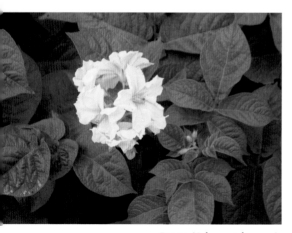

Potato (*Solanum tuberosum*).

of toxins; it was this pathogen that caused the catastrophic Irish potato famine of the late 1840s, which drove many Irish people to immigrate to North America. Boiling in water reduces, but does not eliminate, the alkaloids from green or sprouted potatoes. (If potatoes have "gone green," they may be stored in the dark for two to three weeks until all traces of green have disappeared, then safely eaten.) There is also danger from the berries, which are ten to 20 times as high in toxic alkaloids as normal tubers.

Children are more susceptible to solanine poisoning than adults. Symptoms may be delayed for several hours after ingesting toxic parts. They include severe abdominal pain, diarrhea, fever, sweating, headache, restlessness, delirium, visual disturbances, convulsions, drowsiness, and coma. There may also be urinary retention and kidney failure, but few fatalities in humans have been reported. Livestock have frequently been poisoned, often fatally, from feeding on green, decayed, or sprouting potatoes, peelings, or fruiting plants.

Notes. One of the most dramatic cases of potato poisoning took place in the late 1970s, when 78 schoolboys were poisoned after eating potatoes from a sack that had been stored improperly for several weeks. After a period of eight to ten hours they experienced abdominal pain, followed by diarrhea. Some also suffered restlessness, delirium, visual disturbances, drowsiness, or coma. Three of the boys became seriously ill, but even they recovered completely within about a month.

Symptoms of solanine poisoning are usually delayed, because the alkaloids are not readily absorbed; first they break down to release free alkamines, which are then absorbed, producing symptoms of drowsiness and dulling of the senses.

rhubarb

Rheum rhabarbarum
buckwheat family (Polygonaceae)

Quick check. Common vegetable and garden plant with very large, oval or heart-shaped basal leaves, forming dense clumps. The fleshy, reddish leaf stalks are sour-tasting but edible in moderation; the green leaf blades are highly toxic and potentially fatal if eaten.

Description. Perennial plant from large, fleshy rootstocks. The leaves are mostly basal and very large, with thick, fleshy stalks that may grow 60 cm (2 ft.) or more long (the edible vegetable part of the plant), and green, oval or heart-shaped blades up to 45 cm (18 in.) or more long. The small, numerous, greenish white flowers are produced in dense clusters on tall, hollow stems; the fruits are strongly winged achenes.

Occurrence. Native to Siberia, rhubarb is commonly marketed and widely cultivated in North American gardens for its edible stalks, and also sometimes occurs as an escape. In some areas of the north, where early prospectors and settlers planted it as a food source, it has become well established. Rhubarb stalks are usually harvested in spring before the plant flowers. Related species are sometimes grown as garden ornamentals.

Toxicity. All parts of the plant, but especially the green leaf blades, contain oxalates of calcium or potassium, and oxalic acid, all of which are irritant poisons, and anthranoids are suspected to add to the highly poisonous nature of the leaves. The fleshy, reddish, sour-tasting leaf stalks are a common garden vegetable and are safe to eat in everyday meals and desserts. Many cases of poisoning from eating the green leaves of rhubarb have been reported in both humans and animals. Eating rhubarb leaves was even recommended during World War I in Britain, when food was scarce, and some fatalities resulted. The amount eaten to produce symptoms of poisoning may vary from one individual to another. Cooking does not dispel the toxins.

Symptoms of poisoning, which may begin within an hour of eating the leaves, include severe abdominal pains, nausea, vomiting, weakness, difficulty breathing, burning of the mouth and throat, drowsiness, muscular

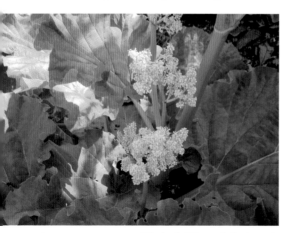

twitching, and in severe cases, convulsions, coma, and death. Even if the patient recovers, liver and kidney damage may be permanent.

Notes. Several other plants in the buckwheat family are known to contain oxalates. Some, such as garden sorrel (*Rumex acetosa*), sheep sorrel, or sourgrass (*R. acetosella*), knotweeds and smartweeds (*Polygonum* spp.), and alpine mountain-sorrel (*Oxyria digyna*), are edible in

Rhubarb (*Rheum rhabarbarum*).

moderation, and the oxalic acid they contain gives them a pleasant, sour taste. However, if eaten in large quantities or over a prolonged period, they can cause poisoning and interfere with the body's calcium metabolism.

snowdrop
Galanthus nivalis and related spp.
lily family (Liliaceae)

Quick check. Spring-blooming bulb with narrow, elongated leaves and single, drooping, white flowers marked with green; bulb causes digestive upset if eaten, but human fatalities unknown.

Description. Snowdrop is an herbaceous perennial growing from a small, membranous-coated bulb, often occurring in dense clumps. The leaves, basal and usually two to three per bulb, appear with the flowers in early spring and die down after the seed capsules ripen. They are long, narrow, smooth-edged, and somewhat fleshy. The nodding flowers are borne singly at the ends of long stalks. The three outer petal-like sepals are pure white and elongated; the inner petals are shorter and green-tipped. A double form is frequently grown. The fruit is a green, globular berry containing several seeds.

Occurrence. Native to Europe and western Asia, snowdrop is commonly cultivated throughout North America as one of the earliest blooming spring flowers. Other species of *Galanthus* are also sometimes grown.

Toxicity. The bulb contains amaryllidaceaen alkaloids, in particular lyco-rine and galanthamine. Eating large quantities of the bulbs can cause nausea, persistent vomiting, and diarrhea, but the plant is apparently not as toxic as its relative daffodil, and no fatalities have been reported.

Notes. Other plants in the amaryllis group of the lily family may also be dangerous, including *Hippeast-rum* spp. (amaryllis) and *Crinum* spp. (cape lily), often grown indoors in winter and outdoors in summer for

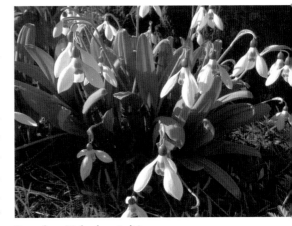

Snowdrop (*Galanthus nivalis*).

their large attractive flowers. Their bulbs, like those of snowdrop, contain lycorine and related alkaloids; however, the concentrations of the toxins are relatively low, and human poisonings from these plants are not common. Galanthamine, one of the more common alkaloids in this group of plants, inhibits cholinesterase activity reversibly and has been suggested as an antidote for atropine poisoning (Frohne and Pfänder 2005). Galanthamine has also become an important therapeutic drug in the treatment of Alzheimer s (it slows neurological degeneration). Furthermore, *Galanthus* has been used in the Caucasus as an apparently effective treatment for poliomyelitis (Heinrich and Teoh 2004).

spurges
Euphorbia spp.
spurge family (Euphorbiaceae)

Quick check. Large group of upright or prostrate herbs or shrubs; most with small, inconspicuous flowers but some with large, showy bracts; most exude a milky juice if cut or bruised; some are toxic and potentially fatal if ingested; sap may irritate eyes and skin.

Description. The more than 1600 species in the genus *Euphorbia* are extremely variable in form, including herbs, shrubs, trees, and succulent, thorny cactus-like types. Many, including cushion spurge (*E. epithymoides*; syn. *E. polychroma*), caper spurge, or moleplant (*E. lathyris*), Mediterranean spurge (*E. characias* ssp. *wulfenii*), and snow on the mountain (*E. marginata*), are grown as garden ornamentals. The last is particularly attractive, with conspicuous white margins around its upper and floral bracts. Other spurges, such as sun spurge, or madwoman's milk (*E. helioscopia*) and the diminutive petty spurge (*E. peplus*), are weedy. Many are grown indoors as house- and greenhouse plants; two of these, christplant (*E. milii*) and poinsettia (*E. pulcherrima*), are discussed in the next chapter. The flowers of most spurges are small, greenish, and inconspicuous, but some (poinsettia, christplant, cushion spurge, snow on the mountain) have large, showy bracts surrounding the flowers. The fruits are three-valved capsules. Many spurges exude a milky latex when cut or bruised.

Occurrence. Spurges are found throughout North America, growing as weeds of roadsides and wastelands, in gardens, and as household ornamentals. Cushion spurge and caper spurge are natives of Europe. Snow on the mountain is native to the Great Plains but thrives in gardens throughout North America. Sun spurge and petty spurge are common weeds.

Toxicity. Many spurges contain an irritant milky latex or sap, which exudes from the plants when cut or crushed. Complex irritant and cocarcinogenic diterpene esters are the main poisonous substances. The toxic properties remain even in dried plants. Human poisoning by spurges has resulted from people mistaking the seed capsules of caper spurge for true capers (which are flower buds of an unrelated plant, *Capparis spinosa*). In one instance, two children were poisoned, one of them fatally, from sucking the juice of sun spurge. In another case, a young woman was fatally poisoned when she attempted to use snow on the mountain as an abortive.

Symptoms of poisoning include intense burning of the mouth, throat, and stomach, salivation, vomiting, convulsions, constriction of

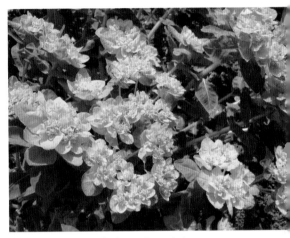

Cushion spurge (*Euphorbia epithymoides*).

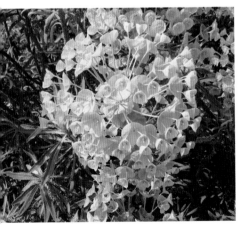

Mediterranean spurge (*Euphorbia characias* ssp. *wulfenii*).

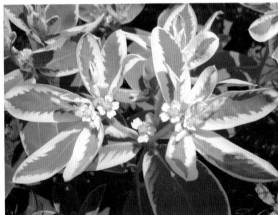

Snow on the mountain (*Euphorbia marginata*).

the pupils, fluid buildup in the lungs, and, in severe cases, coma and death. Even licking the fingers after handling spurge plants can cause severe irritation of the lips and tongue. Spurges frequently cause rashes and blistering on the skin of people touching them. Eye irritation can also develop if the latex comes in contact with the eyes.

Notes. The genus was named for Euphorbus, physician to Juba II, king of Numidia in A.D. 18. These plants have been used in the past as purgatives and emetics, as well as to eliminate warts and freckles, but since their action is drastic, they are seldom used today.

Some members of the spurge family native to North America are well known to indigenous peoples. One is smallseed sandmat, or golandrina (*Chamaesyce polycarpa*), a Pima medicinal plant. Another is arrow poison plant, or Mexican jumpingbean (*Sebastiania bilocularis*), whose juice has been used by the Seri to poison their arrows.

star of Bethlehem

Ornithogalum umbellatum
lily family (Liliaceae)

Quick check. Perennial with onion-like bulbs, grass-like leaves, and star-like, clustered flowers with white petals and greenish sepals; all parts of the plant, especially the bulbs, are toxic and potentially fatal.

Description. An herbaceous perennial growing from a tufted bulb, often occurring in dense clumps. The leaves are narrow and grass-like, with a conspicuous, white midvein. The flowers, in clusters of five to 20, are star-like and six-parted, up to 2.5 cm (1 in.) across, with white petals and greenish sepals. The fruits are three-lobed capsules, each containing a few, dark-colored seeds.

Occurrence. A native of Europe and North Africa, star of Bethlehem, or sleepydick, is frequently grown in North American gardens and can also be found as a weedy escape, especially in the southeastern United States. Other species in the genus are sometimes grown in North American gardens; all should be considered poisonous.

Toxicity. All parts of the plant, especially the onion-like bulbs, are poisonous. More than eight cardenolide toxins have been identified, and there are various unidentified alkaloids as well. Eating the bulbs, leaves, or flowers can lead to pain and cramps, and diarrhea. Slow or irregular heartbeat may also occur. Some deaths from children eating this plant have been reported, and livestock may be poisoned from browsing the plants or bulbs exposed from plowing or frost heave. Juice from the plant can irritate the skin.

Notes. Several other genera of the lily family are poisonous to some extent. Hyacinth (*Hyacinthus orientalis*), widely grown both as an early spring flower in the garden and as a houseplant, has bulbs that are occasionally mistaken for onions; if eaten in any quantity, they can cause stomach cramps, vomiting, and diarrhea. Hyacinth juice can also cause skin irritation. The bright flowers, up to 2.5 cm (1 in.) across and in colors ranging from blue to red, to white, to yellowish, are usually highly scented and are arranged in a dense cylindrical cluster along an upright stem.

Another genus of toxic flowering bulbs frequently encountered in gardens is *Hyacinthoides*. The flowers of English bluebell (*H. non-scripta*), Spanish bluebell (*H. hispanica*), and related species are smaller than those of hyacinth and are commonly light blue, but also pink or white. The bulbs contain glycosides similar in structure to the cardiac glycosides of digitalis. Red squill (*Urginea maritima*) is sometimes cultivated in California and elsewhere as a garden ornamental or for its medicinal and rodenticide properties; its bulb contains similar glycosides.

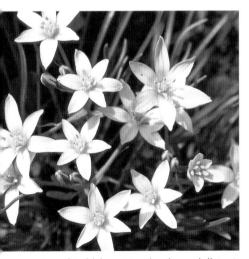
Star of Bethlehem (*Ornithogalum umbellatum*).

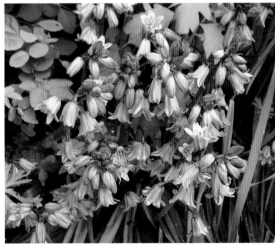
Spanish bluebell (*Hyacinthoides hispanica*).

tobacco

Nicotiana tabacum and related spp.
nightshade family (Solanaceae)

Quick check. Tobacco is widely known in cigarettes and cigars and as a crop plant, with large basal leaves. Some tobacco species, with usually smaller leaves and trumpet-shaped, petunia flowers of various colors, are grown as garden ornamentals; others are wild or naturalized (*Nicotiana rustica*), and one is a small tree (*N. glauca*). All tobaccos should be considered poisonous to consume (smoking tobacco brings its own risks); some have caused fatalities.

Description. In general, the leaves of tobaccos are large, often 15–30 cm (6–12 in.) or more long, simple, hairy, and often sticky; the leaves of cultivated tobacco are large, bright green, hairy, and strong-smelling. The flowers, often strongly fragrant, range from white, yellow, or greenish, to purplish, and usually open at night. The petals are fused into a five-lobed flaring tube. The fruits are dry many-seeded capsules. All tobaccos should be considered poisonous.

Occurrence. Tobacco is grown as a crop plant in many parts of the United States and southern Canada, but many other species of *Nicotiana* occur in North America, some native, some naturalized, and some grown as garden ornamentals. They include annuals and perennials. Flowering tobacco species (*N. alata*, *N. sylvestris*) and cultivars are widely grown as garden flowers and are garden escapes in some areas. Tree tobacco (*N. glauca*), a yellow-flowered shrub or small tree up to 5.5 m (18 ft.) tall, is grown as an ornamental and is also found as an escaped weed in Florida, California, and Hawaii. Desert tobacco (*N. obtusifolia*) grows as a wild annual in the dry soils of the southwestern United States and Mexico.

Toxicity. The most significant toxic species are cultivated tobacco (*Nicotiana tabacum*), longflower tobacco (*N. longiflora*), tree tobacco (*N. glauca*), and desert tobacco (*N. obtusifolia*). Cultivated tobacco contains nicotine, a highly toxic alkaloid and well-known narcotic; it is readily absorbed from ingestion of the leaves, or from inhalation, and in pure form is rapidly fatal in small amounts. Poisoning through intentional or accidental misuse of nicotine and products containing it is a relatively common occurrence. Related species may contain other toxic alkaloids, chemically similar to nicotine.

The long-term health risks of tobacco are well documented. Smoking is implicated as a cause of or contributor to many health problems, including heart disease, cancer of the lungs and throat, and complications in pregnancy and childbirth. Aside from these problems, the direct ingestion of raw or cooked leaves of any *Nicotiana* species can cause severe poisoning when used as a home remedy, or from absorption of nicotine through the skin during commercial tobacco harvesting.

Symptoms of severe nicotine poisoning are nausea, vomiting, abdominal pain, diarrhea, headache, dizziness, confusion, sweating, salivation, rapid, irregular heartbeat, vacillating blood pressure, convulsions, collapse, and possible sudden respiratory failure. Although tobacco plants are distasteful, grazing animals may be poisoned by them under some conditions.

Notes. Children have been poisoned from sucking the flowers of tree tobacco (*Nicotiana glauca*), and the chopped leaves of this species eaten as a salad caused death. A California family was poisoned, one member fatally, when they cooked and ate the leaves of desert tobacco (*N. obtusifolia*) as a potherb.

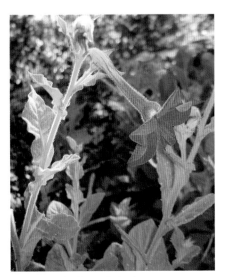

Ornamental tobacco hybrid.

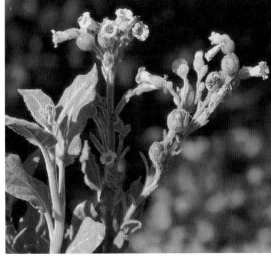

Aztec tobacco (*Nicotiana rustica*).

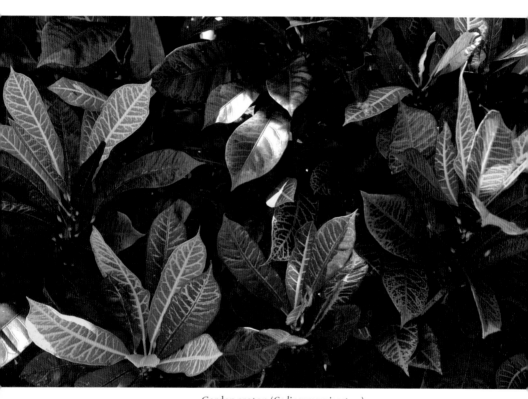

Garden croton (*Codiaeum variegatum*).

CHAPTER 5
Poisonous Houseplants and Subtropical Garden Plants

WOODY PLANTS

avocado
Persea americana
laurel family (Lauraceae)

Quick check. Small to medium-sized tree with large oval, pale green, often drooping leaves; flowers small, greenish yellow; and large, edible fruits. Leaves, bark, unripe fruit, and seeds are toxic to animals and potentially to humans. Keep young children away from leaves and seeds.

Description. Also known as alligator pear, avocados are broad-topped trees up to 20 m (60 ft.) high but much smaller when grown indoors. Leaves are 8–15 cm (3–6 in.) long, oblong to oval, pale green, and somewhat drooping. Flowers are small and greenish yellow, in compact clusters. The edible fruits are well known and widely marketed in North America. They are large (5–20 cm, 2–8 in. long), oval or pear-shaped, and fleshy, with greenish, maroon, or blackish skin, light green, creamy edible flesh, and a single large central seed, rounded at one end, pointed at the other.

Occurrence. Avocado is native to Mexico and Central America and is widely grown as a crop in California, Florida, and other subtropical areas. It is often grown indoors as a potted tree, even in northern regions.

Toxicity. Although the ripe flesh of the avocado fruit is edible and widely used by humans, the leaves, unripe fruit, bark, and seeds have been reported to be toxic, sometimes fatally, to various types of animals, including cattle,

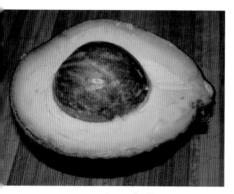

Avocado (*Persea americana*).

horses, goats, rabbits, fish, and canaries. For the last, poisoning resulted from eating ripe fruit. The toxins are as yet unknown but likely to be some kind of cardiotoxin; some varieties, including 'Fuerte' and 'Nabal' (green-skinned strains), are more poisonous than others. A major symptom of avocado poisoning in cattle, goats, and horses is severe mastitis in female animals, with permanent reduction in milk flow. The assumption should be that all parts of the plant (except the flesh of the ripe fruit) may be dangerous for humans until proven otherwise.

Notes. Children often undertake to grow the large, unusual-looking seeds, which sprout easily and grow readily into attractive small trees. In the Philippines, avocado seeds are sometimes used to relieve toothaches.

bird-of-paradise shrub

Caesalpinia gilliesii and related spp.
pea family (Fabaceae)

Quick check. Showy, non-spiny shrub with alternate leaves finely divided into numerous small leaflets; terminally clustered, light yellow flowers with long, red, conspicuous stamens. Bean-like seedpods may be attractive to children and cause serious irritation of the digestive tract but are not known to be fatal to humans.

Description. An upright, or sometimes climbing, shrub or small tree up to 4.5 m (15 ft.) tall. Leaves alternate, and pinnately divided into many small leaflets, which are dotted with black near the margins of the lower surface. The flowers are in terminal clusters and extremely showy. They are large and light yellow, with striking red stamens protruding 8–12 cm (3–5 in.) from the flowers. The fruits are bean-like pods up to 2 cm (0.8 in.) wide and 10 cm (4 in.) long. Several related species (including those classed in the genus *Delonix* (for example, royal poinciana, *D. regia*) are grown as ornamental shrubs and trees in the southern United States. Most have feathery leaves and showy flowers with colors ranging from scarlet to orange-yellow to yellow.

Occurrence. Bird-of-paradise shrub, native to Argentina, is grown as a large container plant in homes and greenhouses of temperate North America and as an outdoor ornamental in subtropical gardens.

Toxicity. The green seedpods contain tannins and are severely irritating to the digestive tract of both humans and animals. Symptoms include nausea, vomiting, and diarrhea. Two children who each ate five pods developed these symptoms within 30 minutes but recovered, with treatment, after about 24 hours.

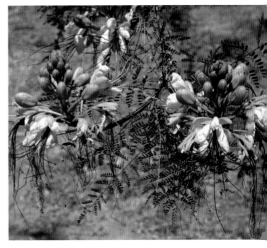

Caesalpinia gilliesii. G. A. Cooper, courtesy of Smithsonian Institution

Notes. The name bird-of-paradise is potentially confusing because it is also applied to another ornamental flowering plant (*Strelitzia* spp.), which, like bird-of-paradise shrub, is grown as a large container plant: it has large, simple, upright leaves with long stalks and large, showy flowers, and is not considered poisonous.

castorbean

Ricinus communis
spurge family (Euphorbiaceae)

Quick check. Bushy, shrub-like, ornamental herb with large, long-stalked, palmately lobed leaves, spiny clustered seedpods, and bean-like seeds usually mottled with white, red, or brown. Seeds violently poisonous, sometimes fatal, especially for children; symptoms may be delayed for hours or days after ingestion.

Description. Large annual with branching stems 4 m (12 ft.) or more tall, often reddish or purplish tinged. The leaves are large (up to about 80 cm, 30 in. across), simple, alternate, long-stalked, and palmately lobed, with five to 11 elongated lobes toothed along the margins. The flowers are inconspicuous and lack petals, but the three-parted fruiting pods are showy, clustered, green or often bright red, and covered with soft spines. The seeds are large

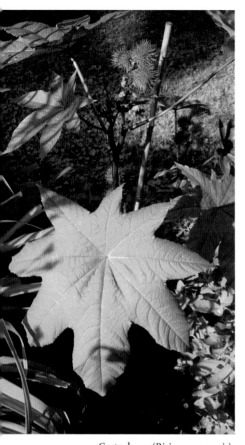

Castorbean (*Ricinus communis*).

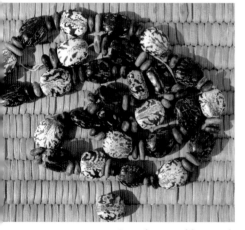

Castorbean necklace, with
dyed blue beans.

and bean-like, glossy black or white, or (usually) mottled black or brown on white.

Occurrence. Native to tropical Africa, where it grows as a woody perennial, castorbean is naturalized in warmer parts of the United States and is grown commercially in California and the southern states for the oil extracted from its seeds. It is often grown as an ornamental, valued either indoors in cooler climates or in yards and gardens in warmer areas for its striking foliage and rapid growth.

Toxicity. The attractive, usually mottled seeds are the most toxic part of the plant; the leaves are less poisonous. The main toxin, a plant lectin, is ricin, a high molecular weight protein that is reputed to be one of the most toxic naturally occurring substances; it inhibits protein synthesis in the intestinal wall. Another lectin, ricinus agglutinin, is known to coagulate and break down red blood cells. Small quantities of the cathartic castor oil are also present. Symptoms of poisoning may not appear for several hours, or even for a few days, after the seeds are eaten. Characteristic symptoms are burning of the mouth and throat, nausea, vomiting, severe stomach pains, diarrhea (sometimes containing blood and mucus), thirst, prostration and shock from massive fluid and electrolyte loss, headache, dizziness, lethargy, impaired vision, possible rapid heartbeat, and convulsions. Two to five hours following ingestion, symptoms of retinal hemorrhaging of the eyes, internal hemorrhaging and fluid buildup in the digestive tract and lungs, and deterioration of the liver and kidneys are evident in serious cases. Death from kidney failure may occur up to 12 days after eating the seeds. Eating one to three seeds can be fatal to a child, two to six to an adult. If swallowed whole, without being chewed, the seeds are unlikely to be harmful, because the hard seed coat prevents the toxin from being released.

Livestock are sometimes fed castorbean products such as husks that have been detoxified with heat or steam, but if the detoxification procedures are inadequate, severe poisoning and death can result. Cattle, sheep, horses, pigs, and poultry have all been poisoned from meal contaminated with castorbean toxins.

Notes. Because this plant is commonly cultivated, children often have access to the seeds, and they are a major cause of poisoning among children. Wherever the plant is grown as an ornamental, the seedheads should be removed before the seeds are allowed to mature. Sometimes necklaces of drilled and strung castorbeans are sold, and these can also be a source of poisoning. Drilling holes in the seeds makes them much more deadly because it exposes the toxin. More than one parent has allowed their baby to suck on a necklace of castorbeans.

Ricin is the FBI's third most poisonous substance known, behind plutonium and botulism toxin. It is considered 6000 times more toxic than cyanide and 12,000 times more toxic than rattlesnake venom (Anon. 1995); only a few hundred millionths of a gram of ricin was used in the 1978 "umbrella murder" of Bulgarian dissident Georgi Markov (see Chapter 1). Periodically, ricin is found in people's possession, and there is always a fear of its use for evil.

Castor oil, which does not itself contain ricin, is used medically as a laxative and industrially as a lubricant and as an ingredient in soaps, varnishes, and paints.

christplant
Euphorbia milii
spurge family (Euphorbiaceae)

Quick check. Very spiny, woody shrub-like plant with a few elongated leaves and flowers borne above red bracts; stem and leaves exude milky juice when cut or bruised. Milky sap an irritant of the skin and digestive tract; spines

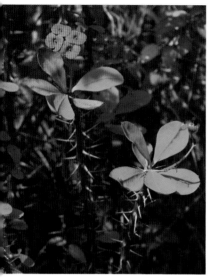

Christplant
(*Euphorbia milii*).

may cause painful injury. Severe human poisoning is rare because the plant is so spiny.

Description. Christplant, or crown of thorns, is a shrub-like plant up to 1.2 m (4 ft.) high, with stems thickly covered by sharp spines up to 2.5 cm (1 in.) long. The leaves are few and scattered, mostly on the young growth, thin and oblong to spoon-shaped, smooth-edged, and up to 5 cm (2 in.) long. The "flowers," borne in clusters, are subtended by two showy red bracts. The fruit is a three-lobed capsule.

Occurrence. Native to Madagascar, this attractive, cactus-like species is frequently cultivated as a house- and patio plant in North America and is grown in gardens in the South.

Toxicity. The milky sap, or latex, which exudes from the stem and leaves of this and related plants, consists of complex terpenes, notably euphorbol. It can produce severe irritation of the mouth and digestive tract, and is corrosive and caustic to the skin and eyes, causing temporary blindness in some cases. These terpenes also have cocarcinogenic properties. Fortunately, no severe cases of poisoning by christplant are on record, probably because it is so prickly that children would not be inclined to eat it. The spines can produce painful injury.

Notes. According to legend, it was a wreath of this plant that was placed as a mock crown on the head of Christ at his crucifixion. Two related spiny shrubs grown as ornamentals in the southern United States and also potentially irritating to the skin and eyes are candelabra cactus (*Euphorbia lactea*) and pencil tree (*E. tirucalli*).

croton, garden

Codiaeum variegatum and related spp.
spurge family (Euphorbiaceae)

Quick check. Shrub or small tree with leathery, laurel-like, often lobed, prominently veined leaves marked with white, yellow, red, or pink. Leaves and stems of many forms contain a highly toxic, irritant, and purgative oil; keep young children away from the brightly colored leaves.

Description. Garden croton, or ornamental croton, is an attractive shrub or small tree, with oval to lance-shaped, often lobed, leaves that are strongly veined and marked with white, yellow, or reddish coloring, with various forms and combinations of variegation. The flowers are small, in elongated racemes, borne in the axils of the upper leaves. Male and female flowers are on separate plants. The fruit is a globose, two-parted capsule.

Occurrence. Native to the South Pacific and Australia, garden croton and its many cultivars are widely cultivated in tropical gardens and as house- and greenhouse plants for their handsome, variegated leaves.

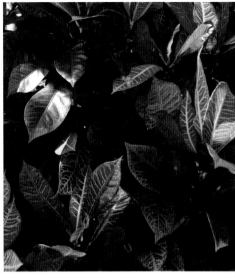

Garden croton (*Codiaeum variegatum*).

Toxicity. Leaves and stems contain irritant diterpene esters and cause dermatitis. Many crotons contain croton oil, predominantly in the seeds but also in the leaves and stems; and the seeds of at least some, probably all, contain crotin, which is similar to ricin, found in castorbean. Fortunately, crotons are distasteful, and cases of poisoning of humans and animals are rare. Nevertheless, because the leaves are so attractive and showy, ornamental crotons should be regarded with great caution, especially around young children.

Notes. Croton oil was commercially extracted from the seed kernels of a species in a closely related genus in the same family, purging croton (*Croton tiglium*). The oil is a drastic purgative and is also highly irritating to the skin, as well as having cocarcinogenic properties; its active compounds consist of a mixture of fatty acid esters of phorbol. Even minute quantities of the pure oil are potentially fatal to humans and domestic animals. Some indigenous *Croton* species are considered toxic; dove weed (*C. setigerus*), was used by various California Native Americans as a fish poison (Moerman 2003).

cycad

Cycas revoluta and related spp.
cycad family (Cycadaceae)

Quick check. Palm-like tree, technically woody, with an evident crown of leathery pinnately compound leaves. Plants are dioecious; the large male or female cones are located at the center of the leaves.

Description. Cycad, or sago palm, grows up to 5 m (16 ft.) high, with a thick trunk and crown of spreading, tough, fern-like (pinnate) leaves. The trunk, which is sometimes sunk into the ground, is clothed with persistent leaf bases. The leaves are dark green, growing up to 1 m (3 ft.) long, and are flattened or V-shaped in cross section. The leaflets, which have a prominent midrib and lack any obvious secondary veins, are coiled (circinate) when young. The plants are dioecious, producing separate male and female inflorescences. The male (pollen-bearing) cones are cylindrical; the female cones are loose and open. The seeds are brownish, ovoid or rounded, produced at the edges of the female cone bracts, usually in pairs.

Occurrence. Subtropical in distribution; naturalized in Florida. Commonly grown indoors in tubs or large containers.

Toxicity. The toxic components of cycad and its relatives, occurring throughout the entire plant, are beta-methylamino-L-alanine (BMAA), a non-proteinogenic amino acid, and methylazoxymethanol, a glycoside of the cyca-

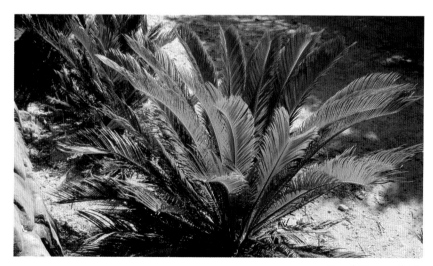

Cycad (*Cycas revoluta*).

sin type (or macrozamin). These toxic principles can produce hydrocyanic acid, but more importantly, the methylazoxymethanol is metabolized to compounds that can alkalize nucleic acids and proteins, producing acute toxic effects in both animals and humans. These compounds are also carcinogenic, producing tumors in the liver and kidneys of animals. BMAA is a neurotoxin and is actually produced by cyanobacteria (bluegreen algae), which live in a symbiotic relationship in specialized coralloid roots of cycads. This toxic compound is biomagnified (concentrated) in the reproductive tissues of cycads, especially in the outermost seed layer. It can affect the nerves and spinal cord, producing amyotrophic lateral sclerosis/parkinsonism-dementia complex (ALS-PDC), a neurodegenerative disease with effects similar to ALS, or Lou Gehrig's disease.

Notes. The most notorious case of cycad poisoning was documented by ethnobotanist Paul Cox and his colleagues (Cox and Sacks 2002; Cox et al. 2003). Flying foxes, large fruit-eating bats of the genus *Pteropus*, forage on the seeds of *Cycas micronesica*, a tree species of cycad in Guam. These bats accumulate the toxins in their flesh at over twice the levels found in the cycad fruits. The bats, in turn, have been a prized food item of the indigenous Chamorro people there, who boil them in shredded coconut and water and eat them whole. The Chamorro population of Guam suffers from ALS-PDC at 50 to 100 times the average worldwide incidence. BMAA has also been found in the brain tissues of Alzheimer's patients from Canada, suggesting alternative pathways for bioaccumulation of this compound in aquatic or terrestrial ecosystems (Cox et al. 2003).

All genera in the cycad family, including *Cycas, Dioon, Encephalartos*, and *Macrozamia*, contain similar poisonous substances. False sago is obtained from *Cycas* stem pith, after prolonged soaking to remove the poisons, but this substance is not recommended for consumption under any circumstances.

fig, edible
Ficus carica and related spp.
mulberry family (Moraceae)

Quick check. Edible fig is a small tree with large, deeply lobed leaves; other species are broadleaved shrubs, vines, or trees, often encountered in homes and places of business as ornamentals; stems and leaves exude a milky juice when cut or bruised; fruits and leaves can cause skin irritation, but severity varies with species.

Description. The common edible fig (*Ficus carica*) has attractive large, deeply lobed leaves. Other species have leaves of various sizes and shapes—some large, some smaller, some shiny and leathery, either deeply or shallowly lobed. All figs share the characteristic of exuding milky white latex from their leaves and stems if cut or bruised.

Occurrence. Approximately 30 of the more than 800 species of *Ficus* are grown as pot and patio plants, indoors and outdoors in warmer areas, throughout temperate North America. The common edible fig (*F. carica*) is native to the Middle East and is widely grown indoors in colder parts of the continent and outdoors in warm, sheltered areas, even in southwestern Canada. Probably the most common indoor species are the large-leaved Indian rubberplant (*F. elastica*), fiddleleaf fig (*F. lyrata*), with large, lyre-shaped leaves, and weeping fig (*F. benjamina*), with smaller, oval, pointed leaves. These species are often used as decorative plants for offices, hotel lobbies, and shopping malls.

Toxicity. One species of fig in particular, fiddleleaf fig, was found to be highly toxic to rats in laboratory experiments and should be considered dangerous for humans until proven otherwise. The leaves, fruits, and sap of several

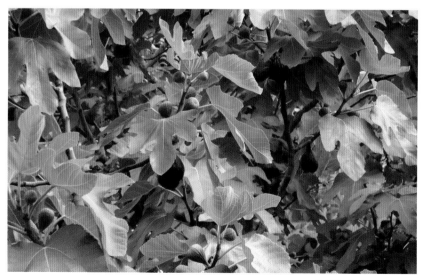

Edible fig (*Ficus carica*).

species of *Ficus* are known to cause irritant dermatitis, or photodermatitis (skin irritation in the presence of UV light). The seriousness of the reaction depends on the species or variety of fig, and effects can vary from person to person. Fig dermatitis, mainly from edible fig, can be quite severe, with blistering and redness of the skin and around the mouth of those who harvest, process, or eat fresh figs or come in contact with their foliage. The initial irritation is sometimes followed by discoloration that can last for years. Some fig species may also cause allergic contact dermatitis, similar to that of poison ivy and poison oak (*Toxicodendron* spp.), and their sap can also be highly irritating to the eyes. The principal irritating compound, contained in the sap, seems to be ficin, an enzyme causing protein breakdown. Some figs also contain ficusin, a psoralen, and 8-methoxypsoralen, both phototoxins.

Notes. In warmer countries where figs are produced commercially, those who dry, pack, or cook them sometimes develop chronic eczema of the hands. Adam and Eve are reputed to have used fig leaves as their rudimentary clothing, but at least one researcher has pointed out that, in view of their irritant properties, they seem to be most unsuitable for this purpose.

lantana

Lantana camara
verbena family (Verbenaceae)

Quick check. Branching, deciduous shrub with yellow to orange (sometimes purple or pinkish) flowers in showy, flat-topped clusters; leaves with pronounced unpleasant odor when crushed. Green unripe fruits and entire plant highly toxic, sometimes fatal.

Description. Also known as red sage or yellow sage, this species is a bushy, sometimes sprawling shrub up to 1.2 m (4 ft.) high as a container plant when grown in greenhouses, or up to 6 m (20 ft.) high in the tropics. The stems are angled, sometimes with short, hooked prickles. The leaves are simple, opposite or whorled, oval-shaped, and coarse, with toothed margins, 2.5–12 cm (1–5 in.) long, and stalked. The plant is unpleasantly aromatic when crushed or touched. The flowers are small, tubular, and four-parted, in attractive, dense, flat-topped clusters up to 5 cm (2 in.) across, and on long stalks. The young flowers at the center are usually yellow, changing to orange, then red as they mature. There are also white- and pink-flowered

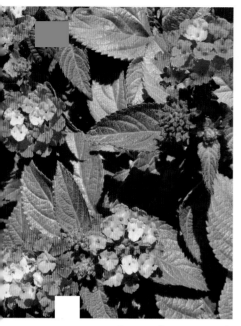

Lantana (*Lantana camara*).

varieties. The fruits are spherical, fleshy, and berry-like, at first green, turning blackish at maturity.

Occurrence. A native of tropical America, lantana is widely grown as a house-, greenhouse, patio, and hanging basket plant throughout temperate North America; it is a common weed and garden ornamental in tropical and subtropical areas. In greenhouses flowering occurs year-round.

Toxicity. Lantana is a chief cause of poisoning in Florida. The green, unripe fruits are the most dangerous. The poisonous agent is presumed to be lantadene A, a phototoxic triterpene that is activated in the presence of sunlight. The ripe fruits are apparently not harmful, but the leaves and green berries are fatally poisonous to animals, even in relatively small amounts. Symptoms of poisoning, which may be delayed up to six hours after ingestion, include weakness and lethargy, vomiting, diarrhea or constipation, loss of appetite, difficulty in walking, visual disturbances, and, in severe cases, circulatory collapse and death. Acute symptoms resemble atropine poisoning. Chronic poisoning produces edema, liver degeneration, gastrointestinal lesions, and hemorrhages in some organs.

Notes. People wishing to grow this attractive houseplant should remove the flower heads as soon as the flowers begin drooping, thus preventing the formation of the toxic fruits. These have caused fatal poisoning of children who are attracted to the shiny, green, unripe "berries."

oleander

Nerium oleander
dogbane family (Apocynaceae)

Quick check. Tall, evergreen shrub with narrow, pointed, leathery leaves having prominent midribs, and large clusters of showy, red, pinkish or white flowers. All parts of the plant, including flower nectar, highly toxic and potentially fatal.

Description. An upright, bushy, evergreen shrub or small tree, compact when grown indoors, up to 8 m (25 ft.) tall when growing outside. The leathery leaves are opposite or in whorls of three, narrow and smooth-edged, 10–20 cm (4–8 in.) long, tapering at the base to a short stem. They are lighter-colored beneath, with prominent yellowish veins and midrib. Leaves of some varieties are variegated white or yellow. The flowers, growing in loose clusters at the tips of the twigs, are large and showy, ranging in color from white to pink to deep red or purplish. They are funnel-like, with five broad or finely cut lobes that spread out and twist to the right; double-flowered varieties are often grown. Fruits are paired, elongated follicles.

Occurrence. Native from the Mediterranean region to Japan, oleander is often grown in temperate North America as a house- or greenhouse plant, or patio tree and is cultivated as a garden ornamental throughout the southern United States.

Toxicity. Oleander is extremely poisonous. All parts of it, smoke from burning it, and water in which flowers have been placed, are toxic. A single leaf is potentially lethal for humans, and eating as little as 0.005% of the animal's weight can be fatal to cattle and other animals. People have been poisoned from using oleander sticks for roasting hot dogs or other meat, and children in particular, from chewing the leaves or sucking the flower nectar. Honey made from the flower nectar is also poisonous.

The toxins are several cardioactive glycosides, especially the cardenolide oleandrin, whose action is similar to that of digitalis. Symptoms of poisoning are nausea, severe vomiting, stomach pain, dizziness, slowed pulse, irregular heartbeat, marked dilation of the pupils, bloody diarrhea, drowsiness, coma, and sometimes respiratory paralysis and death.

Notes. *Nerium indicum* (so closely related as to be considered synonymous by some authorities) is sometimes grown in warm climates, especially in Hawaii, and is also potentially fatally toxic. Yellow oleander (*Thevetia peruviana*), another relative of tropical and subtropical areas, is a shrub or small tree with bright yellow or orange flowers and fleshy fruits, black when ripe and with a central stone. All parts of the plant are dangerous; on the Hawaiian Islands, it is the most frequent cause of severe poisoning in humans. Another related species, yellow allamanda, or golden trumpet (*Allamanda*

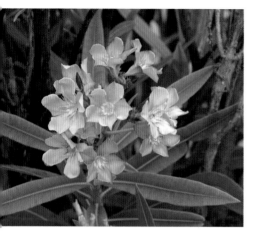

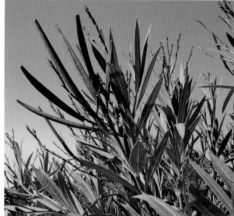

Oleander (*Nerium oleander*).   Oleander fruit.

cathartica), is an ornamental shrub or vine that may cause vomiting and diarrhea but is not known to have caused fatalities. A native of Brazil, this plant has large, glossy, lance-shaped leaves, clusters of showy yellow trumpet-shaped flowers, and prickly capsules. It is commonly cultivated in the southern United States and Hawaii. All parts of the plant, especially the fruit and seeds, and the sap of the stems and leaves, cause mild to severe stomach upset and vomiting.

HERBACEOUS PLANTS
Including common household plant products

alocasias, taros, or elephant's ears
Alocasia spp., *Colocasia* spp., and related genera
arum family (Araceae)

Quick check. Herbaceous perennials with large, long-stalked, arrowhead-shaped leaves usually marked or colored; entire plant contains irritant calcium oxalate crystals, causing intense burning of the mouth and throat if swallowed; not usually fatal.

Description. Perennials growing from rhizomes, with large, long-stalked, entire, scalloped, or lobed, arrowhead-shaped leaves that are often beautifully marked or colored. The flower stalks are shorter than the leaf stalks,

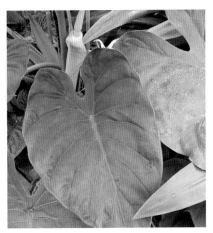

Elephant's ear (*Alocasia macrorrhizos*).

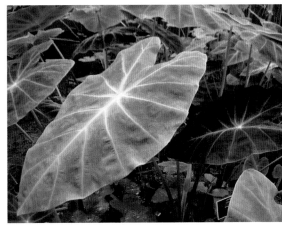

Colocasia esculenta, purple-leaved form.

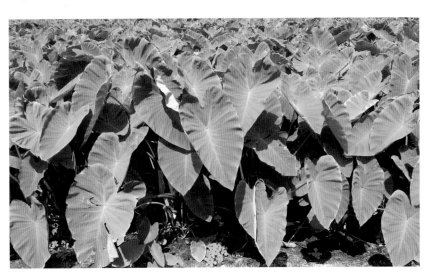

Wild taro, or coco yam (*Colocasia esculenta*).

and the flowering heads consist of a short, greenish, sheathing spathe sub-tending a spadix covered with small, unisexual flowers and terminating in a sterile appendage. Among the most commonly grown species are Chinese taro (*Alocasia cucullata*) and elephant's ear (*A. macrorrhizos*), with large, glossy green leaf blades on stalks up to 1 m (3 ft.) long and 1.2 m (4 ft.) long, respectively; kris plant (*A. sanderiana*), with metallic green, scalloped-edged leaves; arrowleaf elephant's ear, or yautia (*Xanthosoma sagittifolium*), with light green, long-stalked, arrowhead-shaped leaves; and coco yam, or wild taro (*Colocasia esculenta*), with numerous cultivars, some purple-leaved or red-stalked beneath.

Occurrence. These strikingly spectacular, highly visible plants are sometimes found in North American homes, greenhouses, and conservatories, and sometimes as garden escapes in warmer regions. Most species are native to tropical Asia; some are from the New World.

Toxicity. Like other members of the arum family, the genera mentioned here contain sharp, minute crystals, or raphides, of calcium oxalate. If the leaves or any part of the plant are chewed or swallowed, they cause painful irritation and swelling of the mouth and throat. They can also cause skin and eye irritation on contact. Symptoms are similar to those caused by anthurium (which see, later in this section).

Notes. The fleshy underground stems and leaf stalks of some species are a valuable food in parts of the world. *Colocasia esculenta*, the best known, is a popular root vegetable in the tropics; its thick, turnip-like rootstocks, which must be specially prepared to reduce the irritant effect of the calcium oxalate crystals, are a major ingredient of poi, a favorite Polynesian dish. Its starch granules are very small and reputed to more digestible than those of other root crops. The leaves and young shoots of some varieties of taro are eaten as cooked greens.

aloes
Aloe spp.
lily family (Liliaceae)

Quick check. Herbaceous perennials with fleshy, elongated, often spiny-edged leaves in basal clusters; the juice is strongly purgative if ingested, but not fatal.

Description. Many of the approximately 150 species of *Aloe* are grown as house- and greenhouse plants in North America. They are perennials, with basal clusters, or rosettes, of succulent, elongated leaves, which are often sharp-pointed, spiny, or hard-toothed on the edges. The flowers, borne on thin stems above the leaves in dense elongated or umbrella-like clusters, are tubular, and red, pinkish, whitish, or yellow. The fruits are three-angled capsules. Barbados aloe (*Aloe vera*) is probably the most commonly grown species in North America. Its erect or spreading leaves are long, narrow, and pointed, edged with short spines. They are glaucous-green with white spots or markings, thick and fleshy, exuding a mucilaginous gel when cut or broken.

Occurrence. Most aloes are native to tropical Africa (e.g., *Aloe compressa* is a miniature aloe endemic to Madagascar). *Aloe vera* is native to northern Africa but was introduced into the Barbados Islands in the 17th century, hence its common name. Many species are grown in greenhouses in collections of succulent plants, and they are also grown as potted houseplants. In the southern United States they are grown outdoors as garden ornamentals.

Toxicity. The latex in aloe leaves is poisonous if ingested as it contains a powerful purgative known as barbaloin. The quality and quantity of similar glycosides varies from one species to another; *Aloe vera* contains relatively high concentrations and also contains an appreciable amount of chrysophanic acid. These compounds irritate the large intestine and therefore have a strong purgative action, evident six to 12 hours after ingestion. Excessive doses may cause kidney irritation. The anthraquinone compounds color alkaline urine red.

Notes. *Aloe vera*, used for centuries as a skin salve in the treatment of burns, abrasions, and other skin irritations in its native regions, is also grown com-

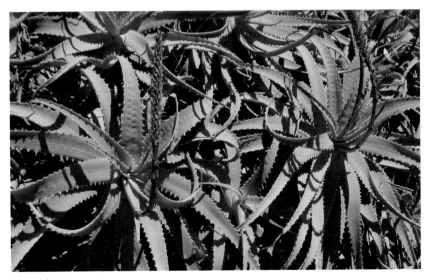

Aloe (*Aloe compressa*).

mercially for its cathartic glycosides and for its mucilaginous gel, which is found in many personal care products such as skin lotions, creams, and shampoos.

angel's-trumpet
Brugmansia ×candida and related spp.
nightshade family (Solanaceae)

Quick check. Leafy, herbaceous perennials as encountered in North America, with large, oval, pale green pointed leaves; flowers large and showy, whitish or pale yellow, trumpet-shaped and usually hanging. Entire plant toxic to humans and animals. Experimentation as potential hallucinogen most common cause of poisoning.

Description. Angel's-trumpet and other brugmansias are found in North America as ornamental indoor shrubs or small trees (up to 10 m, 30 ft., or more) cultivated in warmer regions, with large, trumpet-like flowers. The bark is light brown, and the large leaves, covered with fine hairs, are alternate and 10–30 cm (4–12 in.) long by 15 cm (6 in.) or more wide, with usually coarsely toothed or scalloped margins. The flowers are dramatic: long (up to 50 cm, 20 in.), pendulous, and flaring at the end. There are about six species, and many cultivars, with flower colors ranging from white to orange to red. They emit a delicate, attractive scent. *Brugmansia ×candida* is a hybrid between two Ecuadorian species, *B. aurea* and *B. versicolor*. Angel's-tears is a commonly grown hybrid between *B. versicolor* and *B. suaveolens*. These plants are related to jimsonweeds and thorn-apples (*Datura* spp.).

Occurrence. Brugmansias are native to subtropical South America. They are widely grown in gardens in California, Florida, and other subtropical areas, and often grown indoors as potted trees, even in northern regions.

Toxicity. All parts of *Brugmansia* plants, especially the leaves and seeds, are poisonous, containing tropane alkaloids, most notably hyoscyamine and scopolamine, which is hallucinogenic. Symptoms of poisoning, similar to those of belladonna (*Atropa bella-donna*) and jimsonweed, are evident within a few minutes to several hours after ingestion: intense thirst, dilation of pupils, blurred vision, hallucinations, flushing and dryness of the skin, headache, and nausea; in serious cases, these symptoms are followed by rapid but weak pulse, high temperature (occasionally), high blood pressure, urinary retention, delirium, incoherence, fever, convulsions, coma, and potentially death. Intense symptoms may abate within one or two days, but disturbance of vision may last up to two weeks. Poisoning is often due to people—especially youth—deliberately seeking a hallucinogenic experience from this notorious plant. As well as the direct danger from the plant, they may undertake risky behaviors during intoxication.

Notes. Deaths directly attributed to angel's-trumpet and its relatives are relatively rare, but recovery can be prolonged, and risk of accidents is higher when people are disoriented. The experience of a 15-year-old high school student from Honolulu is typical: in February 2002, the youth was hospitalized in critical condition from consuming several petals of angel's-trumpet flowers from a neighbor's yard. He showed the predominant symptoms of intoxication from this plant (dry mouth, rapid heartbeat, dilated pupils, loss of coordination) and experienced severe hallucinations for 18 hours straight (Ishikawa 2002). Another woman recounted, anecdotally, that about half an hour after being inadvertently splashed with water while hosing off her *Brugmansia* plants (and wiping her face with the hand that turned the leaves as she did so), she experienced dry, burning eyes, blurred vision, and "huge" pupils. At the emergency room, she was diagnosed with atropine poisoning, with additional symptoms of extreme thirst, headache, dizziness, slight nausea, rapid pulse, and elevated blood pressure. She was told to wear dark glasses and sent home to recover (Araillia 2005).

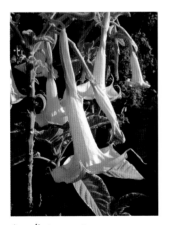

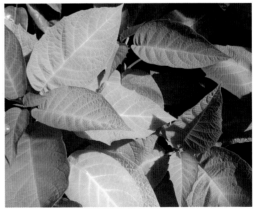

Angel's-trumpet
(*Brugmansia ×candida*).

Angel's-trumpet leaves.

anthuriums

Anthurium andraeanum and related spp.
arum family (Araceae)

Quick check. Large plants with heart-shaped or elliptical leaves and showy "flowers" with a scarlet (or pink) sheath surrounding an elongated spike; entire plant contains calcium oxalate crystals, which irritate the mouth and throat if swallowed; may also irritate skin and eyes.

Description. Herbaceous perennials with clustering, dark green, leathery leaves that are heart-shaped in flamingo-lily (*Anthurium andraeanum*), or lance-shaped in some other *Anthurium* species. The leaf blades are up to 30 cm (1 ft.) long, and the plants up to 60 cm (2 ft.) high. Each showy flower head consists of a shiny, scarlet (occasionally pink or light green), reflexed sheath, or spathe, surrounding a red, yellowish, or greenish, club-like spike, or spadix, which is densely covered with small, bisexual flowers and sometimes curled or spiraled. The fruits are densely clustered, showy berries.

Occurrence. The more than 600 species of *Anthurium* are native to tropical America. Anthuriums, including many hybrids, are grown as house and greenhouse ornamentals in temperate North America, or outdoors in the southern United States. Their exotic flower heads last up to two months, and florists commonly sell them as cut flowers in floral arrangements.

Toxicity. The leaves and stems contain minute, sharp crystals, or raphides, of calcium oxalate, like those found in *Dieffenbachia* and other plants in the arum family. If ingested, the plant causes painful burning and swelling of the lips, mouth, and throat, sometimes with acute inflammation that can restrict breathing. Symptoms may include intense salivation, hoarseness, difficulty in swallowing, loss of speech, and loss of appetite. The initial pain from ingestion almost always inhibits further swallowing. Also, the crystals pass unchanged through the digestive tract and so do not usually cause further complications. The calcium

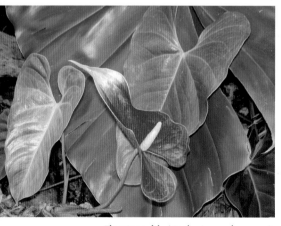

Flamingo-lily (*Anthurium andraeanum*).

oxalate crystals may cause irritation to the skin and eyes. The symptoms may persist for several hours or days.

Notes. Many plants in this family, including several commonly grown houseplants described in this section, contain irritant calcium oxalate crystals. Notwithstanding, these popular ornamentals are often seen in hospital waiting rooms, doctors' offices, schools, restaurants, and shopping malls.

arums

Arum spp.
arum family (Araceae)

Quick check. Large-leaved herbaceous perennials with attractive but bad-smelling "flowers" consisting of a broad, yellowish, whitish, or purplish sheath surrounding a cylindrical spike; bright reddish berries are attractive to children; entire plants, especially berries, toxic and potentially fatal if ingested in quantity.

Description. Stemless plants growing from tuberous roots, with large, long-stemmed oval to triangular or arrow-shaped leaves. The showy but putrid-smelling flower heads are long-stalked and consist of a broad sheath, or spathe, which is greenish, yellowish, cream-colored, or violet, enclosing a dull purple to brownish, cylindrical spike, or spadix. This spadix is crowded with tiny, unisexual flowers, the male flowers situated above the female. The flowering stalk tends to wither rather than fall after maturity. The fruits form a dense cluster of fleshy berries, green at first and ripening to reddish orange or brilliant red after the sheath and leaves die down.

Occurrence. Arums originated in Europe and the Middle East, and a few species are grown for curiosity as houseplants in North America. They are sometimes grown outdoors in the southern United States and in mild climates further

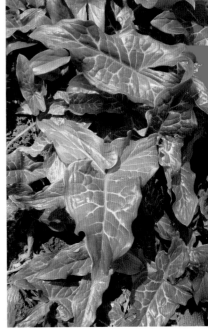

Italian lords and ladies (*Arum italicum*) leaves.

north. Two commonly grown species are Italian lords and ladies (*Arum italicum*), some forms of which have cream-veined foliage, and cuckoo pint (*A. maculatum*).

Toxicity. These plants, like others in the arum family, contain minute, sharp crystals, or raphides, of calcium oxalate. These may irritate the skin and eyes, and, if ingested, the lips, mouth, and throat. The attractive berries are particularly poisonous and are sometimes eaten by children. The acrid juice of the plant usually deters people from eating large amounts, but if sufficient quantities are ingested, it can cause sore throat and digestive irritation and pain, with severe diarrhea, irregular heartbeat, and in extreme cases, coma and death. Fortunately, poisoning is not usually severe. The plant can irritate the eyes and skin on contact. It is also toxic, sometimes fatally, to various types of livestock, but animals seldom willingly eat it because it is so acrid.

Notes. In England, the rootstock of cuckoo pint was used as a source of laundry starch, but it caused chronic irritation of the hands and has been abandoned (it is said that the name lords and ladies originated in Tudor times from the practice of stiffening courtiers' ruffs with the starchy tubers). The baked and powdered root was prepared as a food, Portland arrowroot or Portland sago.

caladiums

Caladium bicolor and related spp.
arum family (Araceae)

Quick check. Herbaceous perennials with showy, variegated, arrowhead-shaped leaves of a wide variety of colors; entire plant contains irritant calcium oxalate crystals, causing intense burning of the mouth and throat if swallowed; not usually fatal.

Description. Perennials growing from underground tubers. The leaves are basal and long-stalked, arising in a clump from the tubers. The blades, large and arrowhead-like, are veined, edged, or splashed with a wide range of very attractive colors. The "flowers" consist of a dense, fleshy spike, or spadix, subtended by a boat-shaped, often showy bract, or spathe. The berries are white.

Occurrence. Caladiums are native to tropical America, and are commonly grown as ornamental house- and greenhouse plants throughout temperate

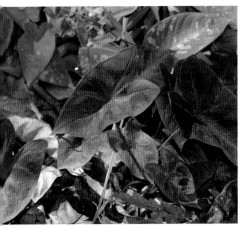

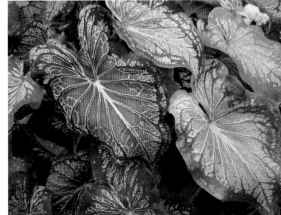

Heart of Jesus (*Caladium bicolor*).   Caladium hybrid.

North America, as well as being cultivated in gardens in subtropical areas. *Caladium bicolor* (heart of Jesus) is among the most common of the approximately one dozen species.

Toxicity. These plants, like other members of the arum family, contain minute, sharp crystals, or raphides, of calcium oxalate, which, if swallowed, cause intense irritation and swelling of the mouth and throat and can also cause skin and eye irritation on contact.

Notes. Most caladiums sold as houseplants in North America are hybrids derived from *Caladium bicolor*; they often have very colorful, often bright red leaves, or white leaves with green veins. Most of the scores of available varieties are sold unnamed. The plants are perennials, but the foliage dies back in the winter.

calla lily
Zantedeschia aethiopica and related spp.
arum family (Araceae)

Quick check. Large herbaceous perennial with smooth, arrowhead-shaped leaves and showy white-sheathed "flowers"; entire plant contains irritant calcium oxalate crystals that cause intense burning and inflammation of the mouth and throat if ingested; seldom fatal.

Description. Calla lily is a robust, rhizomatous perennial up to 1 m (3 ft.)

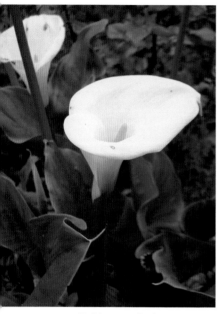

Calla lily (*Zantedeschia aethiopica*).

high, with smooth-edged, shining, arrowhead-shaped leaves that are basal, clustered, and long-stalked. The "flowers" consist of a showy, flaring white spathe 13–25 cm (5–10 in.) long surrounding a fragrant, yellow, club-like spike of tiny true flowers; the many hybrids are variously colored. The fruits are berry-like.

Occurrence. Calla lily, native to South Africa, is grown as a large, potted house- and greenhouse plant throughout North America and as an outdoor garden plant in the southern United States, where it is sometimes found as a garden escape. Other species are sometimes grown.

Toxicity. Calla lily, like other members of the arum family, contains irritant crystals of calcium oxalate, which, if ingested, cause intense burning and swelling of the mouth and throat and can also cause skin and eye irritation on contact. An unidentified toxic protein has also been reported.

Notes. Calla lily (*Zantedeschia aethiopica*) is sometimes confused with the native water arum (*Calla palustris*), a plant of the same family growing in wet, boggy areas throughout much of the United States and Canada and sometimes planted around ponds in gardens.

chili pepper

Capsicum annuum and related spp.
nightshade family (Solanaceae)

Quick check. Herbaceous perennial with smooth-edged, elliptical or oval leaves, whitish flowers, and smooth, rounded or elongated fruits that are usually bright red (sometimes yellow or purple) when mature; the fruits contain varying amounts of capsaicin and derivatives, which can cause painful inflammation and burning of the mouth, mucous membranes, skin, and eyes.

Description. Perennial with simple, alternate, elliptical or oval, somewhat thin leaves. The small, star-shaped flowers are borne in the branch axils and are whitish, usually with a purplish tinge. The fruits are pod-like and many-seeded, with a smooth, fleshy skin. They vary in form—elongated, pointed, or rounded; upright or drooping—and are variously colored (white, green, yellowish, or purplish) during ripening, usually bright red (sometimes yellow, orange, or purple) at maturity. Some varieties have sweet-tasting fruits; these are the common green, red, and yellow sweet or bell peppers used in salads and cooking in North American households. Others—mostly the smaller, elongated types—are the chili peppers, or cayenne peppers. They are hot and biting to the taste and are used as flavoring, particularly in Mexican and Southeast Asian dishes. Paprika is from yet another variety of *Capsicum annuum*. The pepper used in tabasco sauce is from a related species, tabasco pepper (*C. frutescens*).

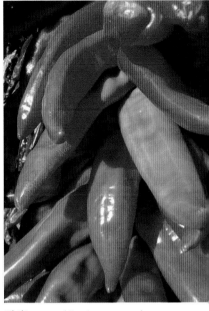

Chili pepper (*Capsicum annuum*).

Occurrence. The wild ancestor to the chili peppers is native to Central and South America. Chili peppers are cultivated in the southern United States and Mexico and elsewhere in the world for their hot, spicy fruits; some forms grow wild in the South. Many varieties are grown as potted ornamental houseplants, which may die back within one season.

Toxicity. The fruits and seeds of chili peppers, especially some of the more pungent varieties, contain the compound capsaicin. The degree of "heat" is measured in Scoville units: the hottest peppers available in North American markets can be near 1,000,000 Scoville units, which would be incredibly painful. Although capsaicin in higher amounts can be painful, it is usually harmless. It can cause irritation of the lips and mouth if ingested, however, and if large amounts are eaten, chili peppers may cause digestive upset and diarrhea. They may also cause painful inflammation and burning of the mucous membranes and skin on contact. A major danger is if the acrid juice from the fruits gets into the eyes; it can cause acute inflammation, and pain, with heavy tear production. This can happen simply from inadvertent rubbing of the eye with the hands if one has been handling chili peppers in cooking. Smoke from cooking the peppers may also irritate the eyes.

Notes. Capsaicin interacts with vanilloid receptor proteins, which mediate pain signals, and has been used as an analgesic to treat cluster headache sufferers and people with chronic pain conditions. Capsaicin cream and other products are sometimes effective against pain that is unresponsive to other treatments (Brinker 1999). Chili peppers are used in pepper spray, and *Capsicum annuum* has topped the list for the number of inquiries and cases of poisoning in the United States (Frohne and Pfänder 2005).

dumbcanes

Dieffenbachia spp.
arum family (Araceae)

Quick check. Tall herbaceous perennials with large, usually mottled leaves; entire plant contains irritating calcium oxalate crystals, excruciatingly painful to the mouth and throat if eaten, and causing inability to speak, potentially lasting several days; seldom fatal.

Description. Perennial plants 1–2 m (3–6 ft.) tall, with green, unbranched stems having conspicuous, evenly spaced, horizontal leaf scars. The leaves are large, oblong, and smooth-edged, with clasping or sheathing stalks. The veins are prominent, and the blades are usually blotched with whitish, light green, dark green, or yellow-green markings. The calla-like flowers, when they occur, are of a typical arum form, with a greenish or whitish sheath surrounding a spadix. *Dieffenbachia seguine* and its cultivars are most frequently encountered: leaves are dark green, up to 45 cm (18 in.) long, and striped or mottled with white bars. Also very popular is *D. picta* (now considered by most taxonomists to be synonymous with *D. seguine*); its smaller leaves range from nearly all green to practically all cream except for a green margin. Plants are grown primarily for their decorative leaves.

Occurrence. Native to tropical America, several species of dumbcanes, or dieffenbachias, and their cultivars are grown as indoor ornamentals in North America, especially in areas of low light intensity, or outdoors in the warmest regions. They are even found in preschools and health care centers, where their toxic, irritant properties and the risk they pose to children are apparently not well known.

Toxicity. Dieffenbachias contain minute needle-like crystals, or raphides, of calcium oxalate, which penetrate the tissues of the mouth and throat if the plant is eaten. The concentration of these oxalates varies considerably from one variety to another. The plants contain special "ejector cells" on the surface of their leaves that, on contact, shoot the raphides out, causing them to penetrate the tissue, along with quantities of oxalic acid. This dual action produces both mechanical and chemical injury, resulting in severe burning and inflammation of the throat and mouth, and heavy salivation. In severe cases, swelling of the throat and tongue may cause temporary loss of speech (hence, dumbcane), and choking, which has occasionally been fatal. Nausea, vomiting, and diarrhea are additional symptoms, perhaps due to the presence of other, unknown toxins. Symptoms may persist for a week or more. These plants also cause irritation to the skin and eyes.

Notes. Dieffenbachias, which originate from Brazil and the West Indies, were used in the past as a means of human torture, especially of slaves.

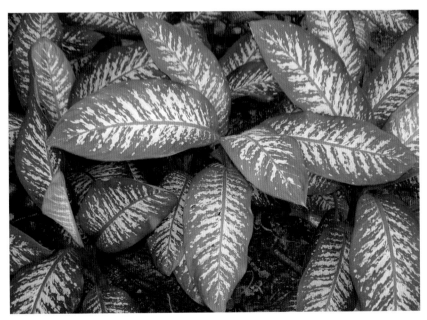

Dumbcane (*Dieffenbachia seguine*).

glorylily

Gloriosa superba
lily family (Liliaceae)

Quick check. Herbaceous perennial from a tuberous rootstock, with showy yellow or red lily-like flowers with swept-back petals; all parts extremely poisonous, potentially fatal.

Description. Glorylily, or flame lily, is a slender, climbing plant or vine up to 1.5 m (5 ft.) long, growing from a thick, tuberous rootstock. The leaves are alternate or almost opposite, lanceolate or elliptical, and up to 15 cm (6 in.) or more long, each with a tendril-like tip. The large, striking flowers are yellow at first, changing to orange and then to bright crimson; they are borne on long stalks, and each has six tepals (petals and sepals that are like), which are crinkled along the edges and spreading, or reflexed, with the stamens and single green pistil exserted. The fruit is a large, oblong capsule, containing bright red seeds. 'Rothschildiana' is among the most widely known of this plant's many cultivars.

Occurrence. Native to tropical Africa and Asia, glorylily is frequently grown in gardens of the southern United States, and as a container plant, mainly in greenhouses but occasionally outdoors in pots in more temperate areas, elsewhere in North America.

Toxicity. The entire plant is toxic, particularly the tubers. It contains the alkaloid colchicine and other compounds related to those found in autumn cro-

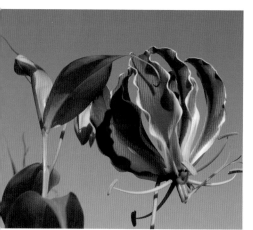

Glorylily (*Gloriosa superba*).

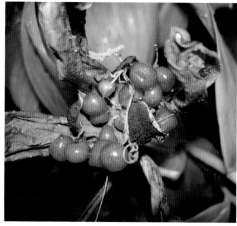

Glorylily fruit.

cus. Symptoms of poisoning include intense burning and numbness of the mouth and throat, thirst, nausea, and vomiting. Abdominal pain and severe diarrhea may follow after a delay of two or more hours. Bloody urine, reduced urine output, difficulty in breathing, convulsions, and sometimes death may also result.

Notes. Glorylilies are known around the world as poisonous to both humans and animals. The bulbs are sold in nurseries, often without warnings about their toxicity.

Jerusalem cherry
Solanum pseudocapsicum
nightshade family (Solanaceae)

Quick check. An herbaceous to somewhat woody evergreen with dark green leaves, white flowers, and attractive, round, yellow or red fruits; entire plant, and especially the fruits toxic and potentially fatal.

Description. Bushy, erect, evergreen up to 1.2 m (4 ft.) tall, with shiny, dark green, oblong, lance-shaped leaves up to 10 cm (4 in.) long. The flowers are white and solitary, about 1.2 cm (0.5 in.) across. The cherry-sized berries are bright red or yellow, and long-lasting.

Occurrence. A native of the Old World, Jerusalem cherry makes an attractive and highly ornamental potted houseplant, especially during the Christmas season. It is often purchased in nurseries when the berries are green, so their ripening can be enjoyed. It is also grown as an outdoor patio plant, or year-round garden plant in warmer regions. Occasionally it occurs as a garden escape.

Toxicity. The entire plant contains a toxic steroid alkaloid, solanocapsine, which acts on the heart. It also contains solanine and related alkaloids, as do other *Solanum* species, including nightshades. The attractive, brightly colored fruits are especially dangerous, and eating three or four has proven fatal to children. Symptoms of poisoning, which may not appear until several hours after ingestion, include

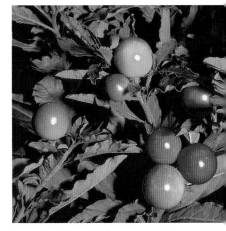

Jerusalem cherry (*Solanum pseudocapsicum*).

scratchy feeling in the throat, abdominal pain, fever, nausea, vomiting, salivation, severe diarrhea, and headache. In the worst cases, lowered or irregular heart rate, difficulty in breathing, restlessness, confusion, delirium, hallucinations, convulsions, kidney failure, and coma followed by death may occur. Recovery from poisoning may be slow, with symptoms persisting for several days.

Notes. Several varieties of Jerusalem cherry are grown, including some variegated forms. Another showy relative, strawberry groundcherry, or Chinese lantern (*Physalis alkekengi*), is often included in dried flower arrangements for its bright red or orange, papery fruiting calyces. Its berries, enclosed within the "lanterns," contain solanine when unripe and may cause digestive upset if eaten. The ripe berries of this and related species, however, are nontoxic. Sweet and flavorful, they are sometimes made into jams and preserves.

mistletoes
Phoradendron spp. and related genera
mistletoe family (Viscaceae)

Quick check. Semi-parasitic plants growing in dense clusters on deciduous and evergreen trees; widely used as traditional Christmas decorations; white berries and green plants produce severe digestive upset when ingested in quantity; rarely fatal.

Description. Mistletoes are semi-parasites of several genera of deciduous and evergreen trees, both flowering and cone-bearing. The mistletoes of Christmas are mainly *Phoradendron* species, especially *P. tomentosum*. They have smooth-edged, oblong, leathery green leaves in opposite pairs. The tiny, inconspicuous flowers ripen into clusters of showy, whitish or pinkish, translucent berries. The seeds are sticky and are often spread from one tree to the next by birds. Dwarf mistletoes (*Arceuthobium* spp.), smaller plants in the same family, with broom-like aerial shoots, are parasitic on coniferous trees;

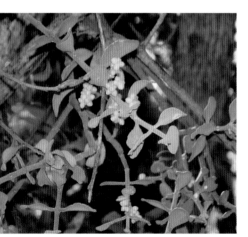

Mistletoe (*Phoradendron* sp.).

they are a major forest pest, responsible for extensive damage in wood production in North America.

Occurrence. *Phoradendron* mistletoes grow in large, dense clusters on deciduous trees. Various species occur from Oregon and California east to New Jersey and Florida. In their fruiting stage, mistletoes are harvested and distributed commercially throughout North America for use as Christmas decorations. European mistletoe (*Viscum album*) has been introduced locally in some areas, particularly California.

Toxicity. The entire plant, especially the leaves and stems, contains toxic polypeptides and lectins, such as phoratoxin, which inhibit protein synthesis in the intestinal wall. The biochemistry is fairly complex, including alkaloids and cardenolides from the host plants. Eating only a few mistletoe berries may cause minor abdominal pain and diarrhea, but ingesting large quantities of the berries, or drinking tea made from the leaves, can produce severe irritation of the digestive tract, including vomiting, diarrhea, and acute cramping. Lowered heart rate, similar to but less severe than that produced by digitalis, may also occur. Mistletoe has on rare occasions been fatal.

Notes. An old Christmas tradition, its origins probably extending back to early European pagan ceremonies, is that any person caught standing beneath mistletoe must forfeit a kiss. Nowadays, to prevent poisoning in children (and to increase the shelf life of mistletoe in marketing), plastic berries are often substituted for real ones by commercial florists.

Mistletoe species have been widely used in folk medicine over the course of human history. Recently, European mistletoe has been involved in research to treat immune system disorders, including HIV/AIDS. It is also being investigated as a therapeutic agent in the treatment of cancer, nervous disorders, pain management, and menstrual problems (Evans 2005).

nutmeg

Myristica fragrans
nutmeg family (Myristicaceae)

Quick check. Brown, ovoid, spicy seed, or grated brown powder, widely used as a culinary spice; nutmeg is harmless in small amounts but if ingested in larger doses (i.e., greater than 10 g, or 0.4 oz) it can cause acute poisoning and death.

Description. Nutmeg is the large, woody brown seed of a tropical evergreen tree, which yields two spices commonly found in North American homes: nutmeg and mace, the thin, net-like, reddish or yellowish covering of the seed. These spices can be purchased and stored whole, to be grated or ground as required, or bought and stored in ground form. The nutmeg tree is tall, with alternate, yellowish brown leaves that are elliptical or lanceolate, and up to 13 cm (5 in.) long. The flowers are small and inconspicuous, male and female borne on separate individuals. The fruit is globular, about the size of a golf ball, reddish or yellowish, and splitting into two valves, each containing a nutmeg enclosed in a hard shell.

Occurrence. Whole or ground nutmeg is often found on the spice shelf of North American homes. Occasionally nutmeg trees are grown in conservatories and botanical gardens in North America. Nutmeg is native to India, Australia, and the South Pacific, and there are about 80 different species in the genus.

Toxicity. Nutmeg contains volatile oils, which give it its spicy scent and flavor; however, if excessive amounts are inhaled or ingested, it can cause acute poisoning. The volatile oils are irritating to all tissues. Myristicin, elemicin, and safrol are the toxins. In large quantities (over 10 g, or 0.4 oz), powdered nutmeg or mace affects the central nervous system and produces hallucinations and unpleasant side effects, including headache, dizziness, drowsiness, nausea, stomach pain, excessive thirst, rapid pulse, delirium, anxiety, double vision, and sometimes acute panic and coma. Most cases of nutmeg poisoning occur when people try to use it as a readily obtainable hallucinogenic drug. People who have taken it agree that it causes an agonizing hangover.

Notes. Many other common household herbs and spices, including cinnamon, cloves, eucalyptus, mint, black pepper, rosemary, sage, and sassafras, contain volatile oils that could be harmful in large or concentrated doses. Moderation is the key to using these substances.

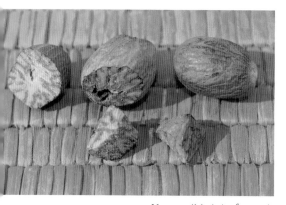

Nutmeg (*Myristica fragrans*).

philodendrons and monsteras

Philodendron spp. and *Monstera* spp.
arum family (Araceae)

Quick check. Climbing or trailing vines or large, leafy plants with heart-shaped leaves, sometimes deeply cut or lobed; entire plants contain irritant calcium oxalate crystals, which cause intense burning of the mouth and throat if ingested; seldom life-threatening.

Description. Climbing vines or large, leafy plants with hard stem bases, many growing up to 18 m (60 ft.) or more high in the wild, clinging to the trunks of trees by means of aerial roots. When grown as potted indoor plants, they are usually much shorter but can still attain a considerable length. The foliage and plant characteristics vary from one species to another, but in general the leaves are leathery and glossy or velvety, bright green to reddish, heart- to arrowhead-shaped, and in some types, deeply lobed or cut (e.g., *Philodendron bipinnatifidum*). The leaf stalk forms a sheath around the stem. The plants seldom flower; when they do, male and female flowers are produced separately on the same individual plant. The flower heads are anthurium-like, with a leafy spathe subtending a long, slender spadix. One of the most commonly grown species is heartleaf philodendron, or sweetheart plant (*P. cordatum*); with thin, trailing stems and heart-shaped, pointed leaves up to 13 cm (5 in.) long, it is usually grown in hanging pots. Some cultivars produce red, burgundy, or cream-and-green variegated leaves. Tarovine (*Monstera deliciosa*) has large, interesting leaves that are deeply cut along the edges and perforated with irregularly placed holes (hence its other common names, split-leaf philodendron, or Swiss-cheese plant).

Occurrence. The genera *Philodendron* and *Monstera* contain more than 200 species native to the tropical rain forests of Central and South America, several of which are grown as potted ornamentals in North American homes. They are among the most popular of all houseplants, and in the southern United States they are also sometimes grown outdoors.

Toxicity. Philodendrons, like other members of the arum family, contain minute, sharp crystals of calcium oxalate in their leaves, roots, stems, flowers, and unripe fruits. If swallowed, these raphides cause intense irritation and swelling of the mouth and throat, and can also cause skin

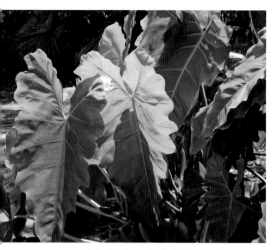

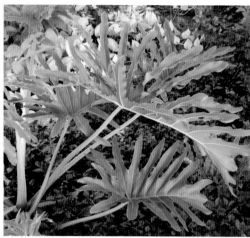

Philodendron (*Philodendron* sp.).

Elephant ear philodendron (*Philodendron bipinnatifidum*).

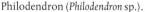

and eye irritation on contact. The plants also contain unidentified toxic proteins.

Notes. The trailing or climbing heartleaf philodendron is a particular hazard to young children and pets because they can easily reach and chew on the hanging stems and leaves. Be especially watchful of babies as they learn to crawl or stand. More than one mother has discovered her newly mobile baby with a philodendron leaf in its mouth, pulled from a plant that only a week before had been out of reach.

The fleshy fruit of tarovine is edible, giving rise to other names for it, including Mexican breadfruit and fruit salad plant. The fruit takes a year or so to ripen and must be fully mature before it can be eaten.

poinsettia

Euphorbia pulcherrima
spurge family (Euphorbiaceae)

Quick check. Low, bushy potted plant or large shrub with bright red, pink, or white floral bracts; entire plant exudes a milky juice when cut or bruised. Ingesting the plant may produce stomach upset; milky juice may irritate the skin.

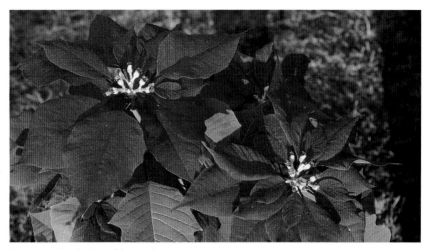

Poinsettia (*Euphorbia pulcherrima*).

Description. Poinsettia, or Christmas flower, is a low and bushy plant with a woody base when grown as a potted houseplant; when growing freely outdoors in warm areas or planted out in a greenhouse, poinsettia is a large, woody shrub up to 3 m (10 ft.) or more high. Indoors it is much smaller, and usually densely leafy. The leaves, 8–15 cm (3–6 in.) or more long, are alternate, bright green, oval or elliptical, smooth-edged or shallowly lobed, and slightly hairy beneath. The familiar "flowers" of Christmas time are actually brightly colored bracts surrounding an open cluster of small yellow and red flowers, which mature into small capsules. The most common color of the flower bracts is bright vermilion-red, but white, pink, and variegated forms are also seen.

Occurrence. A native of Mexico and Central America, poinsettia is widely encountered in North America each December, as a potted seasonal ornamental. In warmer areas of the southern United States, it is grown outdoors in containers or in gardens as a shrub or hedge plant.

Toxicity. The milky juice, which is exuded when the plant is cut or bruised, has the same irritant effect as that of other *Euphorbia* species, but it appears to be less potent than in other members of this genus. Much attention has centered on poinsettias and their possible toxicity. In recent years, hundreds of cases of children ingesting parts of poinsettias have been reported;

in most of these, however, no symptoms (or only minor ones) were experienced, the most severe being vomiting, abdominal pain, and diarrhea. Chemical studies have shown the plant to be lacking the irritant diterpenes found in other euphorbias. Handling poinsettias, however, can be irritating to the skin, especially for those working in nurseries or florist shops.

Notes. Poinsettia is a short-day flowering plant, and growing it for the North American December holiday market is a major industry. Modern plant breeding has developed shorter, bushier, longer-flowering hybrids, which will bloom year after year if allowed short days and long, dark nights in the fall.

rosarypea

Abrus precatorius
pea family (Fabaceae)

Quick check. Climbing tropical vine whose small, attractive, usually red seeds are used as beads in novelty jewelry; seeds are highly toxic if broken or chewed when ingested; may be fatal.

Description. The plant is weedy, a slender, twining vine growing 3 m (10 ft.) tall, with pinnately compound leaves composed of many small leaflets, and red, lavender, or white pea-like flowers in small clusters. The fruiting pods are flat, broad, and hairy, about 4 cm (1.5 in.) long, each containing four to

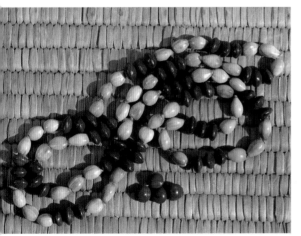

eight shining, hard seeds about 6 mm (0.25 in.) long, which are brilliant scarlet, and black at the base.

Occurrence. Native to India, this plant has spread to most tropical and subtropical regions and is a common weed in Florida, the Caribbean, Hawaii, and Guam. The attractive but deadly seeds often find their way into households, in the form of beads on imported rosaries and necklaces, inside rattles, and as good luck charms.

Necklace of rosarypea (*Abrus precatorius*) seeds (red) and Job's tears (*Coix lacryma-jobi*) seeds (white).

Toxicity. The hard-coated mature seeds, if swallowed whole, usually pass through the digestive tract without harm. However, if chewed, broken, or immature, they release a lectin, abrin, which inhibits protein synthesis in growing cells of the intestinal wall and agglutinates red blood cells. Symptoms of poisoning occur after a latent period of many hours, or sometimes as much as three days, depending on the number of seeds swallowed, and the amount of chewing they underwent. Nausea, vomiting, diarrhea, severe abdominal pain, dilation of the pupils, and ulcerating and bleeding of the mouth and digestive tract are major symptoms. Loss of intestinal function and liver damage may occur, and in severe cases, convulsions, coma, and death. A single, well-chewed seed can be fatal for a child, even with treatment. Seeds drilled to make beads are dangerous because the inner part is thus exposed.

Notes. In addition to their toxic principles, the seeds also contain abrusosides, which are much sweeter than sugar. The common name refers to the popular use of the seeds for rosaries in some parts of the world. The epithet is also derived from this use, originating from the Latin *precator* ("one who prays"). The plant and its seeds have a wide variety of other local and colloquial names, most pertaining to the use of the seeds as beads: crab's eyes, red bead, coral bead, prayer beads, love bean, Indian bead, and Seminole bead.

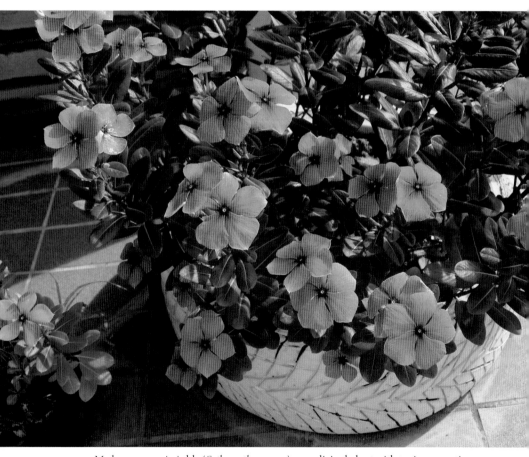

Madagascar periwinkle (*Catharanthus roseus*), a medicinal plant with toxic properties..

APPENDIX 1
Fruits, Vegetables, and Beverage Plants

Listed alphabetically by common name. Almost all are harmless when used in normal quantities under normal circumstances and are potentially toxic only when misused.

AKEE (*Blighia sapida*). The covering around the unripe fruit, the fruit wall, and the seeds of this tropical fruit contain hypoglycin, which can cause acute low blood sugar; sometimes fatal. In Jamaica, where this fruit commonly grows, akee poisoning (or vomiting sickness) has been common in times of food shortage. The ripe fruit is a favorite food.

ALMOND (*Prunus dulcis*). Bitter oil contains a cyanide-producing compound amygdalin, most of which is removed in commercially produced oils.

APPLES (*Malus* spp.). Seeds contain a cyanide-producing compound; harmful if seeds are eaten in quantity.

APRICOT (*Prunus armeniaca*). Kernels contain a cyanide-producing compound; harmful if kernels are eaten in quantity.

ASPARAGUS (*Asparagus officinalis*). Young shoots may cause skin irritation; berries not edible. The rhizome is used as an herbal medicine in various ways. It contains saponins and other potentially harmful compounds; it should not be used for inflammatory kidney diseases and may cause allergic skin reactions.

AVOCADO (*Persea americana*). Seeds, leaves, stems poisonous.

BAMBOO (*Bambusa* spp. and other genera). Young shoots of many species contain cyanogenic compounds in very high concentrations, but boiling or drying the shoots eliminates virtually all the prussic acid.

BANANA and PLANTAIN (*Musa* ×*paradisiaca* and related spp.). Fruit peel, and to a much lesser extent, the fruit pulp, contains amines (serotonin, tyramine, dopamine, norepinephrine), which cause an increase in blood pressure in animals.

BEAN, FAVA, or BROADBEAN (*Vicia faba*). Eating fresh fava beans cooked or uncooked, causes severe hemolytic anemia in susceptible people, particularly in those of the northern Mediterranean countries, who have an inherited deficiency of a particular enzyme (glucose-6-phosphate dehydrogenase). Fava beans also contain a phytotoxin or lectin, and a glycoside, vicine.

BEAN, HYACINTH (*Lablab purpureus*; syn. *Dolichos lablab*). Contains a cyanide-producing glycoside; must be thoroughly cooked (with two to four water changes).

BEAN, KIDNEY (*Phaseolus vulgaris*). Known to contain lectins.

BEAN, LIMA (*Phaseolus lunatus*). Some strains (not usually found in North America) contain dangerous quantities of a cyanide-producing glycoside.

BEET (*Beta vulgaris*). Greens are high in soluble salts of oxalic acid and can cause calcium deficiency if eaten in high quantities in a calcium-poor diet.

BRASSICAS (*Brassica* spp.). The hot, pungent taste and odor of these and other mustards, and of mustard oils, is due to the presence of glucosinolate compounds, which are called goitrogens because they interfere with the uptake of iodine by the thyroid gland, and in extreme cases can lead to goiter. There is little evidence that these plants, when used as vegetables and condiments in moderation, cause problems for people with adequate iodine in their diets.

BROCCOLI (*Brassica oleracea* var. *botrytis*). See BRASSICAS

BRUSSELS SPROUTS (*Brassica oleracea* var. *gemmifera*). See BRASSICAS

BUCKWHEAT (*Fagopyrum esculentum*). Plant contains phototoxic phenolic compounds; can cause photosensitivity in susceptible individuals.

CABBAGE (*Brassica oleracea*). See BRASSICAS

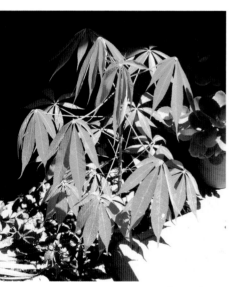

Cassava (*Manihot esculenta*).

CASHEW (*Anacardium occidentale*). Raw nuts and kernels contain a cyanide-producing compound, but commercial processing removes this; oil may cause irritation in susceptible individuals.

CASSAVA (*Manihot esculenta*). Raw or improperly prepared tubers and tuber peelings contain a cyanide-producing compound; potentially fatal.

CAULIFLOWER (*Brassica oleracea*). See BRASSICAS

CELERY (*Apium graveolens*). Plants, especially those contaminated with the mold *Sclerotinia sclerotiorum*, produce phototoxins (psoralens, which are furanocoumarin compounds), sometimes causing serious dermatitis of workers handling celery.

CHARD, SWISS (*Beta vulgaris* ssp. *cicla*). See BEET

CHERRIES (*Prunus* spp.). Leaves, bark, and seed kernels contain a cyanide-producing compound.

CHILI PEPPER (*Capsicum annuum*). Fruits and seeds contain the compound capsaicin.

CHOCOLATE, COCOA (*Theobroma cacao*). Contains caffeine. See COFFEE

COFFEE (*Coffea arabica*). Contains caffeine, a purine alkaloid, which has a stimulating effect on the central nervous system. Large quantities can lead to dizziness, pains, vomiting, rapid pulse, and lowered blood pressure. Chronic poisoning from continued high doses may result in headaches, restlessness, insomnia, tremors, and constipation.

CRESS, GARDEN (*Lepidium sativum*). Contains glucosinolates. See BRASSICAS

EGGPLANT (*Solanum melongena*). Plants, unripe fruits, and overripe fruits contain solanine and related compounds. See POTATO

ELDERBERRIES (*Sambucus* spp.). Bark, twigs, leaves, and seeds contain cyanide-producing glycoside; ripe berries the only edible part.

FIGS (*Ficus* spp.). Sap contains skin irritant.

FLAXES (*Linum* spp.). Seeds contain cyanide-producing glycosides, varying considerably in concentration depending on genetic strain, season, and climate; these are usually a problem only when linseed cake or meal is fed in quantity to livestock.

HORSERADISH (*Armoracia rusticana*). Contains glucosinolates. See BRASSICAS

KALE, CHINESE (*Brassica alboglabra*). See BRASSICAS

KIWI (*Actinidia chinensis*). Contains proteolytic enzymes; excessive use could irritate mucous membranes.

KOHLRABI (*Brassica oleracea* var. *gongylodes*). See BRASSICAS

MACE (*Myristica fragrans*). Contains myristicin, a potent and dangerous hallucinogen, but harmful only in large amounts. See NUTMEG

MANGO (*Mangifera indica*). Sap from the stem at the base of the fruit contains a poison ivy-like toxin; carefully wash fruit, and do not eat the skin.

MINT, including PEPPERMINT (*Mentha ×piperita* and related spp.). Its aromatic oil contains menthol, which can be harmful to susceptible individuals in high doses.

MUSTARDS (*Brassica* spp.). Contain glucosinolates. See BRASSICAS

NUTMEG (*Myristica fragrans*). Contains myristicin, a potent and dangerous hallucinogen, but harmful only in large amounts.

ONION (*Allium cepa* and related spp.). Onions, chives (*A. schoenoprasum*), and garlic (*A. sativum*) contain several sulfur-containing volatile oils, which cause irritation to the eyes and nose, and may also cause skin irritation.

Eaten in large amounts over a period of time, onions can cause anemia, jaundice, and digestive disturbances in humans. They are also harmful to cattle and horses.

PAPAYA (*Carica papaya*). Contains proteolytic enzymes, which may cause irritation of mucous membranes with excessive use.

PARSNIP (*Pastinaca* spp., including *P. sativa*, wild parsnip). Contains phototoxic furanocoumarins; contact with foliage in sunlight can cause skin irritation, blistering, and discoloration.

PEA, FIELD (*Pisum sativum*). Plant contains lectins, substances that agglutinate red blood cells and may, in large doses, interfere with the body's immune system.

PEACH (*Prunus persica*). Bark, leaves, and seed kernels contain a cyanide-producing compound.

PEANUT (*Arachis hypogaea* and related spp.). Many people are allergic to peanuts; peanuts contaminated with certain molds (mainly *Aspergillus flavus*) contain aflatoxins, which are potent carcinogens.

PEPPER, BLACK (*Piper nigrum*). Contains myristicin and safrole. See NUTMEG

PEPPERMINT (*Mentha* ×*piperita*). See MINT

PINEAPPLE (*Ananas comosus*). Contains proteolytic enzymes, which may cause irritation of mucous membranes with excessive use.

POTATO (*Solanum tuberosum*). Greens, sprouts, and green tubers contain solanine and other toxic alkaloids.

RADISH (*Raphanus sativus*). Contains glucosinolates. See BRASSICAS

RAPESEED (*Brassica napus* and related spp.). Seeds and oil contain erucic acid and glucosinolates. Note: canola oil is from rapeseed varieties genetically developed in Canada, which are very low in erucic acid and glucosinolates and therefore safe to consume. See BRASSICAS

RHUBARB (*Rheum rhabarbarum*). Stalks contain oxalic acid; leaves very poisonous.

RUTABAGA (*Brassica napus* and related spp.). Contains glucosinolates. See BRASSICAS

RYE (*Secale cereale*). This and other cereal grains may become contaminated with ergot (*Claviceps* spp.) and cause poisoning.

SAGE (*Salvia officinalis*). Contains thujone, which is toxic in high doses.

SOYBEAN (*Glycine max*). Raw beans contain several enzyme inhibitors, proteins inhibiting the digestion of other proteins, and hemagglutinins, substances that agglutinate red blood cells; these are largely destroyed by cooking.

SPINACH (*Spinacia oleracea*). High in soluble salts of oxalic acid and can cause calcium deficiency if eaten in high quantities in a calcium-poor diet.

TEA (*Camellia sinensis*). Contains caffeine, a purine alkaloid, which has a stimulating effect on the central nervous system. See COFFEE

TOMATO (*Solanum lycopersicum*). Plant contains an alkaloid similar to solanine; leaves and vines can cause headache, abdominal pain, vomiting, and diarrhea.

TURNIP (*Brassica septiceps* and related spp.). Contains glucosinolates. See BRASSICAS

WALNUT (*Juglans regia* and related spp.). Blackened hulls and moldy nuts have poisoned dogs eating them from the ground underneath the trees.

WASABI (*Wasabia japonica*). Well-known Japanese condiment; contains glucosinolates. See BRASSICAS

WATERCRESS (*Nasturtium officinale*). Contains glucosinolates. See BRASSICAS

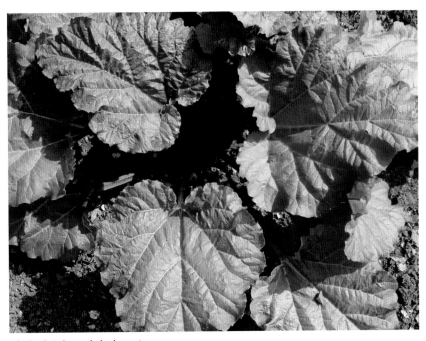

Rhubarb (*Rheum rhabarbarum*).

Wild Edible Plants

All the plants listed here have potentially toxic properties or toxic parts. Some of these are still perfectly edible if used with caution or in moderation; others (some described in detail in Chapter 3) are no longer recommended as edible.

ARROWGRASS (*Triglochin maritima* and related spp.). Young vegetative leaf bases of *T. maritima* eaten by some northwestern indigenous peoples (Turner 1995), but the plants under some conditions contain cyanide-producing glycosides and have caused illness and death in livestock.

BEECHNUT, EUROPEAN, and AMERICAN BEECHNUT (*Fagus sylvatica* and *F. grandifolia*). Roasted nuts edible, but raw seed kernels contain a saponin-like substance and an alkaloid-like compound, fagin. If eaten in quantity (50 or more nuts), the kernels of the European beech, and possibly American beech as well, can produce headache, abdominal pain, vomiting, diarrhea, and extreme fatigue, symptoms that develop within an hour of eating the nuts and last up to five hours.

BRACKENFERN (*Pteridium aquilinum*). Contains several toxic and carcinogenic substances; eating the young shoots or rhizomes of this species not recommended.

BROOM, SCOTCH (*Cytisus scoparius*). Flowers sometimes used in wine making, and roasted seeds as a coffee substitute, but the plant contains alkaloids and may cause digestive upset; use not recommended.

BUCKEYES (*Aesculus* spp.). Some Native peoples used the thoroughly leached and roasted seeds as an emergency food, but the entire plant should be considered toxic.

CHERRIES, WILD (*Prunus* spp.). Bark, foliage, and seed kernels contain a potent cyanide-producing glycoside.

CHOKECHERRY (*Prunus virginiana*). Bark, foliage, and seed kernels contain a potent cyanide-producing glycoside.

CLOVERS (*Trifolium* spp.). Clover flowers and leaves are sometimes eaten or made into teas, and the rhizomes of some species are also eaten. However, clovers should be used with caution and only in moderation, because they contain a number of toxic compounds, including infertility-causing estrogens, cyanide-producing glycosides, goitrogens, nitrates, and substances that can cause photosensitivity or coagulate the blood.

COWPARSNIP (*Heracleum maximum*). Young leafstalks and budstalks peeled and eaten in spring by many indigenous peoples in North America (Turner 1995, 1997; Kuhnlein and Turner 1987). However, plants contain several phototoxic furanocoumarins that can cause poison ivy–like dermatitis and discoloration of the skin if the plants are touched or handled followed by exposure to ultraviolet radiation from sunlight.

DOCKS (*Rumex* spp.). Leaves and stems used as potherb, but should be used only in moderation; contain soluble oxalates, which can interfere with calcium uptake.

ELDERBERRIES (*Sambucus* spp.). Bark, twigs, leaves, and seeds contain cyanide-producing glycoside; ripe berries the only edible part.

FERNLEAF BISCUITROOT (*Lomatium dissectum*). Taproots and very young shoots eaten by some Native peoples in northwestern North America, but use not recommended; roots contain high concentrations of furanocoumarins, and used as fish poison.

JACK IN THE PULPITS (*Arisaema* spp.). Contains calcium oxalate crystals.

KENTUCKY COFFEETREE (*Gymnocladus dioicus*). Contains cytisine, a quinolizidine alkaloid with action similar to nicotine.

LABRADOR TEA and **WESTERN LABRADOR TEA** (*Ledum palustre* and *L. glandulosum*). Contain andromedotoxins; apparently safe in weak tea solution but should not be made too strong.

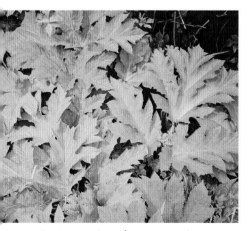

Cowparsnip (*Heracleum maximum*).

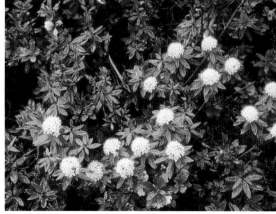

Western Labrador tea (*Ledum glandulosum*).

LAMBSQUARTERS (*Chenopodium album*). High content of soluble oxalates, which can cause reduction of calcium when eaten in excess; may also cause phototoxicity when eaten in large quantities.

LAUREL, CALIFORNIA (*Umbellularia californica*). Leaves contain as much as 4% dry weight as irritating oils, mainly umbellulone, a volatile oil. Inhaling this aromatic substance can cause headache and unconsciousness in some people.

LUPINES (*Lupinus* spp.). Roots of some species eaten by indigenous peoples, but the plants contain lupine alkaloids; use not recommended.

MALLOWS (*Malva* spp.). Greens and green fruits eaten, but plants known to cause livestock poisoning if eaten in quantity; toxin unknown.

MARSH MARIGOLDS (*Caltha* spp.). Plants contain irritant protoanemonin; should never be eaten raw; considered poisonous by some indigenous peoples (Moerman 2003).

MAYAPPLE (*Podophyllum peltatum*). Only fully ripe fruits edible.

MILKWEEDS (*Asclepias* spp.). Young shoots and green fruits of *A. speciosa* and *A. syriaca* have been eaten as potherbs, but all species should be treated with caution.

MOUNTAIN ASHES, or **ROWANS** (*Sorbus* spp.). Fruits used to make jellies and wine, but seeds should be strained out; contain cyanogenic glycosides.

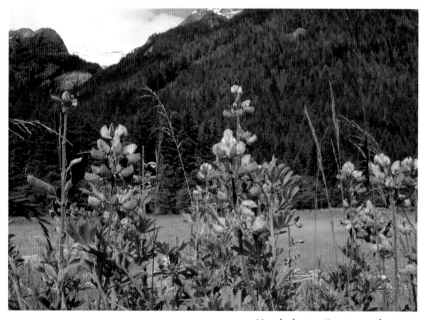

Nootka lupine (*Lupinus nootkatensis*).

MULBERRY, RED (*Morus rubra*). Unripe fruits and milky sap in leaves and stems cause hallucinations and digestive upset.

OAKS (*Quercus* spp.). Leaves and shoots highly toxic to livestock. Acorns contain tannins of the gallotannin class; for food use, they must be leached in running water to remove bitter tannins.

ONIONS, WILD (*Allium* spp.). Use in moderation; some species can cause digestive upset and some species have caused breakdown of red blood cells in livestock.

ORACHES, or **SALTBUSHES** (*Atriplex* spp.). May be phototoxic if eaten in excessive amounts; at least one species (*A. canescens*) is considered poisonous by indigenous peoples (Moerman 2003).

PAWPAW (*Asimina triloba*). Fruits may cause skin irritation.

PIGWEEDS, or **AMARANTHS** (*Amaranthus* spp.). Plants may accumulate oxalates and nitrates; known to cause fluid accumulation around the kidneys of livestock eating the plants.

POKEWEED, AMERICAN (*Phytolacca americana*). Roots and raw leaves and fruits have caused fatal poisoning. Fully cooked greens and berries have been eaten in the past, but use not recommended because of presence of cell-destroying mitogens.

PURSLANE (*Portulaca oleracea*). Plant may accumulate oxalates and nitrates; use only in moderation.

SASKATOON SERVICEBERRY (*Amelanchier alnifolia* and related spp.). Fruits safe and edible, but leaves, bark, and seeds contain cyanide-producing glycosides and can be toxic (seeds present in fruits are not harmful with normal use).

SASSAFRAS (*Sassafras albidum*). Considered unsafe for medicinal or beverage use (root bark is used as tea). Its volatile oil contains safrole, which is known to cause tumors in rats; hence, the use of safrole for flavoring has been banned by the U.S. Food and Drug Administration.

SEDUMS (*Sedum* spp.). Various species contain oxalic acid and soluble oxalates; use only in moderation.

SKUNKCABBAGE, WESTERN (*Lysichiton americanus*). Entire plant contains needle-like calcium oxalate crystals; rhizomes eaten by some northwestern indigenous peoples, but must be prepared specially and cooked for a long time.

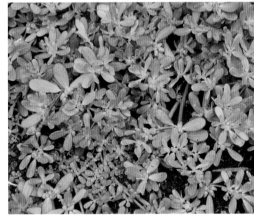

Purslane (*Portulaca oleracea*).

SOAPBERRY, or **RUSSET BUFFALOBERRY** (*Shepherdia canadensis*). Berries contain bitter, sudsing saponins that allow them to be whipped up with water into a favorite confection of indigenous peoples of British Columbia (Turner 1995); no reports of poisoning from their use, but should be used only in moderation.

SORREL, SHEEP (*Rumex acetosella*). Plant contains oxalic acid and soluble oxalates; use only in moderation.

SWEETFLAG and **CALAMUS** (*Acorus americanus* and *A. calamus*). Volatile oil, especially in triploid forms of these plants, contains beta-asarone, which causes illness and tumor growth in rats; calamus oil has now been withdrawn from use as a flavoring ingredient in many countries, and use as a vegetable, flavoring, or condiment is not recommended.

SWEETVETCH, ALPINE (*Hedysarum alpinum*). Also known as Eskimo potato, licorice root, Alaska carrot, or bearroot; the roots are widely eaten but easily confused with a toxic relative, Mackenzie's sweetvetch (*H. boreale* ssp. *mackenziei*), also known as wild sweet pea, boreal sweetvetch, or brown bear's Indian potato, a plant well known among indigenous peoples of the north for its poisonous qualities (Moerman 2003).

WALNUT, BLACK (*Juglans nigra*). Hulls and moldy nuts are toxic to livestock.

WATERPARSNIP (*Sium suave* and related spp.). Indigenous peoples consider the parsnip-like roots edible (Kuhnlein and Turner 1991), but accidents have occurred when people have confused these plants with the highly toxic water hemlocks (*Cicuta* spp.).

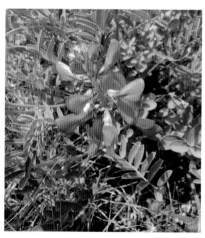 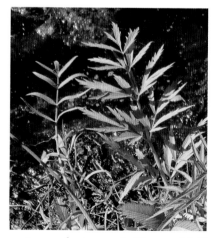

Mackenzie's sweetvetch (*Hedysarum boreale* ssp. *mackenziei*).

Leaves of waterparsnip (*Sium suave*) (left) and the deadly Mackenzie's water hemlock (*Cicuta virosa*) (right) at Bella Coola, B.C.

WILDGINGERS (*Asarum* spp.). Volatile oil contains asarone, which can cause illness and tumor growth in rats in high concentrations.

WOODSORRELS (*Oxalis* spp.). Plants contain oxalic acid and soluble oxalates; use only in moderation.

WORMWOODS (*Artemisia* spp.). Especially absinthe (*A. absinthium*), the main flavoring ingredient in the spirit of the same name. This alcoholic drink, popular in the late 19th and early 20th centuries in France and now enjoying a revival in the European Union, was blamed for profoundly affecting the mental and physical state of those under its influence. Scientists believe that the thujone in the absinthe is similar to marijuana in its effects on the mind; wormwoods and other plants containing high concentrations of thujone should be regarded with extreme caution and should not be used as an herb or flavoring.

YAUPON (*Ilex vomitoria*). Used as a tea, but causes vomiting in high concentrations.

APPENDIX 3
Skin and Eye Irritants

Plants cause several types of skin irritation, or dermatitis. Some types are mechanical, caused by injury from thorns, barbs, or spines. Others, such as those caused by buttercups, spurges, and stinging nettles, are from irritant chemicals present in the juice, sap, or hairs. In other cases, an allergic reaction results from a person being sensitized to a particular plant. Some plants, such as poison ivy and its relatives, are allergy-causing in most individuals after an initial exposure. Allergic reactions are possible with many herbal medicines; use any with caution. Some plants are phototoxic. These cause the skin to be hypersensitive to sunlight, and skin irritation occurs after exposure to these plants with subsequent exposure to sunlight (see discussion in Chapter 1). Many of the plants listed also cause eye irritation or injury if allowed to come in contact with the eyes.

ALLAMANDA, YELLOW (*Allamanda cathartica*). All parts.

ALSTROEMERIA (*Alstroemeria aurea* and related spp.). All parts.

ANEMONES (*Anemone* spp., *Pulsatilla* spp.). Leaves, flowers.

ANGELICA (*Angelica archangelica*). Roots, leaves potentially phototoxic.

ARUMS (many genera in Araceae). Leaves, stems, roots.

ASPARAGUS (*Asparagus officinalis*). Young shoots and rhizome may cause allergic skin reactions.

BARBERRIES (*Berberis* spp.). Spines.

BLACKTHORN, or SLOE PLUM (*Prunus spinosa*). Spines.

BLEEDING HEARTS (*Dicentra* spp.). All parts.

BLOODROOT (*Sanguinaria canadensis*). Sap.

BLUE COHOSH (*Caulophyllum thalictroides*). Roots.

BORAGES (*Borago* spp.). Prickly hairs.

BOX, COMMON (*Buxus sempervirens*). Leaves.

BURDOCKS (*Arctium* spp.). Burs.

BUTTERCUPS (*Ranunculus* spp.). Leaves, flowers.

CACTUS (*Opuntia* spp. and other genera). Barbed spines and bristles.

CARDINALFLOWER (*Lobelia cardinalis*). Sap, leaves.

CASHEW (*Anacardium occidentale*). Oil, nutshells; strongly allergenic.

CASTORBEAN (*Ricinus communis*). Plant.

CEDAR. Western redcedar (*Thuja plicata*) and Alaska cedar, or yellowcedar (*Cupressus nootkatensis*): boughs, wood allergenic.

CELANDINE (*Chelidonium majus*). Red sap.

CELERY (*Apium graveolens*). Phototoxic (especially when contaminated with the mold *Sclerotinia sclerotiorum*).

CENTURY PLANTS (*Agave* spp.). Sap.

CHILI PEPPER (*Capsicum annuum*). Fruits and seeds. Keep away from eyes and mucous membranes; potentially allergenic.

CHRYSANTHEMUMS (*Chrysanthemum* spp.). Plant.

CITRUS FRUITS (*Citrus* spp.). Peel, thorns; occasional photosensitization.

CLEMATIS (*Clematis* spp.). Leaves.

COCKLEBUR, ROUGH (*Xanthium strumarium*). Plant.

COMFREYS (*Symphytum* spp.). Hairs on leaves, stems.

COWPARSNIP (*Heracleum maximum*). Sap of leaves, stems phototoxic; potentially serious.

CROTONS, GARDEN (*Codiaeum* spp.). Plant.

DEVILSCLAW (*Proboscidea parviflora* and related spp.). Fruits with sharp curved claws.

DEVILSCLUB (*Oplopanax horridus*). Spiny stems can cause serious allergy.

DITTANY, or **GASPLANT** (*Dictamnus albus*). Plant phototoxic.

DOCKS (*Rumex* spp.). Plants phototoxic.

FALSE HELLEBORE, GREEN (*Veratrum viride* and related spp.). Leaves.

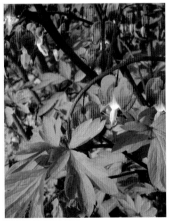

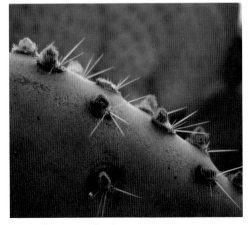

Showy bleeding heart
(*Dicentra spectabilis*).

Cactus (*Opuntia* sp.) spines.

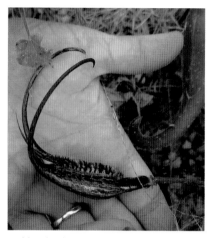
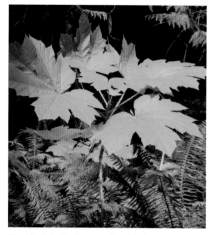

Golden devilsclaw (*Proboscidea althaeifolia*).   Devilsclub (*Oplopanax horridus*).

FEVERFEW (*Tanacetum parthenium*). Commonly allergenic with skin contact.

FIGS (*Ficus* spp.). Sap.

FINGER ROT (*Cnidoscolus urens* var. *stimulosus*). Stinging hairs; very painful, potentially serious.

FOUR O'CLOCK, or **MARVEL OF PERU** (*Mirabilis jalapa*). Plant.

FRANGIPANI, or **TEMPLETREE** (*Plumeria rubra*). Sap.

GINKGO (*Ginkgo biloba*). Seeds.

GOLDENASTER, HAIRY FALSE (*Heterotheca villosa*). Entire plant said to cause skin irritation similar to ant bites (Moerman 2003).

GOOSEBERRIES (*Ribes* spp.). Spines.

GRASSES. Awned grass fruits and bracts can become embedded in the fur, ears, eyes, and nostrils of pets and livestock; sometimes inadvertently swallowed; can cause choking. Many species, including cheatgrass (*Bromus tectorum*); needle and thread, or needlegrass (*Stipa* spp., *Hesperostipa* spp.); Fendler threeawn grass (*Aristida purpurea* var. *longiseta*); foxtail barley (*Hordeum jubatum*); and wild oat (*Avena fatua*).

HAWTHORNS (*Crataegus* spp.). Thorns.

HELIOTROPES (*Heliotropium* spp.). Leaves.

HERCULES' CLUB (*Aralia spinosa*). Bark, spines.

HOGWEED, GIANT (*Heracleum mantegazzianum*). Sap of leaves, stems phototoxic; potentially serious.

HOLLIES (*Ilex* spp.). Prickly leaves.

HONEYLOCUST (*Gleditsia triacanthos*). Long, sharp spines.

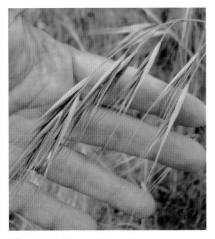

Cheatgrass (*Bromus tectorum*).

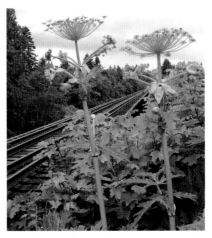

Giant hogweed (*Heracleum mantegazzianum*).

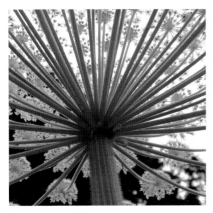

Giant hogweed flower.

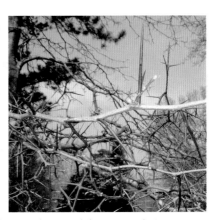

Honeylocust (*Gleditsia triacanthos*).

HOP (*Humulus lupulus*). Leaves.

HYACINTH (*Hyacinthus orientalis*). Plants, bulbs.

HYDRANGEAS (*Hydrangea* spp.). Occasional reports of allergic skin irritation due to handling.

INDIAN-TOBACCO (*Lobelia inflata*). Juice, leaves.

IRISES (*Iris* spp.). Juice or sap.

IVY, ENGLISH (*Hedera helix*). Leaves.

JACK IN THE PULPITS (*Arisaema* spp.). Leaves, roots.

JIMSONWEED (*Datura stramonium*). Leaves, flowers.

JUNIPERS (*Juniperus* spp.). Boughs, wood allergenic.

KNOTWEEDS (*Polygonum* spp.). Leaves phototoxic.

LADY'S SLIPPERS (*Cypripedium* spp.). Leaves.

LILY OF THE VALLEY, EUROPEAN (*Convallaria majalis*). Leaves, roots.

MANCHINEEL (*Hippomane mancinella*). Milky juice; potentially serious.

MANGO (*Mangifera indica*). Sap from fruit stem allergenic.

MARIGOLDS (*Tagetes* spp.). Plants phototoxic.

MARSH ELDERS (*Iva* spp.). Plants phototoxic.

MAYAPPLE (*Podophyllum peltatum*). Roots.

MESQUITES (*Prosopis* spp.). Spines.

MULBERRY, RED (*Morus rubra*). Leaves, stems.

OLEANDER (*Nerium oleander*). Leaves.

OSAGE ORANGE (*Maclura pomifera*). Milky juice.

PALMS, DATE (*Phoenix* spp.). Leaf stalk thorns, sharp-tipped leaves.

PAPAYA (*Carica papaya*). Sap.

PARSNIP, WILD (*Pastinaca sativa*). Leaves phototoxic.

PAWPAW (*Asimina triloba*). Fruits.

PINE, SCOTS (*Pinus sylvestris*). Needle oil.

POINSETTIA (*Euphorbia pulcherrima*). Sap.

POISON HEMLOCK (*Conium maculatum*). Leaves.

POISON IVY (*Toxicodendron radicans* and *T. rydbergii*). Severely allergenic.

POISON OAK (*Toxicodendron diversilobum* and *T. pubescens*). Severely allergenic.

POISON SUMAC (*Toxicodendron vernix*). Severely allergenic.

POISONTREE, FLORIDA (*Metopium toxiferum*). All parts; severely allergenic.

PRIMROSES (*Primula* spp.). Commonly allergenic.

PRIVET, EUROPEAN (*Ligustrum vulgare*). Leaves.

PUNCTUREVINE (*Tribulus terrestris*). Spiny fruits.

QUEEN ANNE'S LACE (*Daucus carota*). Leaves phototoxic.

RAGWORTS (*Senecio* spp.). Leaves phototoxic.

ROSES (*Rosa* spp.). Spines.

RUSSIAN THISTLE (*Salsola kali*). Spines.

SCARLET PIMPERNEL (*Anagallis arvensis*). Leaves.

SMARTWEEDS (*Polygonum* spp.). Leaves phototoxic.

SPURGES (*Euphorbia* spp.). Milky juice, spines of some species; potentially serious.

STINGING NETTLE (*Urtica dioica* and related spp.). Stinging hairs; very painful.

SWEETCICELYS, or **SWEETROOTS** (*Osmorhiza* spp.). Spine-like fruits can become embedded in skin or ears of pets; if swallowed can cause choking.

TANSY, COMMON (*Tanacetum vulgare*). Plant phototoxic.

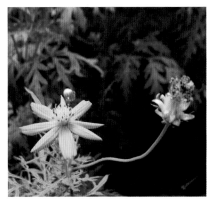

Marigold (*Tagetes* sp.).

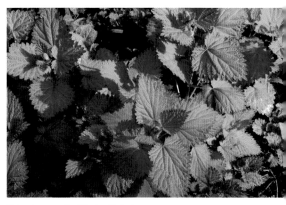

Stinging nettle (*Urtica dioica*).

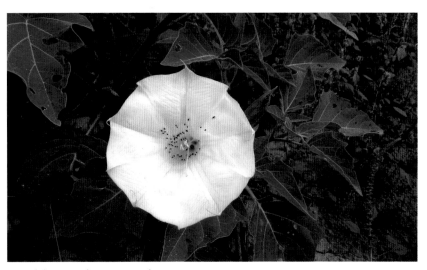

Sacred thorn-apple (*Datura wrightii*).

THORN-APPLES (*Datura* spp.). Leaves, flowers.

TOMATO (*Solanum lycopersicum*). Plant.

TRUMPET CREEPER (*Campsis radicans*). Leaves, flowers; potentially serious.

TRUMPETFLOWER, EVENING (*Gelsemium sempervirens*). Leaves, stems.

TULIPS (*Tulipa* spp.). Tuliposides in the leaves, bulbs cause skin irritation, especially among those collecting, sorting, and packing them.

WOOD NETTLE (*Laportea canadensis*). Stinging hairs; very painful.

YARROW (*Achillea millefolium*). Plant phototoxic.

YUCCAS (*Yucca* spp.). Sharp, pointed leaves.

APPENDIX 4
Honey Poisons

Honey is flower nectar that has been gathered, modified, concentrated, and stored by honeybees. Poisoning by honey is rare, either because bees often avoid flowers of poisonous plants, or because the bees themselves are poisoned directly before honey can be produced. Commercial honey producers are careful to ensure that poisonous honey does not reach the market; the main danger is in eating home-produced honey where the bees' nectar sources have not been monitored. Flowers of the following plants found in North America are known to yield poisonous honey.

AZALEAS (*Rhododendron* spp.)
BOG ROSEMARYS (*Andromeda* spp.)
BUCKEYES (*Aesculus* spp.)
BUTTERCUPS (*Ranunculus* spp.) and other Ranunculaceae
HENBANES (*Hyoscyamus* spp.)
JIMSONWEED (*Datura stramonium*)
LAURELS (*Kalmia* spp.)
MILKVETCHES (*Astragalus* spp.)
OLEANDER (*Nerium oleander*)
PIERIS, JAPANESE (*Pieris japonica*)
RAGWORT, TANSY (*Senecio jacobaea*)
RHODODENDRONS (*Rhododendron* spp.)
SPURGES (*Euphorbia* spp.)
THORN-APPLES (*Datura* spp.)
TRUMPETFLOWER, EVENING (*Gelsemium sempervirens*)

APPENDIX 5
Milk Poisons

The following toxic plants are known to taint milk of browsing or grazing dairy cows and/or goats. In addition to these species, many other toxic plants can reduce milk yield. In only a few cases (e.g., in white snakeroot) has a definite link been established between tainted milk and poisoning in people or animals drinking it. Note that plants that accumulate selenium, such as milkvetch (*Astragalus* spp.), aster (*Aster* spp.), and orache (*Atriplex* spp.), can cause toxicity to nursing offspring of animals grazing plants with excessive amounts of selenium (Panter and James 1990). When known, the toxicant excreted through milk is also listed.

AUTUMN CROCUS (*Colchicum autumnale*)

BITTERWEED (*Picris sprengeriana*). Sesquiterpene lactones.

BRACKENFERN (*Pteridium aquilinum*)

BRASSICAS (*Brassica* spp.). Glucosinolates.

BUTTERCUPS (*Ranunculus* spp.)

COMFREYS (*Symphytum* spp.). Pyrrolizidine alkaloids.

FESCUE, TALL (*Schedonorus phoenix*). Pyrrolizidine alkaloids.

FIDDLENECKS (*Amsinckia* spp.). Pyrrolizidine alkaloids.

FOOL'S PARSLEY (*Aethusa cynapium*)

GARLICS (*Allium* spp.)

GOLDEN CHAIN TREE (*Laburnum anagyroides*)

GYPSYFLOWER (*Cynoglossum officinale*). Pyrrolizidine alkaloids.

HELIOTROPES (*Heliotropium* spp.). Pyrrolizidine alkaloids.

HELLEBORES (*Helleborus* spp.)

HENBANE, BLACK (*Hyoscyamus niger*)

HORSERADISH (*Armoracia rusticana*). Glucosinolates.

HORSETAILS (*Equisetum* spp.)

IVY, ENGLISH (*Hedera helix*)

LUPINES (*Lupinus* spp.). Quinolizidine alkaloids.

MEADOWFOAMS (*Limnanthes* spp.). Glucosinolates.

OAKS (*Quercus* spp.)

PENNYCRESS, FIELD (*Thlaspi arvense*). Glucosinolates.

POISON HEMLOCK (*Conium maculatum*). Piperidine alkaloids.

POTATO (*Solanum tuberosum*). Solanine (greens, sprouts, and green tubers).

RADISH (*Raphanus sativus*). Glucosinolates.

RAGWORT, TANSY (*Senecio jacobaea* and related spp.). Pyrrolizidine alkaloids.

RATTLEBOX, SHOWY (*Crotalaria spectabilis* and related spp.). Pyrrolizidine alkaloids.

RAYLESS GOLDENRODS (*Bigelowia* spp.). Tremetol or tremetone.

RUBBERWEEDS (*Hymenoxys* spp.). Sesquiterpene lactones.

SNAKEROOT, WHITE (*Ageratina altissima*). Tremetol or tremetone.

TOBACCOS (*Nicotiana* spp.). Piperidine alkaloids.

VIPER'S BUGLOSSES (*Echium* spp.). Pyrrolizidine alkaloids.

WATERCRESS (*Nasturtium officinale*). Glucosinolates.

WOODSORRELS (*Oxalis* spp.)

YEWS (*Taxus* spp.)

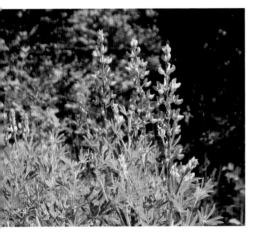

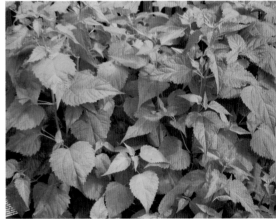

Arctic lupine (*Lupinus arcticus*).   White snakeroot (*Ageratina altissima*).

APPENDIX 6
Medicinal Herbs

Information on the questionable safety of the plants listed here is derived mainly from Blumenthal (2000), Duke (1997), and Tyler (1987). The reader is referred to these authoritative books on medicinal herbs for details of these and other potentially harmful herbs. In particular, Blumenthal (2000) provides a list of known side effects of commonly used herbal medicines, and a list of herbs that should be avoided during pregnancy and/or lactation. The comments generally pertain to internal consumption of the herbs, or solutions containing them. Although many of these herbs may be used without harm when prescribed by properly trained and experienced herbalists, none should be taken without extreme care and awareness of their potential dangers. Those suggested to be "very dangerous" should not be used at all in most circumstances.

James Duke (1997) provides excellent advice for the safe use of herbal medicine. He cautions pregnant women to avoid not only the herbs noted here but also coffee (caffeine), alcoholic beverages, and tobacco. His advice to those wishing to take herbal medicines: *Make sure of the diagnosis* ("Diagnosis is a separate art [. . .] best left to physicians."); *Watch out for side effects* (cut back on your dosage or stop taking the herb if you have an unpleasant reaction); *Be alert for allergic reactions* (call 911 immediately if you experience difficulty breathing within 30 minutes or so of trying a new herb: you may have the most severe form of allergic reaction, anaphylaxis, which can be rapidly fatal unless treated promptly); and *Beware of interactions* (as with pharmaceutical medicines, herbal medicines sometimes interact badly with each other and with certain foods). An example of a potential interaction is between monamine oxidaze (MAO) inhibitors and wine, cheese, and many other foods. St. Johnswort is an herbal MAO inhibitor, and the same interactions should be considered for those taking St. Johnswort as for any pharmaceutical MAO inhibitor drug.

Duke (1997) also warns that herbal medicines can vary tremendously in their active compounds and potency, from one genetic strain to another, under different growing conditions, from different growth stages of the same plant or species, and with different harvesting and processing methods. For this reason, he recommends purchasing standardized medicinal herbs when possible, especially for those inexperienced in herbal medicines.

Tyler (1997), Blumenthal (2000, 2006b), and Blumenthal et al. (2003) point out that most approved herbal medicines, when used in a responsible and informed way, are safe and effective. Many of the cautions provided here would equally apply to prescription drugs. Some problems can arise when people are using herbal products that may be adulterated, or are not standardized, or if they have specific allergies or sensitivities. A recent survey showed that over 70% of Canadians regularly take vitamin supplements, herbal products, and homeopathic medicines, all falling under the category of "natural health products." Health Canada (2008) has developed a licensing system for natural health products approved for marketing, which takes safety and quality into consideration. Under this system, in effect since 2004, hundreds of herbal preparations—including many covered in this appendix and other parts of this book—have been approved, from arnica and angelica to wormwood and yarrow.

AKEE (*Blighia sapida*). Plant considered very dangerous for herbal use.

ANGELICA (*Angelica archangelica* and related spp.). Tyler (1987) considers this plant safe when used as flavoring but unsafe if used medicinally in more concentrated form. The root, used as an infusion to treat digestive problems, contains furanocoumarins, which sensitize the skin to UV light; do not use with prolonged sun bathing or exposure to intense sunlight. Do not use during pregnancy or lactation.

APRICOT (*Prunus armeniaca*). Kernels or pits are a source of the drug laetrile, which Tyler (1987) considers dangerous and ineffective as an anticancer agent; Duke (1985) too rates it as potentially dangerous.

ARBORVITAE, or WHITE CEDAR (*Thuja occidentalis*). Not recommended during pregnancy.

ARNICA, MOUNTAIN (*Arnica montana*). Plant should be used with great caution. It is applied externally to sore muscles, sprains, bruises, and wounds. It has antimicrobial and anti-inflammatory properties, and reduces pain and inflammation. However, according to Blumenthal (2000), prolonged treatment of damaged skin often causes edematous dermatitis, with formation of pustules; prolonged use can also cause eczema; in treatments using high concentrations of arnica preparations, toxic skin reactions with vesicles or even necroses may result.

AUTUMN CROCUS (*Colchicum autumnale*). Plant considered very dangerous for herbal use.

BARBADOS NUT (*Jatropha curcas*). Plant considered very dangerous for herbal use.

BARBERRIES (*Berberis* spp.). Barberry root not recommended during pregnancy.

BELLADONNA (*Atropa bella-donna*). Plant considered very dangerous for herbal use.

BITTER GOURD (*Momordia charantia*). Not recommended during pregnancy.

BLESSED THISTLE (*Cnicus benedictus*). Not recommended during pregnancy and lactation.

BROOM, SCOTCH (*Cytisus scoparius*). Plant potentially unsafe for herbal use.

BUCKTHORN, GLOSSY (*Frangula alnus*). Bark used as an ingredient in laxative preparations; cramp-like discomforts of the gastrointestinal tract can occur in some cases, and long-term use can disturb the body's electrolyte balance, potentially causing potassium deficiency (Blumenthal 2000). Not recommended during pregnancy and lactation.

BUSHMINTS (*Hyptis* spp.). Not recommended during pregnancy.

CANAIGRE DOCK (*Rumex hymenosepalus*). Root has high tannin content and is therefore potentially carcinogenic in long-term herbal use (Tyler 1987); Duke (1985) also rates it as potentially unsafe.

CASCARA (*Frangula purshiana*). Bark used as an ingredient in laxative preparations; cramp-like discomforts of the gastrointestinal tract can occur in some cases, and long-term use can disturb the body's electrolyte balance, potentially causing potassium deficiency, according to Blumenthal (2000). Not recommended during pregnancy and lactation.

CASTORBEAN (*Ricinus communis*). Entire plant, especially seeds, considered very dangerous for herbal use.

CEDAR, WESTERN RED (*Thuja plicata*). Not recommended during pregnancy.

CHAPARRAL, or **CREOSOTE BUSH** (*Larrea tridentata*). Tyler (1987) considers leaves and twigs unsafe for use as an alternative and anticancer agent. Rated relatively safe by Duke (1985).

CHASTETREE (*Vitex agnus-castus*). Not recommended during pregnancy.

CHERVILS (*Anthriscus* spp.). Not recommended during pregnancy.

CHILI PEPPER (*Capsicum annuum*). Do not apply to injured or broken skin; keep away from eyes and mucous membranes.

CHINABERRYTREE (*Melia azedarach*). Plant very dangerous for human use.

CINNAMON BARK (*Cinnamomum* spp.). Not recommended during pregnancy and lactation.

COHOSH, BLACK, or **BLACK BANE-BERRY** (*Actaea racemosa*; syn.

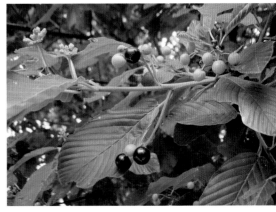

Cascara (*Frangula purshiana*).

Cimicifuga racemosa). Plant widely used medicinally for general illness, kidney ailments, malaria, rheumatism, sore throat, menstrual irregularities, and childbirth; may cause gastric problems, and is not recommended during pregnancy or lactation. Said to be a "safe and effective alternative for hormone replacement therapies in the treatment of menopause" (Foster 1999; Blumenthal 2006c, d; Milot and Blumenthal 2006). Although there is alleged liver toxicity associated with this plant, American Botanical Council states that there is "no attributable risk associated with the use of properly manufactured black cohosh preparations" (ABC note to members, 31 October 2007).

COHOSH, BLUE (*Caulophyllum thalictroides*). Plant potentially unsafe for herbal use.

COLTSFOOT (*Tussilago farfara*). Tyler (1987) considers leaves and flower heads unsafe for use as a demulcent and against coughs; may contain liver-damaging pyrrolizidine alkaloids (Bergner 1989). Rated relatively safe by Duke (1985).

COMFREY, COMMON (*Symphytum officinale*). Tyler (1987) considers plant potentially unsafe as a general healing agent when taken internally; may contain pyrrolizidine alkaloids, which can cause permanent and irreversible liver damage (Bergner 1989).

CYCAD, or SAGO PALM (*Cycas revoluta*). Plant considered very dangerous for herbal use.

DAFFODIL (*Narcissus tazetta*). Plant considered very dangerous for herbal use.

DAPHNE (*Daphne mezereum*). Plant and berries considered very dangerous for herbal use.

DATURAS (*Datura* spp.). Plants considered very dangerous for herbal use.

DONG QUAI (*Angelica sinensis*; syn. *A. polymorpha*). Duke (1985) and Tyler (1987) consider root potentially unsafe for herbal use.

ECHINACEA (*Echinacea angustifolia, E. pallida, E. purpurea*). Can cause short-term reactions: fever, chills, nausea, vomiting; in rare cases, allergic reactions may occur. Not recommended during pregnancy.

ELEUTHERO, or SIBERIAN GINSENG (*Eleutherococcus senticosus*). Root used to treat fatigue, chronic inflammatory conditions; people with high blood pressure should not use.

EPHEDRA, or MA HUANG (*Ephedra distachya, E. sinica*, and related spp.). Major ingredient in dietary supplements; contains alkaloids l-ephedrine, d-pseudoephedrine and others. Used for respiratory tract diseases, bronchial asthma, nasal congestion, common cold, hay fever. Do not use during pregnancy or lactation, or in combination with digitalis or other cardiac glycosides, or in cases of anxiety, restlessness, high blood pressure, glaucoma

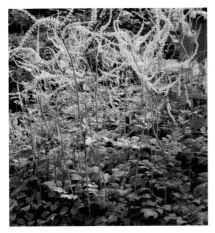

Black cohosh (*Actaea racemosa*).

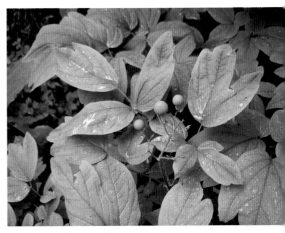

Blue cohosh (*Caulophyllum thalictroides*).

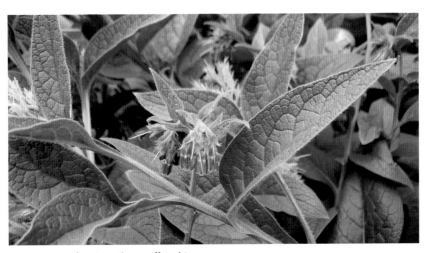

Common comfrey (*Symphytum officinale*).

or impaired circulation of cerebrum; in higher doses, can cause drastic increases in blood pressure, irregular heartbeat and other effects. Occasional deaths from overdoses (Eisenberg 1997); banned by the U.S. Food and Drug Administration in 2004 on the grounds that it does not present a significant health benefit to outweigh the reported increased risk of heart attack, stroke, and death.

EUCALYPTUS OIL (*Eucalyptus* spp.). Used to treat coughs and sore throats, and externally for rheumatic complaints and in inhalants; may in rare cases cause nausea, vomiting, and diarrhea. Do not use in cases of gastrointestinal

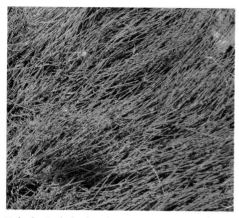

Ephedra (*Ephedra distachya*).

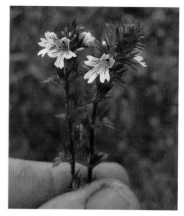

Drug eyebright (*Euphrasia stricta*).

tract inflammation or liver disease; do not apply externally to face or nose of infants or children.

EVENING PRIMROSE (*Oenothera* spp.). Evening primrose oil not recommended during pregnancy.

EYEBRIGHT, DRUG (*Euphrasia stricta*; syn. *E. officinalis*). Tyler (1987) considers plant unsafe and ineffective for treatment of eye diseases. Duke (1985) rates it as relatively safe.

FALSE HELLEBORE, GREEN (*Veratrum viride*). Root used with great care in indigenous medicine; entire plant considered very dangerous for herbal use.

FENNEL (*Foeniculum vulgare*). Not recommended in large quantities during pregnancy.

FENUGREEK (*Trigonella foenum-graecum*). Not recommended in large quantities during pregnancy, or while taking blood thinners.

FEVERFEW (*Tanacetum parthenium*). Not recommended during pregnancy.

FOOL'S PARSLEY (*Aethusa cynapium*). Plant considered very dangerous for herbal use.

FOXGLOVE, PURPLE (*Digitalis purpurea*). Plant considered very dangerous for herbal use.

GARLIC (*Allium sativum*). Not recommended during lactation.

GINSENG (*Panax* spp.). Not recommended during pregnancy.

GLORYLILY, or FLAME LILY (*Gloriosa superba*). Plant considered very dangerous for herbal use.

GOLDEN CHAIN TREE (*Laburnum anagyroides*). Plant considered very dangerous for herbal use.

GOTU KOLA (*Centella asiatica*). Safety and efficacy of herbal use questionable.

GYPSYFLOWER, or HOUND'S TONGUE (*Cynoglossum officinale*). Dangerous for internal use; contains pyrrolizidine alkaloids.

HELIOTROPES (*Heliotropium* spp.). Dangerous for internal use; contain pyrrolizidine alkaloids.

HELLEBORE, BLACK (*Helleborus niger*). Plant considered very dangerous for herbal use.

HENBANE, BLACK (*Hyoscyamus niger*). Plant considered very dangerous for herbal use.

HERNANDIAS (*Hernandia* spp.). Not recommended during pregnancy.

HOREHOUND (*Marrubium vulgare*). Not recommended during pregnancy or lactation.

HORSE CHESTNUT (*Aesculus hippocastanum*). Used to treat problems with veins: cramps, swelling, leg pains, varicose veins, edema in lower limbs; not generally harmful if used as prescribed.

HORSERADISH (*Armoracia rusticana*). Not recommended during pregnancy or lactation.

HYDRANGEAS (*Hydrangea* spp.). Safety and efficacy of herbal use questionable according to Tyler (1987), but Duke (1985) considers it relatively safe.

INDIAN-TOBACCO (*Lobelia inflata*). Entire plant potentially dangerous for herbal use.

JIMSONWEED (*Datura stramonium* and related spp.). Plant considered very dangerous for herbal use.

JUNIPER (*Juniperus communis* and related spp.). Used for indigestion, and sometimes for bladder and kidney conditions, but safety of berries for use as diuretic questionable; do not use during pregnancy or if there is inflammation of the kidneys; prolonged usage or overdosing may cause kidney damage.

KAVA (*Piper methysticum*). Used for treating nervous anxiety, stress, and restlessness; do not use for endogenous depression, or during pregnancy and lactation. Extended use may cause yellow discoloration of skin, hair, and nails. Rare allergic reactions. Some countries have banned kava because of alleged risk of liver toxicity, but there is no convincing proof of inherent toxicity (Schmidt 2007).

LAUREL, MOUNTAIN (*Kalmia latifolia* and related spp.). Plant considered very dangerous for herbal use.

LICORICE (*Glycyrrhiza glabra* and related spp.). Not recommended during pregnancy or lactation. Do not use for liver disorders, or with kidney problems. Prolonged use or higher doses may result in sodium and water retention and potassium loss; potential sensitivity to digitalis glycosides.

LIFE ROOT (*Packera aurea*). Plant considered very dangerous for herbal use; contains pyrrolizidine alkaloids.

MALE FERN (*Dryopteris filix-mas*). Formerly well known as an effective remedy against tapeworms but has caused problems and occasionally deaths from overdosing or in hypersensitive patients and has been entirely supplanted by synthetic vermifuges, which are more predictable in their effects (Frohne and Pfänder 2005).

MANDRAKE (*Mandragora officinarum*). Plant considered very dangerous for herbal use.

MAYAPPLE (*Podophyllum peltatum*). Not recommended during pregnancy.

MEADOWSWEET (*Filipendula ulmaria*). Do not use if person is allergic to salicylate or aspirin or is using blood thinner medication.

MERCURY, ANNUAL (*Mercurialis annua*). Plant considered very dangerous for herbal use.

MISTLETOES (*Phoradendron* spp., *Viscum* spp.). Leaves considered unsafe for herbal use.

MONKSHOODS (*Aconitum* spp.). Plants considered very dangerous for herbal use.

MOTHERWORT (*Leonurus cardiaca*). Not recommended during pregnancy.

MOUNTAINMINTS (*Pycnanthemum* spp.). Not recommended during pregnancy.

MUGWORTS (*Artemisia* spp.). Not recommended during pregnancy.

MYRRHS (*Commiphora* spp.). Not recommended during pregnancy.

NUX-VOMICA, or STRYCHNINE TREE (*Strychnos nux-vomica*). Plant considered very dangerous for herbal use.

OLEANDER (*Nerium oleander*). Plant considered very dangerous for herbal use.

ORANGE, BITTER (*Citrus aurantium*). Peel used as an appetite stimulant; may cause skin reaction in sunlight, especially for fair-skinned people.

PARSLEY (*Petroselinum crispum*). Herb and root, not recommended during pregnancy as herbal medicine; considered safe as culinary herb.

PENNYROYAL (*Mentha pulegium*). Herbal use of leaves or oil considered unsafe; not recommended during pregnancy. At least one attributed death (Eisenberg 1997).

PEONY (*Paeonia officinalis*). Plant considered very dangerous for herbal use.

PERIWINKLE (*Vinca minor*). Plant considered very dangerous for herbal use.

PERIWINKLE, MADAGASCAR (*Catharanthus roseus*). Source of vincristine and vinblastine, important anticancer alkaloid drugs, but potentially dangerous for herbal use.

PINE, SCOTS (*Pinus sylvestris*). Needle oil used as fragrance and flavor in cough and cold medicine, decongestant, and analge-

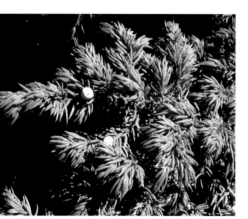

Juniper (*Juniperus communis*).

sic ointments. Do not use with bronchial asthma or whooping cough; may cause irritation of skin and mucous membranes.

POINSETTIA (*Euphorbia pulcherrima*). Plant considered very dangerous for herbal use.

POISON HEMLOCK (*Conium maculatum*). Plant considered very dangerous for herbal use.

POKEWEED, AMERICAN (*Phytolacca americana*). Plant considered very dangerous for herbal use; do not use during pregnancy.

ROSARYPEA (*Abrus precatorius*). Seeds and entire plant very dangerous for herbal use.

ROSEMARY (*Rosmarinus officinalis*). Not recommended in large quantities during pregnancy.

RUES (*Ruta* spp.). Not recommended during pregnancy.

RYEGRASS, DARNEL (*Lolium temulentum*). Plant considered very dangerous for herbal use.

SAGE (*Salvia officinalis*). Used to treat indigestion or excessive perspiration, and externally for nose and throat mucous membrane inflammations. Do not use internally during pregnancy. With prolonged ingestion of pure sage oil or alcohol extracts of oil, epileptiform convulsions can occur, but sage leaves are safe when used in moderation as flavoring.

SAGEBRUSH, BIG (*Artemisia tridentata* and related spp.). Used medicinally by indigenous peoples, but considered unsafe to take internally, or in any concentration; not recommended especially during pregnancy.

SANDBOX TREE (*Hura crepitans*). Plant considered very dangerous for herbal use.

SENNA (*Senna alexandrina*). Leaf and pods used to treat constipation. May cause occasional cramping and discomfort. Prolonged or heavy use may affect electrolyte balance and result in potassium loss. Do not use during pregnancy or in combination with cardiac glycosides or heart medications.

SHEPHERD'S PURSE (*Capsella bursa-pastoris*). Not recommended in large quantities during pregnancy.

SOUTHERNWOOD (*Artemisia abrotanum*). Not recommended during pregnancy.

SPURGES (*Euphorbia* spp.). Plants considered very dangerous for herbal use.

SQUILL, RED (*Urginea maritima*). Plant considered very dangerous for herbal use.

ST. JOHNSWORT (*Hypericum perforatum*). Used to treat mild depression, anxiety; used externally for muscle pain, burns, and pain from acute injuries; can cause photosensitivity (skin irritation in bright sunlight or UV light), especially in fair-skinned individuals, but according to Blumenthal (2000) and Schultz et al. (1998), this would likely occur only at 30 to 50 times the recommended daily dose. Not recommended during pregnancy.

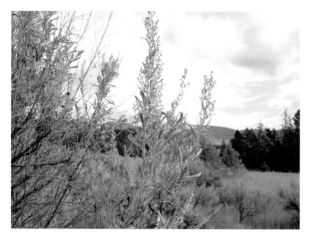

Big sagebrush (*Artemisia tridentata*).

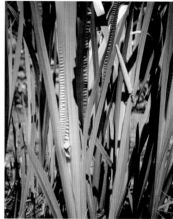

Calamus (*Acorus calamus*).

SWEETFLAG and **CALAMUS** (*Acorus americanus* and *A. calamus*). Rhizomes considered potentially unsafe for herbal use, due to the presence of high levels of beta-asarone in some strains.

TABASCO PEPPER (*Capsicum frutescens*). Used topically to relieve painful muscle spasms, as topical analgesic, counterirritant, rubefacient; do not apply to injured or broken skin; keep away from eyes and mucous membranes; some people may have allergies to these preparations.

TANSY, COMMON (*Tanacetum vulgare*). Entire plant toxic, causing serious illness and occasional fatalities when misused as herbal tea, flavoring, or medicinal essential oil; use in herbal medicine, especially during pregnancy, not recommended. Oil of tansy contains varying amounts of thujone, a volatile oil that in high doses can cause convulsions and psychotic effects in people. Tansy is also poisonous to grazing animals.

THORN-APPLE, SACRED (*Datura wrightii* and related spp.). Plant considered very dangerous for herbal use.

THYME (*Thymus vulgaris*). Not recommended in large quantities during pregnancy.

TOBACCOS (*Nicotiana tabacum* and related spp.). Plants considered very dangerous for herbal use.

TRUMPETFLOWER, EVENING (*Gelsemium sempervirens*). Plant considered very dangerous for herbal use.

TURMERIC (*Curcuma longa*). Not recommended in large quantities during pregnancy.

UVA-URSI, or **KINNIKINNICK** (*Arctostaphylos uva-ursi*). Used to treat mild urinary tract infections and inflammation. May cause nausea and vomiting in

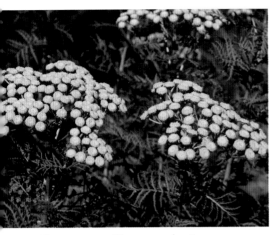

Common tansy (*Tanacetum vulgare*).

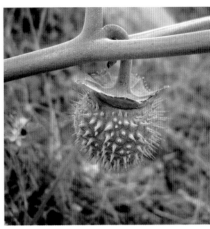

Sacred thorn-apple (*Datura wrightii*).

those with sensitive stomachs. Do not use during pregnancy and lactation. Do not use with substances that cause acidic urine; this will reduce the antibacterial effect (Blumenthal 2000).

WATER HEMLOCKS (*Cicuta* spp.). Plants considered very dangerous for herbal use.

WATERCRESS (*Nasturtium officinale*). Not recommended in large quantities during pregnancy.

WILLOWS (*Salix alba* and related spp.). Bark used to treat fever, rheumatic ailments, headaches, arthritis; possible interactions with aspirin and other salicylates, but no known toxicity.

WORMWOOD (*Artemisia absinthium* and related spp.). Leaves and tops considered

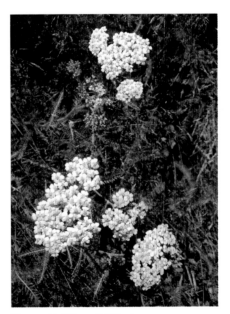

Yarrow (*Achillea millefolium*).

unsafe for use as deworming agent or tonic, for mind-altering action, or as flavor, according to Tyler (1987); not recommended in large quantities during pregnancy.

YARROW (*Achillea millefolium*). Not recommended during pregnancy. Potentially phototoxic; contains a range of alkaloids, flavonoids, and glycosides and volatile oil complex.

Glossary

ACHENE. Small, dry indehiscent one-seeded fruit with tight, thin outer wall.

ALGAL BLOOM. Rapid growth of algae (or cyanobacteria) in water, resulting in visible coating or coloring of the water.

ALTERNATE. Leaves, buds, or branches arising first on one side of the stem and then on the other (compare OPPOSITE).

ANNUAL. Plant growing from seed, flowering, producing seeds, and dying all in a single growing season.

ANNULUS. In mushrooms, the membranous remnant of partial veil found on mature stems of some species.

ANTHER. Male, or pollen-bearing structure of a flower, usually borne on a stalk, or filament (see also STAMEN).

APICAL. At the tip of a branch or stem.

ARBORESCENT. Of tree-like habit.

ARIL. Fleshy covering around a seed.

AXIL. Angle formed between the stem axis and attached leaf or other appendage.

BERRY. Simple, fleshy, usually indehiscent (not splitting open) fruit with one or more seeds (e.g., gooseberry, tomato).

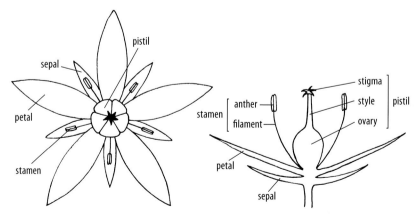

Parts of a typical, regular, five-parted flower. Left—top view; right—side view.

BIENNIAL. Plant growing from seed and living for two years, with flowering and seed production usually occurring in the second year (e.g., purple foxglove).

BISEXUAL. Having both sexual reproductive structures (male and female) produced on the same plant.

BRACT. Modified leaf; some bracts growing near a flower may be more showy than the flower itself (e.g., poinsettia, where the red "flower" parts are actually bracts).

BULB. Modified short, underground stem surrounded by a row of fleshy leaves with thickened bases (e.g., onion).

CALYX. Sterile outer whorl of flower parts composed of sepals, usually covering an unopened flower bud.

CAPSULE. Dry, dehiscent (splitting open) fruit in the form of a case containing seeds.

CARPEL. One of the units comprising a pistil or ovary (female part) in a flower; a simple pistil has one carpel, a compound pistil two or more united carpels.

CATKIN. Spike-like inflorescence (flower cluster) usually containing scaly bracts.

CHAFF. Small, thin, dry, membranous scales or bracts, such as around the grains of grasses.

CLASPING. Partially or completely surrounding a stem, as the bases of some leaves.

COMPOUND LEAF. Two or more leaflets attached to the leaf stalk (e.g., walnut, horse chestnut, or lupine).

CONVEX. Regularly rounded; broadly obtuse. Said of a cap of mushrooms.

CORM. Swollen, usually spherical or rounded underground stem capable of producing a new plant.

COROLLA. The ring of petals in a flower, usually the most conspicuous part of the flower.

CROWN. The region of a plant where the root and shoot join; the branching part of a tree.

CRUSTOSE. Lichen growth form in which the thallus (main structure of lichen) adheres closely to the substrate on which it grows.

CUP. In some mushrooms, a cup-like remnant of the universal veil found at the stem base (see also VOLVA).

CYLINDRIC. A shape having the same diameter throughout; tube-like.

DEHISCENT. Opening by valves or along regular lines, as in ripe seed capsules or some anthers.

DRUPE. Type of fleshy fruit generally containing one seed (e.g., cherry).

ENTIRE LEAF. Leaf whose margins are smooth (compare SERRATED).

EVERGREEN. Having foliage that remains green and functional through more than one growing season.

FIBRILLOSE (stringy). Composed of parallel fibers, especially of the cap of some species of mushrooms.

FIBRILS. Minute hairs.

FOLLICLE. Dry fruit of one carpel that splits along one suture line (e.g., columbine fruit segment).

FROND. Leaf of a fern or palm, or similar leaf-like structure.

FRUTICOSE. Lichen growth form in which the thallus (main structure of lichen) is generally erect and branching.

GENUS (pl., GENERA). A group of closely related plants containing one or more species.

GILLS. Radiating vertically aligned plate-like spore-bearing structures found on the undersurface of the cap of some mushrooms.

GLABROUS. Smooth, not hairy.

HERB. Vascular plant with little, if any secondary growth; not woody. Also a term for plants used as culinary seasoning or for medicinal purposes.

HERBACEOUS. Having the characteristics of an herb; not woody.

HYBRID. Plant with parents which are genetically distinct. The parent plants may be different cultivars, varieties, species, or genera; the hybrid usually exhibits a mixture of traits of its parents.

HYPHAE (sing., HYPHA). Minute tubular structures forming the mycelium and fruiting bodies of fungi.

INDEHISCENT. Not opening, or not opening by valves or along regular lines, as some fruits and anthers.

INFLORESCENCE. Term for cluster or grouping of flowers on an axis or stalk; also, the mode of arrangement of the flower(s) on a plant.

INVOLUTE. Inrolled margin.

KEEL. The two united, lowermost petals of flowers belonging to the pea, or legume family.

LATEX. Sap produced or exuded by plants.

LIGULATE. Strap-shaped, or tongue-shaped.

LUMINESCENCE. Emission of light from a living organism.

MYCELIUM. Mass of hyphae making up the main growing body of a fungus; typically embedded in soil, wood, etc.

NODE. Place on the stem where one or more leaves or branches are attached.

NUT. Hard, (usually) one-seeded fruit.

NUTLET. A small or diminutive nut, similar to an achene but with a harder, thicker wall.

OPPOSITE. Leaves, buds, or branches which are borne in pairs along the stem (compare ALTERNATE).

PALMATE LEAF. Five or more lobes arising from one point in a hand-like arrangement (e.g., typical maple leaf).

PARASITE. Organism that derives its nutrients and energy from a living host.

PEDICEL. Stalk bearing reproductive structures (flower stem).

PERENNIAL. Plant living from year to year for three years or more under normal conditions.

PINNATE LEAF. A compound leaf in which the leaflets are arranged along the central axis in a feather-like arrangement (e.g., elderberry or walnut leaf).

PISTIL. Female flowering structure, typically consisting of an ovary (containing one or more eggs, later to be fertilized and grow into seeds), a neck-like style, and a stigma which receives pollen from the male flowering structure, or anther. Pistils and anthers may be contained within the same flower or in separate flowers.

PROSTRATE. Lying flat on the ground.

RACEME. Unbranched, elongated inflorescence (flower cluster) with stalked flowers, the earliest blooming at the bottom, the least mature at the top.

RAY FLOWER. Ligulate flower, with corolla flattened and strap-like above a very short tube (e.g., the outer "petal" of a daisy, actually part of a single flower in a composite head).

RECEPTACLE. Part of the floral axis supporting floral parts.

RED TIDE, RED WATER. Concentration of toxic species of algae that cause a reddish coloration in water.

RHIZOME. Creeping, often fleshy underground stem from which new plants may arise.

RING. See ANNULUS

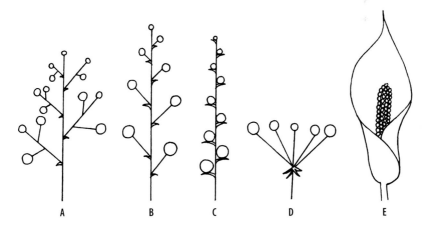

Some common types of flower arrangements: **A** panicle (loose cluster); **B** raceme (elongated cluster with stalked flowers); **C** spike (elongated cluster with stalkless flowers); **D** umbel (umbrella-like cluster); **E** arum type, with spathe surrounding club-like spadix.

RUNNER. Creeping above-ground stem which may produce small plantlets along its length; also called a stolon.

SCLEROTIUM (pl., SCLEROTIA). Resting body of some fungi, composed of a hardened mass of hyphae usually rounded in shape.

SERRATE LEAF. Toothed around the margin.

SESSILE. Lacking a stem or a stalk.

SIMPLE LEAF. One leaf blade attached to a leaf stalk (compare COMPOUND LEAF).

SPADIX. Fleshy flower spike bearing many tiny florets; the type of flower spike found in members of the arum family, usually enclosed or subtended by a leafy sheath or spathe.

SPATHE. Large, often colored or leafy bract surrounding the spadix in members of the arum family.

SPECIES. Plants that are genetically similar and breed true from seeds; also fungi and animals which interbreed and have distinctive traits.

SPICATE. Spike-like.

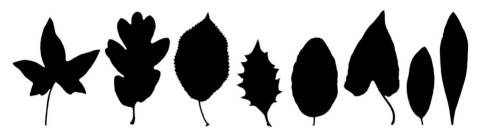

Common simple leaf types (not to scale). Left to right: palmately lobed (English ivy); pinnately lobed (oak); toothed or serrated margin (cherry); spiny margin (holly); smooth or entire margin, oval-shaped (snowberry); heart-shaped, or cordate (morning-glory); ellipse-shaped (privet); inversely lance-shaped, or oblanceolate (daphne laurel).

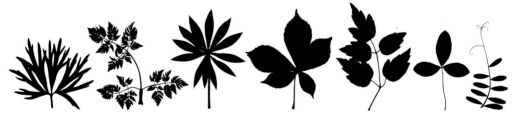

Common compound leaf types (not to scale). Left to right: deeply lobed, palmately compound (monkshood); finely divided (three times pinnately compound (poison hemlock); palmately compound, smooth-margined leaflets (lupine); palmately compound, toothed leaflets (horse chestnut); pinnately compound, coarsely toothed leaflets (clematis); three-parted (laburnum); pinnately compound, with terminal tendril (vetch).

SPIKE. Unbranched, elongated inflorescence (flower cluster) in which the flowers are sessile (stalkless).

SPIKELET. A secondary spike.

STAMEN. Male reproductive organ of a flower, consisting of a pollen-bearing structure (anther) borne on a stalk, or filament.

STEM, STIPE. Stalk-like portion of a mushroom's fruiting body; main stalk of any plant.

STIPULE. One or a pair of appendages at the base of a petiole, or leaf stalk, of some plants.

STOLON. See RUNNER

STRIATE. Having lines or minute grooves; common in mushrooms on the upper surface of the cap near its margin, or on the stem.

SUCCULENT. Plants having thick, fleshy leaves and/or stems.

TAPROOT. Strong, sometimes swollen or fleshy root that grows vertically into the soil.

TENDRIL. Thread-like stem or leaf tip that tends to grow in a spiral and clings to any nearby support (e.g., pea vines).

THALLUS. Having a simple plant or fungus body without differentiation into leaves or leaf-like structures.

THALLOSE. In lichens, having a simple, flattened thallus.

TOMENTOSE. Densely matted with a covering of soft hairs.

TUBER. Swollen underground stem, such as produced by dahlias and potatoes, which can sprout and produce new plants.

UMBEL. Umbrella-shaped inflorescence (flower cluster) in which the pedicels (stalks or flowers or flower clusters) radiate from a common point, like the ribs of an umbrella.

UMBO. Raised conical mound on the center of the cap of some mushrooms.

UNDULATE. Wavy.

UNISEXUAL. Having only one type of sexual structure (either male or female) produced by any one individual.

UNIVERSAL VEIL. Tissue surrounding a developing mushroom button (see also **VOLVA**).

VARIEGATED LEAF. Green leaf which is blotched, edged, or spotted with yellow, white, cream, or red (e.g., many caladium and dieffenbachia leaves)

VOLVA. In some mushrooms, remnants of the universal veil, the membranous covering enclosing certain mushrooms (e.g., amanitas) especially at their early growth stage, which may be reduced to cup-like structure at the base of the stalk with maturity.

WHORL. Leaves, petals, or branches arranged in a ring manner.

References

Ainsworth, G. D. 1952. *Medical Mycology*. Pitman, New York.

Allegro, J. M. 1970. *The Sacred Mushroom and the Cross*. Hodder and Stoughton, London.

American Association of Poison Control Centers. http://www.aapcc.org/

Ammirati, J. F., J. A. Traquair, and P. A. Horgen. 1985. *Poisonous Mushrooms of the Northern United States and Canada*. University of Minnesota Press, Minneapolis.

Anon. 1989. *Amanita phalloides* poisoning. *Mycofile*. The Newsletter of the Vancouver Mycological Society 1033 (January).

Anon. 1995. Ricin, deadly toxin from castor bean. *HerbalGram* 37:10.

Araillia. 2005. Angel trumpet warning. Wed., 27 July, Village GardenWeb, Brugmansia forum. http://forums.gardenweb.com/forums/load/brug/msg0715250623664.html?43

Arnold, H. L. 1944. *Poisonous Plants of Hawaii*. Tongg Publishing Co., Honolulu.

Baer, H. 1979. The poisonous Anacardiaceae. In Kinghorn, *Toxic Plants*.

Baginski, S., and J. Mowszowica. 1963. *Krajowe Rosliny Trujace*. Panstwowe Wydawnictwo Naukowe, Lodz, Poland.

Bandoni, R. J., and A. F. Szczawinski. 1976. *Guide to Common Mushrooms of British Columbia*. British Columbia Provincial Museum Handbook No. 24, Victoria.

Bas, C. 2000. Una visione più ampia sulle *Amanita*. *Boll. Gruppo Micologico G. Bresadola (Trento)* 43(2):9–12.

Bayne, H. M. 2000. FDA publishes new draft guidance for botanical drug products. *HerbalGram* 50:68–69.

Benjamin, D. R. 1995. *Mushrooms: Poisons and Panaceas*. W. H. Freeman and Company, New York.

Bergner, P. 1989. Comfrey, coltsfoot, and pyrrolizidine alkaloids. *Medical Herbalism* 1(1):1, 3–5.

Beug, M. W. 2000. Poisonous and hallucinogenic mushrooms. Web educational program, prepared for the North American Mycological Association,

The Evergreen State College ePress, Olympia, Wash. Illustrated "slide" show. http://academic.evergreen.edu/projects/mushrooms/phm/index.htm

———. 2004. Mushroom poisonings reported in 2004. Mushroom Poisoning Case Registry/North American Mycological Association Toxicology Committee. http://www.sph.umich.edu/~kwcee/mpcr/2004Case.htm http://www.sph.umich.edu/~kwcee/mpcr/index.htm

Bhatt, R. P., R. E. Tulloss, K. C. Semwal, K. C. Bhatt, J. M. Moncalvo, and S. L. Stephenson. 2003. Amanitaceae reported from India. A critically annotated checklist. *Mycotaxon* 88:249–270.

Blumenthal, M., ed. 2000. *Herbal Medicine: The Complete German Commission E Monographs*. American Botanical Council, Austin, Tex.

Blumenthal, M. 2005. St. John's wort extract shown as effective as and safer than Paxil. *HerbalGram* 68:23.

———. 2006a. Sativex—cannabis-based medicine reduces pain in MS patient. *HerbalGram* 69:34.

———. 2006b. AHPA adopts new and revised trade recommendations for herb industry self-regulation. *HerbalGram* 69:56–58.

———. 2006c. Australian TGA [Therapeutic Goods Administration] publishes liver warning policy for black cohosh. *HerbalGram* 71:60–61.

———. 2006d. Black cohosh safety. Editorial, *HerbalGram* 72:6.

Blumenthal, M., T. Hall, A. Goldberg, T. Kunz, K. Dinda, J. Brinckmann, B. Wollschlaeger. 2003. *The ABC Clinical Guide to Herbs*. American Botanical Council, Austin, Tex.

Boesi, A., and F. Cardi. 2006. Tibetan herbal medicine: traditional classification and utilization of natural products in Tibetan *Materia Medica*. *HerbalGram* 71:38–48.

Brett, M. 2006. Body pulled from lake. *Penticton Herald*, 25 September.

Brinker, F. J. 1983. *An Introduction to the Toxicology of Common Botanical Medicinal Substances*. National College of Naturopathic Medicine, Portland, Ore.

———. 1999. Variations in effective botanical products: the case for diversity of forms for herbal preparations as supported by scientific studies. *HerbalGram* 46:36–50

Bruce, E. A. 1927. *Astragalus campestris* and other stock poisoning plants of British Columbia. Canada Department of Agriculture Bulletin 88, Ottawa.

Buck, R. W. 1961. Mushroom poisoning since 1924 in the United States. *Mycologia* 53:538.

Burrows, G. E., and R. J. Tyrl. 2006. *Handbook of Toxic Plants of North America*. Blackwell Publishing, Oxford.

Busia, K., and F. Heckels. 2006. Jimson weed: history, perceptions, traditional uses, and potential therapeutic benefits of the genus *Datura*. *HerbalGram* 69:40–50.

Canada Department of Agriculture. 1968. *Poison Ivy*. Publication No. 820, Ottawa.

Cavaliere, C. 2007. Intravenous milk thistle compound used to save victims of poisonous mushrooms. *HerbalGram* 74:16.

Cavaliere, C., and M. Blumenthal. 2006. UK expert committee upholds kava ban. *HerbalGram* 72:59.

Ciegler, A. 1975. Mycotoxins: occurrence, chemistry, biological activity. *Lloydia* 38:21–35.

Chi-Kit, W., T. Johns, and G. H. N. Towers. 1980. Phototoxic and antibiotic activities of plants of the Asteraceae used in folk medicine. *Journal of Ethnopharmacology* 2:279–290.

Claus, E. P., V. E. Tyler, and L. R. Brady. 1970. *Pharmacognosy*. Lea and Febiger, Philadelphia.

Cooper, M. R., and A. W. Johnson. 1984. *Poisonous Plants in Britain and Their Effects on Animals and Man*. Ministry of Agriculture Fisheries and Food, Reference Book 161. Her Majesty's Stationery Office, London.

———. 1998. *Poisonous Plants and Fungi in Britain: Animal and Human Poisoning*. The Stationery Office, London.

———. 2003. *Poisonous Plants and Fungi: An Illustrated Guide*, 2d ed. The Stationery Office, London.

Cornell University Poisonous Plants Informational Database. http://www.ansci.cornell.edu/plants/

Couplan, F., and E. Styner. 2006. *Guide des plantes sauvages comestibles et toxiques*. Delachaux et Niestlé, Paris.

Cox, P. A., S. A. Banack, and S. J. Murch. 2003. Biomagnification of cyanobacterial neurotoxins and neurodegenerative disease among the Chamorro people of Guam. *PNAS* 100(23):13380–13383.

Cox, P. A., and O. W. Sacks. 2002. Cycad neurotoxins, consumption of flying foxes, and ALS-PDC disease in Guam. *Neurology* 58:956–959.

Crawford, S. 2007. *Ethnolichenology of* Bryoria fremontii: *wisdom of elders, population ecology, and nutritional chemistry*. M.Sc. thesis, Department of Biology and School of Environmental Studies, University of Victoria, British Columbia.

Crum, H. 1973. Mosses of the Great Lakes forest. *Contributions University of Michigan Herbarium* 10:1–404.

Der Marderosian, A., and F. C. Roia, Jr. 1979. Literature review and clinical management of household ornamental plants potentially toxic to humans. In Kinghorn, *Toxic Plants*.

DeVries, J. W., M. W. Trucksess, and L. S. Jackson, eds. 2002. *Mycotoxins and food safety* (Proceedings of an American Chemical Society symposium held in Washington, D.C., 21–23 August 2000). Advances in Experimental Medicine and Biology, Kluwer Academic Publishers, New York.

DeWolf, G. P. 1974. Guide to potentially dangerous plants. *Arnoldia* 34(2):45–91.

Diaz, J. H. 2005. Evolving global epidemiology, syndromic classification, general management, and prevention of unknown mushroom poisonings. *Critical Care Medicine* 33(2):419–426.

Duke, J. A. 1985. *CRC Handbook of Medicinal Herbs*. CRC Press, Inc., Boca Raton, Fla.

———. 1997. *The Green Pharmacy*. Rodale Press, Emmaus, Pa.

Eisenberg, D. M. 1997. Advising patients who seek alternative medical therapies. *Annals of Internal Medicine* 127(1):61–69.

Emboden, W. 1979. *Narcotic Plants: Hallucinogens, Stimulants, Inebriants, and Hypnotics, Their Origins and Uses*, rev. ed. Collier Books, New York.

Etkin, N. L. 2006. *Edible Medicines: An Ethnopharmacology of Food*. University of Arizona Press, Tucson.

Evans, J. 2005. Mistletoe: good for more than free kisses. *HerbalGram* 68:50–59.

Faulstich, H. 1980. Mushroom poisoning. *Lancet* 2:794–795.

Faulstich, H., B. Kommerell, and T. Wieland, eds. 1980. *Amanita Toxins and Poisoning*. Verland Gerhard Witzstrock, Baden-Baden, Germany.

Fernald, M. L., A. C. Kinsey, and R. C. Rollins. 1958. *Edible Wild Plants of Eastern North America*. Harper and Row, New York.

Floersheim, G. L. 1987. Treatment of human amatoxin mushroom poisoning: myths and advances in therapy. *Medical Toxicology* 2:1–9.

Foster, S. 1999. Black cohosh, *Cimicifuga racemosa*: a literature review. *HerbalGram* 45:35–50.

Fowler, M. H. 1980. *Plant Poisoning in Small Companion Animals*. Ralston Purina Co., St. Louis, Mo.

Frohne, D., and H. J. Pfänder. 2005. *Poisonous Plants: A Handbook for Doctors, Pharmacists, Toxicologists, Biologists and Veterinarians*, 2d ed, trans. from the German 5th ed. (2004) by Inge Alford. Timber Press, Portland, Ore.

Fuller, T. C., and E. McClintock. 1986. *Poisonous Plants of California*. University of California Press, Berkeley.

Fyles, F. 1920. *Principal Poisonous Plants of Canada*. Dominion of Canada, Department of Agriculture, Ottawa.

Gardner, D. R., and L. F. James. 1999. Pine needle abortion in cattle: analysis of isocupressic acid in North American gymnosperms. *Phytochemical Analysis* 10:132–136.

Groves, J. W. 1979. *Edible and Poisonous Mushrooms of Canada*. Agriculture Canada Publication No. 1112, Ottawa.

Haard, R., and K. Haard. 1977. *Poisonous and Hallucinogenic Mushrooms*, 2d ed. Cloudburst Press, Seattle.

Hall, R. L. 1973. Toxicants occurring naturally in spices and flavors. In National Academy of Sciences, *Toxicants Occurring Naturally in Foods*.

Hardin, J. W., and J. M. Arena. 1974. *Human Poisoning from Native and Cultivated Plants*, 2d ed. Duke University Press, Durham, N.C.

Hatfield, G. M. 1979. Toxic mushrooms. In Kinghorn, *Toxic Plants*.

Hatfield, G. M., and L. R. Brady. 1975. Toxins of higher fungi. *Lloydia* 38(1):36–55.

Hawksworth, D. L. 1991. The fungal dimension of biodiversity: magnitude, significance, and conservation. *Mycological Research* 95:641–655.

Health Canada/Santé Canada. 2008. Information on licensed natural health products. http://www.hc-sc.gc.ca/dhp-mps/prodnatur/applications/licen-prod/listapprnhp-listeapprpsn_eng.php

Hebda, R. J., N. J. Turner, S. Birchwater, M. Kay, and the Elders of Ulkatcho. 1996. *Ulkatcho Food and Medicine Plants*. Ulkatcho Band, Anahim Lake, B.C.

Hedrick, U. P., ed. 1972. *Sturtevant's Edible Plants of the World*. Dover Publications, Inc., New York.

Heinrich, M., and J. L. Teoh. 2004. Galanthamine from snowdrop—the development of a modern drug against Alzheimer's disease from local Caucasian knowledge. *Journal of Ethnopharmacology* 92:147–162.

Hessayon, D. G. 1985. *The Indoor Plant Spotter*. Pbi Publications, Britannica House, Herts, England.

Hill, R. J. 1986. *Poisonous Plants of Pennsylvania*. Pennsylvania Department of Agriculture, Harrisburg.

Hotson, J. W., and E. Lewis. 1934. *Amanita pantherina* of western Washington. *Mycologia* 26:384.

Howards, R. A. 1974. *Poisonous Plants*. Arnoldia, Harvard University, Jamaica Plain, Mass.

Hulbert, L. C., and F. W. Oehme. 1984. *Plants Poisonous to Livestock: Selected Plants of the United States and Canada of Importance to Veterinarians*. Kansas State University Printing Service, Manhattan.

International Programme on Chemical Safety. 2008. Retrieved in February from the IPCSINTOXDatabank, Poisons Information Monographs. http://www.inchem.org/documents/pims/fungi/fungi.htm

Ishikawa, S. 2002. Teen hospitalized after eating plant. *The Honolulu Advertiser*, 22 February.

Johns, T. 1996. *The Origins of Human Diet and Medicine*. University of Arizona Press, Tucson.

Johns, T., and I. Kubo. 1988. A survey of traditional methods employed for the detoxification of plant foods. *Journal of Ethnobiology* 8(1):81–129.

Kallas, J. 2004a. Wild sweet pea—a few of my favorite things. *The Wild Food Adventurer* (10 December):1–7.

———. 2004b. Lathyrism—what's all the fuss about? *The Wild Food Adventurer* (10 December):1, 8–14.

Keeler, R. F. 1979. Toxins and teratogens of the Solanaceae and Liliaceae. In Kinghorn, *Toxic Plants*.

Keeler, R. F., K. R. Van Kampen, and L. F. James, eds. 1978. *Effects of Poisonous Plants on Livestock*. Symposium on Poisonous Plants, Utah State University. Academic Press, New York.

Kent, D. A., G. A. Willis, and K. Lepik, eds. 1997. *Poison Management Manual*, 4th ed. Vancouver, British Columbia Drug and Poison Information Centre.

Kinghorn, A. D., ed. 1979. *Toxic Plants*. Columbia University Press, New York.

Kinghorn, A. D. 1979. Cocarcinogenic irritant Euphorbiaceae. In Kinghorn, *Toxic Plants*.

Kingsbury, J. M. 1964. *Poisonous Plants of the United States and Canada*. Prentice-Hall, Inc., Engelwood Cliffs, N.J.

———. 1967. *Deadly Harvest: A Guide to Common Poisonous Plants*. George Allen and Unwin Ltd., London.

———. 1979. The problem of poisonous plants. In Kinghorn, *Toxic Plants*.

Knight, A. P. 2005. *A Guide to Poisonous House and Garden Plants*. Teton NewMedia, Jackson, Wyo. http://www.tetonnm.com/phptoc.html

Knight, A. P., and R. G. Walter. 2001. *A Guide to Plant Poisoning of Animals in North America*. Teton NewMedia, Jackson, Wyo.

Kramer, J. 1977. *A Complete Guide to Indoor Trees*. Coles Publishing Co. Ltd., Toronto.

Krochmal, A., L. Wilkins, D. van Lear, and M. Chien. 1974. Mayapple (*Podophyllum peltatum* L.). United States Department of Agriculture Research Paper NE-296. Northeastern Forest Experiment Station, Upper Darby, Pa.

Kuhnlein, H. V., and N. J. Turner. 1987. Cow-parsnip (*Heracleum lanatum* Michx.): an indigenous vegetable of Native people of northwestern North America. *Journal of Ethnobiology* 6(2):309–324.

———. 1991. *Traditional Plant Foods of Canadian Indigenous Peoples: Nutrition, Botany and Use*. Vol. 8. In S. Katz, ed., *Food and Nutrition in History and Anthropology*, Gordon and Breach Science Publishers, Philadelphia.

Kuo, M. 2006a. *Amanita smithiana*. Retrieved in March from the Mushroom

Expert.com Web site. http://www.mushroomexpert.com/amanita_
    smithiana.html

———. 2006b. The American matsutake: *Tricholoma magnivelare*. Retrieved in
    October from the MushroomExpert.com Web site. http://www.
    mushroomexpert.com/tricholoma_magnivelare.html

Lampe, K. F., and M. A. McCann. 1985. *AMA Handbook of Poisonous and Injurious
    Plants*. American Medical Association, Chicago.

Langenheim, J. H. 2003. *Plant Resins: Chemistry, Evolution, Ecology, and Ethnobot-
    any*. Timber Press, Portland, Ore.

Lantz, T., K. Swerhun, and N. J. Turner. 2004. Devil's club (*Oplopanax horridus*):
    an ethnobotanical review. *HerbalGram* 62:33–48.

Lavoie, J. 2007. Crypto threat ignored, says researcher. *Times Colonist*, Victoria,
    B.C., 5 October.

Lebot, V. 2006. The quality of kava consumed in the South Pacific. *HerbalGram*
    71:34–37.

Leeuwenberg, A. J. M., ed. 1987. *Medicinal and Poisonous Plants of the Tropics*.
    Pudoc Wageningen, The Netherlands.

Levy, B. 1999. U.S. and U.N. studies support medicinal marijuana research.
    HerbalGram 46:14–15.

Levy, C. K., and R. B. Primack. 1984. *A Field Guide to Poisonous Plants and Mush-
    rooms of North America*. The Stephen Greene Press, Brattleboro, Vt.

Lewis, W. H. 1979a. Poke root herbal tea poisoning. *Journal of the American Medi-
    cal Association* 242:2759.

———. 1979b. Snowberry (*Symphoricarpos*) poisoning in children. *Journal of the
    American Medical Association* 242:2663.

Lewis, W. H., P. Vinay, and V. E. Zenger. 1983. *Airborne and Allergenic Pollen of
    North America*. The Johns Hopkins University Press, Baltimore.

Lewis, W. H., and M. P. F. Elvin-Lewis. 2003. *Medical Botany*, 2d ed. John Wiley
    and Sons, Hoboken, N.J.

Lincoff, G. H. 1981. *The Audubon Society Field Guide to North American Mushrooms*.
    Alfred A. Knopf, New York.

———. 2005. Recent poisonings from edible mushrooms! A report on a few
    new kinds of mushroom poisoning gleaned from Hanna Tschekunow's
    NYMS talk on mushroom poisoning at the Museum of Natural History, 13
    March. http://www.nemf.org/files/lincoff/lookalikes/Recent_mushroom_
    poisonings.html

———. 2007. The 50 best edible mushrooms in the world. Slide show pro-
    gram, 17 January. http://www.fungusfed.org/body/GaryLincoff_011707.
    htm

Lincoff, G. H., and D. H. Mitchel. 1977. *Toxic and Hallucinogenic Mushroom Poisoning: A Handbook for Physicians and Mushroom Hunters*. Van Nostrand Reinhold Co., New York.

Macinnis, P. 2004. *Poisons: From Hemlock to Botox and the Killer Bean of Calabar*. Arcade Publishing, New York.

Madlener, J. C. 1977. *The Seavegetable Book*. Clarkson N. Potter, Inc., New York.

Main, D. C., and A. R. Butler. 2006. Probable *Malva parviflora* (small flowered mallow) intoxication in sheep in Western Australia. *Australian Veterinary Journal* 84(4):134–135.

McKenny, M., and D. E. Stuntz. 1987. *The New Savory Wild Mushroom*, rev. and enlarged by J. F. Ammirati. University of Washington Press, Seattle.

McLean, A., and H. H. Nicholson. 1958. *Stock Poisoning Plants of the British Columbia Ranges*. Publication No. 1037. Canada Department of Agriculture, Ottawa.

McPherson, A. 1979. Pokeweed and other lymphocyte mitogens. In Kinghorn, *Toxic Plants*.

Meijer, W. 1974. *Podophyllum peltatum*, May apple: a potential new cash-crop plant of eastern North America. *Economic Botany* 28:68–72.

Miller, J. A. 1973. Naturally occurring substances that can induce tumors. In National Academy of Sciences, *Toxicants Occurring Naturally in Foods*.

Miller, O. K. 1980. *Mushrooms of North America*. E. P. Dutton & Co., Inc., New York.

Millspaugh, C. F. 1974. *American Medicinal Plants*. Originally published in 1892 under the title *Medicinal Plants*; reprinted by Dover Publications, Inc., New York.

Milot, B. 2004. Ivy extracts show benefit in pediatric bronchial asthma. *HerbalGram* 62:28–29.

Milot, B., and M. Blumenthal. 2006. Safety and efficacy of Remifemin black cohosh extract in alleviating symptoms of menopause confirmed in large clinical trial. *HerbalGram* 69:31.

Mitchell, J., and A. Rook. 1979. *Botanical Dermatology*. Greengrass Ltd., Vancouver, B.C.

Moerman, D. 2003. Native American ethnobotany: a database of foods, drugs, dyes and fibers of Native American peoples, derived from plants. University of Michigan, Dearborn. http://herb.umd.umich.edu/

Morton, A. G. 1981. *History of Botanical Science*. Academic Press, New York.

Morton, J. F. 1958. Ornamental plants with poisonous properties. *Proceedings of the Florida State Horticultural Society* 71:372–380.

———. 1962. Ornamental plants with toxic and/or irritant properties. *Proceedings of the Florida State Horticultural Society* 75:484–491.

————. 1971. *Plants Poisonous to People*. Hurricane House, Miami.

Naegele, T. A. 2006. *Cicuta maculata*. Web excerpt from *Edible and Medicinal Plants of the Great Lakes Region* (Thunder Bay Press, rev. ed., 2004). http://permaculture.info/index.php/Cicuta_maculata

National Academy of Sciences. 1973. *Toxicants Occurring Naturally in Foods*. National Academy of Sciences, Washington, D.C.

National Safety Council. 1975. Poison ivy, poison oak, and poison sumac. Data sheet 304, revision A. *National Safety News* (September):99–102.

Oliff, H. S. 2004. More research on St. John's wort and interactions: effect on immunosuppressive drug, tacrolimus, and no effect on asthma drug, theophylline. *HerbalGram* 64:21–22.

Panter, K. E., and L. F. James. 1990. Natural plant toxicants in milk: a review. *Journal of Animal Science* 68(3):892–904.

Patterson, D. S. P. 1982. Mycotoxins. *Environmental Chemistry* 2:205–233.

Patwardhan, V. N., and J. W. White. 1973. Problems associated with particular foods [includes discussion on honey toxins]. In National Academy of Sciences, *Toxicants Occurring Naturally in Foods*.

Pelizzari, V., E. Feifal, M. M. Rohrmoser, G. Gstraunthaler, and M. Moser. 1994. Partial purification of a toxic component of *Amanita smithiana*. *Mycologia* 86:555–560.

Pieroni, A. 1999. Toxic plants as food plants in the traditional uses of the eastern Apuan Alps region, northwest Tuscany, Italy. In Guerci, A., ed., *Il cibo e il corpo: dal cibo alla cultura, dalla cultura al cibo* (Food and body: from food to culture, from culture to food). Erga Edizioni, Genoa.

Powell, R. A., and R. P. Adams. 1973. Seasonal variation in the volatile terpenoids of *Juniperus scopulorum* (Cupressaceae). *American Journal of Botany* 60(1):1041–1050.

Prieto, J. M., M. C. Recio, R. M. Ginner, S. Máñex, and J. L. Rios. 2003. Pharmacologial approach to the pro- and anti-inflammatory effects of *Ranunculus sceleratus* L. *Journal of Ethnopharmacology* 89:131–137.

Ralphs, M. H., R. Creamer, D. Baucom, D. R. Gardner, S. L. Welsh, J. D. Graham, C. Hart, D. Cook, and B. L. Stegelmeier. 2008. Relationship between the endophyte *Embellisia* spp. and the toxic alkaloid swainsonine in major locoweed species (*Astragalus* and *Oxytropis*). *Journal of Chemical Ecology* 34:32–38.

Rengstorff, D. S., R. W. Osorio, and M. Bonacini. 2003. Recovery from severe hepatitis caused by mushroom poisoning without liver transplantation. *Clinical Gastroenterology and Hepatology* 1(5):392–396.

Richardson, D. H. S. 1975. *The Vanishing Lichens*. David and Charles, London.

Rumack, B. H., and E. Salzman, eds. 1978. *Mushroom Poisoning: Diagnosis and Treatment*. CRC Press, Inc., Boca Raton, Fla.

Schantz, E. J. 1973. Seafood toxicants. In National Academy of Sciences, *Toxicants Occurring Naturally in Foods*.

Scheel, L. D. 1973. Photosensitizing agents. In National Academy of Sciences, *Toxicants Occurring Naturally in Foods*.

Schmidt, M. 2007. Kava: quality criteria for kava. *HerbalGram* 73:44–49.

Schneider, D. 1986. Poisonous plants. *Canadian Geographic* 106(2):60–65.

Schultes, R. E., and A. Hofmann. 1980. *The Botany and Chemistry of Hallucinogens*. Charles C. Thomas, Springfield, Ill.

Seiger, R. E. 2003. Trial key to Pacific Northwest *Lepiota* and allies. Prepared for the Pacific Northwest Key Council, Puget Sound Mycological Society, Seattle. http://www.svims.ca/council/Lepiota.htm

Singh, Y. N., and M. Blumenthal. 1997. Kava: an overview. Special Review, *HerbalGram* 39:33–55.

Smith, A. L. 1921. *Lichens*. Cambridge University Press, London.

Soper, J. H., and M. L. Heimburger. 1982. *Shrubs of Ontario*. Royal Ontario Museum, Toronto.

Stamets, P. E. 1978. *Psilocybe Mushrooms and Their Allies*. Homestead Book Company, Seattle.

———. 1996. *Psilocybin Mushrooms of the World*. Ten Speed Press, Berkeley, Calif.

Suter, A., S. Bommer, and J. Rechener. 2006. Treatment of patients with venous insufficiency with fresh plant horse chestnut seed extract: a review of clinical trials. *Advanced Therapy* 23(1):179–190.

Sütlüpmar, N., A. Mat, and Y. Satganoglu. 1993. Poisoning by toxic honey in Turkey. *Archives of Toxicology* 67(2):148–150.

Sweet, M. 1962. *Common Edible and Useful Plants of the West*. Naturegraph Company, Healdsburg, Calif.

Szczawinski, A. F., and N. J. Turner. 1980. *Wild Green Vegetables of Canada*. National Museum of Natural Sciences, National Museums of Canada, Ottawa.

Trestrail, J. H. 1993. Gyromitrin-containing mushrooms: a form of gastronomic roulette. *McIlvainea* 11(1):45–50.

Towers, G. N. 1979. Contact hypersensitivity and photodermatitis evoked by Compositae. In Kinghorn, *Toxic Plants*.

Tu, A. T., ed. 1988. *Handbook of Natural Toxins*. Vol. 3, *Marine Toxins and Venoms*. Marcel Dekker, New York.

Tulloss, R. E. 1990. *Amanita crenulata*: history, taxonomy, distribution, and poisonings. *Mycotaxon* 39:393–405.

————. 2000. Le amanita nel mondo: bellezza, pericolo e diversità. *Boll. Gruppo Micologico G. Bresadola (Trento)* 43(2):13–21.

Tulloss, R. E., and J. E. Lindgren. 1992. *Amanita smithiana*: taxonomy, distribution, and poisonings. *Mycotaxon* 45:373–387.

————. 2005. *Amanita aprica*: a new toxic species from western North America. *Mycotaxon* 91:193–205.

Tulloss, R. E., C. L. Ovrebo, and R. E. Halling. 1992. Studies on *Amanita* (Amanitaceae) from Andean Colombia. *Mem. New York Bot. Gard.* 66:1–46.

Tulloss, R. E., and Z. Yang. 2007. Studies in the Genus *Amanita* Pers. (Agaricales, Fungi), Herbarium Rooseveltensis Amanitarum, Roosevelt, N.J. http://eticomm.net/~ret/amanita/mainaman.html

Turner, N. J. 1977. Economic importance of black tree lichen (*Bryoria fremontii*) to the Indians of western North America. *Economic Botany* 31:461–470.

————. 1982. Traditional use of devil's-club (*Oplopanax horridus*; Araliaceae) by Native peoples in western North America. *Journal of Ethnobiology* 2:17–38.

————. 1984. Counter-irritant and other medicinal uses of plants in Ranunculaceae by Native peoples in British Columbia and neighbouring areas. *Journal of Ethnopharmacology* 11:181–201.

————. 1995. *Food Plants of Coastal First Peoples*. Royal British Columbia Museum, Victoria, and University of British Columbia Press, Vancouver.

————. 1997. "Le fruit de l'ours": Les rapports entre les plantes et les animaux das les langues et les cultures amérindiennes de la Côte-Ouest" ("The bear's own berry": ethnobotanical knowledge as a reflection of plant/animal interrelationships in northwestern North America). In *Recherches amérindiennes au Québec*, vol. 27 (3–4). Special Edition on *Des Plantes et des Animaux: Visions et Pratiques Autochtones*, P. Beaucage, ed. Université de Montréal, Québec.

————. 1998. *Plant Technology of British Columbia First Peoples*, rev. ed. Royal British Columbia Museum, Victoria, and University of British Columbia Press, Vancouver.

————. 2004. *Plants of Haida Gwaii*. X̲aadaa Gwaay guud gina k̲'aws (Skidegate), X̲aadaa Gwaayee guu giin k̲'aws (Massett). Sono Nis Press, Winlaw, B.C.

————. 2006. *Food Plants of Interior First Peoples*, new ed. Royal British Columbia Museum, Victoria.

————. 2008. The food/medicine/poison triangle: implications for traditional ecological knowledge systems of indigenous peoples of British Columbia, Canada. In R. K. Singh, J. Pretty, N. J. Turner, V. Reyes-García, and K. Swiderska, eds., *Opportunities from Biocultural Diversity: Traditional Foods, Local Knowledge and Biodiversity Conservation*. Indian Council of Agricultural Research, New Delhi.

Turner, N. J., R. Bouchard, and D. I. D. Kennedy. 1980. *Ethnobotany of the Okanagan-Colville Indians of British Columbia and Washington.* British Columbia Provincial Museum Occasional Paper No. 21, Victoria.

Turner, N. J., and A. Davis. 1993. "When everything was scarce": the role of plants as famine foods in northwestern North America. *Journal of Ethnobiology* 13(2):1–28.

Turner, N. J., L. M. J. Gottesfeld, H. V. Kuhnlein, and A. Ceska. 1992. Edible wood fern rootstocks of western North America: solving an ethnobotanical puzzle. *Journal of Ethnobiology* 12(1):1–34.

Tyler, V. E. 1987. *The Honest Herbal: A Sensible Guide to Herbs and Related Remedies,* rev. ed. George F. Stickley Co., Philadelphia.

———. 1997. "When will there come a savior…?" *HerbalGram* 41:27–28, 56.

Upton, R., ed. 1997. St. John's wort, *Hypericum perforatum.* Insert, American Herbal Pharmacopoeia and Therapeutic Compendium. *HerbalGram* 40 (July):1–32.

U.S. Department of Agriculture, NRCS. 2008. The PLANTS Database. National Plant Data Center, Baton Rouge, LA 70874-4490. http://plants.usda.gov

U.S. Food and Drug Administration. 2000. Center for Drug Evaluation and Research, Guidance for Industry Botanical Drug Products (draft, 3 August).

———. 2006. FDA Poisonous Plant Database, Center for Food Safety and Applied Nutrition, Office of Plant and Dairy Foods (March update). http://www.cfsan.fda.gov/~djw/plantox.html

Wasson, R. 1968. *Soma: Divine Mushroom of Immortality.* Harcourt, Brace and World, New York.

Woloshuk, C. 2006. NC1025: Mycotoxins: Biosecurity and Food Safety (NC129). Botany and Plant Pathology, Purdue University, West Lafayette, Ind. http://www.btny.purdue.edu/NC1025/

Wyllie, T. D., and L. G. Morehouse, eds. 1978. *Mycotoxic Fungi, Mycotoxins and Mycotoxicoses,* vol. 2. Marcel Dekker, New York.

Index

Photographs are indicated by **boldfaced** page numbers.